Irish Guide to Complementary and Alternative Therapies

Paperback Parade
BOOK MARKET
Exchange for Half Price

LUCY COSTIGAN has had a long and wide association with the areas of psychotherapy and complementary therapies. She is a member of the Institute for Reality Therapy in Ireland, the Irish Association of Hypno-analysts, and the National Federation of Spiritual Healers. She also holds a Maynooth Diploma in Counselling Skills, a UCD certificate in Women's Studies, an advanced diploma in clinical hypnotherapy from the Irish School of Ethical and Analytical Hypnotherapy, and a Ki massage diploma from the Irish Health Culture Association. Other areas of study have included art therapy, family therapy, gestalt, colour therapy, psychosynthesis, and movement and dance therapy. She has also worked with the Samaritans and the Simon Community. Lucy runs her own counselling, hypnotherapy and spiritual healing practice in Dublin, and in her native town of Wexford.

This book is dedicated to my parents,
Michael and Catherine:
For all the love, guidance, understanding
and friendship you gave to me over a lifetime,
and for your continued support,
even from the other side.

Irish Guide to Complementary and Alternative Therapies

Lucy Costigan

WOLFHOUND PRESS

First published in 1997 by
Wolfhound Press Ltd
68 Mountjoy Square
Dublin 1, Ireland

British Library Cataloguing in Publication Data
A catalogue record for this book is available from the British Library.

ISBN 0-86327-584 2

Members of the public are advised to check with the relevant societies
whether practitioners are registered and insured. No responsibility will be
accepted by the author or publisher for any form or instance of malpractice by
practitioners listed in this book.

Note to Therapists
If you are a therapist and have not been included in the directory section at the
back of the book, please send your details to Wolfhound Press, 68 Mountjoy
Square, Dublin 1, and we will endeavour to include you in the next edition.

Cover Design: Slick Fish Design
Typesetting: Wolfhound Press
Printed in the Republic of Ireland by Colour Books, Dublin.

Contents

Acknowledgements

No man — or woman — is an island. No book could ever be written without the support and encouragement of family, friends and colleagues.

I'd like to say a big 'thank you' to my family. These are the people who love, nurture, and inspire me, and who provide me with a natural form of healing on a day-to-day basis. Thanks to my brother Anthony, to my sister Theresa, to my brother-in-law Sean (Cullen), to my special nephews Michael, Damien, and Paul, and to my 'golden' niece Sharon. Thanks also to my brother Val, and to all the other members of the Costigan clan, for your special support, and for all the many moments shared over a myriad of lifetimes.

To my cousin Raymond (McGovern), thank you for the many hours of proofreading and editing, and for all of your helpful suggestions.

Thanks to my dear friends Andrew (Rea), Carmel (Larkin), Maura (O'Connor), Isabel (MacMahon), Clara (Martin), Paddy (Meyler), and Phena (Gallagher), not only for the help and enthusiasm that you gave to me over the past hectic months, but for the years of philosophising, which is the nourishment that I thrive on, and to each of you for your unique connection and love.

Thanks to my friend and mentor, Brendan (O'Callaghan), who has been the instigator in helping me to find my own unique path in life. Thanks Brendan, for kindling the spark!

I wish to thank Ailbhe Smith, head of Women's Studies at UCD, who first advised me to seek publication for my project *Women and Therapy*, which I completed as part of my certificate course. This has led directly to the present publication.

Thank you to my friend Paul (Howe), for your help with some of the technical aspects of the book, and for your support.

Thanks to all the practitioners, organisations and individuals who have contributed to this book. Many people have willingly given of their precious time to help with research and to share

their experiences of therapy. Thank you all for your encouragement and friendly advice.

Thanks to Emer Ryan, Susan Houlden, Jenna Dowds,
Seamus Cashman, and the staff of Wolfhound Press, for all your
advice and helpful assistance.

Introduction

What is Therapy?

Therapy can be defined as the treatment of physical or mental disorders, by means other than surgery. The word 'alternative' has been popularly used for some time to refer to therapies that are not part of the orthodox medical or psychiatric system. Most therapists, however, prefer to use the term 'complementary'. They see their therapy, not as a system of treatment which exists in isolation, but rather as a therapeutic aid to healing, which can be used in conjunction with medical treatment or with any other form of therapy.

Therapy in the 1990s

Therapy is a very familiar concept in the Ireland of the 1990s. Television programmes, newspaper articles, countless books and leaflets advertise, explain, discuss, challenge and inform us of the latest techniques and developments in a wide range of therapies. It is no longer unusual for a next-door neighbour to mention that she is attending an acupuncturist, or for a friend to say that he is attending a spiritual healer to help with some long-standing ailment. From time to time we ourselves may choose to sample the healing and relaxing benefits of massage and aromatherapy, at the hands of a trained therapist.

People are increasingly turning to therapies in times of crisis or trauma. Many of our communities are not as intimate and supportive as they once were. Organised religion does not play the same central role as it did in former times. When relationships fail, when there is a sudden death in the family, or when life lacks meaning and fulfilment, people have come to view therapy as a means of expressing their pain and bewilderment. It offers a way of coming to terms with losses and upheavals, and of learning to create a new life, with the help of a caring therapist. Many therapies can help us to cope with the day-to-day stresses and strains of life, can ease and soothe, nourish and heal our bodies, our minds and our spirits. In the majority of cases we are not practising anything new. Almost all of these

therapies have been with us for thousands of years, in all societies of the world. We are merely rediscovering a way of healing
that is holistic, safe, and effective, when practised by dedicated,
professional therapists.

Although the medical system of treatment has a very important place, some of us have become disenchanted with the
amount and variety of synthetic drugs being used to treat
everything from asthma to sciatica. Many are also disillusioned
with the lack of time spent taking case histories, and the lack of
interest in our lifestyles and our emotional lives, which may be
contributing to our illnesses. Holistic therapies treat the person
at every level: physical, psychological, emotional and spiritual.
Homoeopathic and herbalist remedies offer us treatment holistically with natural substances, which do not have unpleasant
long-term side effects. People with painful symptoms may look
to the expertise of the acupuncturist, the massage therapist, the
osteopath, the chiropractor, or other practitioners, to be treated
holistically, without recourse to drugs. When offering a diagnosis, these therapists will take into account the person's diet,
lifestyle, emotions and family history.

Choosing a Therapist

It is important to seek details of a therapist's training and qualifications and to find out whether they are members of any
professional body. If there is any doubt as to whether the person
is a member of a particular organisation, you are quite entitled
to contact the relevant organisation to ascertain membership.
Also, it is important to ask whether the therapist is governed by
a code of conduct, and whether professional indemnity and
public liability insurance have been taken out.

When you first contact the therapist, either by phone or in
person, you might like to ask questions regarding the length of
training and how long the therapist has been in practice.
Therapists who have studied their chosen area thoroughly will
be only too happy to tell you where they obtained their training
and experience. Before making an appointment, it is best to ask
the cost of therapy, the estimated number of sessions that you
may be required to attend, and the frequency of sessions. It is
important to go by your own feelings when talking with the

therapist, as the rapport between you and the therapist is central to all therapy. If you find that the therapist is rather brusque, or seems to be hurrying you, or is in any way insensitive to your queries or needs, this is not a good indication of the quality of treatment you can expect during therapy.

Although most therapists whom I have met during my years of involvement as a student, a client, and a therapist have been genuinely sensitive and caring people, this cannot be taken for granted. The level of sensitivity, dedication, commitment and expertise of the therapist is of the utmost importance to the effectiveness of therapy. Feeling accepted, listened-to, safe, respected and understood, and being treated with warmth and empathy, are as important as the kind of therapy that is being practised. Although the techniques and the theories are useful tools to focus and guide the therapist, it is only through integrating these with the therapist's own life-experience, and genuine love of others, that healing can be facilitated. This connection between two unique individuals who truly value and see the humanity of each other is at the heart of all healing.

About the Book

The main aim of this book is to represent each therapy in a comprehensive way, taking into account the limited amount of space available. There are thirty-six main therapies included, each of which is explained in some detail. Chapters comprise an introduction to the therapy, benefits of the therapy, case studies, and a suggested reading list. There are nineteen lesser-known therapies included, which are also briefly described. Details of training and a directory of practitioners in Ireland — or in some cases the address and contact number of an organisation that will make referrals to qualified therapists — are contained in the Directory section at the back. There are also directories of healing centres, residential centres and helplines in Ireland.

The book has been written with the following in mind:

- Members of the public who require or are interested in complementary medicine, to help them to find the method and treatment that most suits their individual needs

- Those who wish to undertake professional training in the complementary healthcare area

- Practitioners, both medical and complementary, who may wish to refer their patients or clients to therapists who offer other forms of therapy.

The various therapies are listed in alphabetical order. As each therapy is holistic, it can affect the person at all levels — physical, psychological, emotional and spiritual — which leads to a difficulty in trying to categorise therapies. For example, acupuncture treats the person at the physical, spiritual and emotional levels, and the first level treated is the physical, as needles are inserted into the body to induce healing at all levels. Yet it is the unblocking of the qi — at an energy or spiritual level — which brings about healing.

Where possible, there is a list of therapists who have undergone training in their chosen area, or who are registered with a professional body. There is an outline of the requirements of some organisations regarding acceptance of practitioners for full membership. These organisations have reputable standards and many have a code of ethics. The book can act as a guide in the selection of a therapist, for anyone seeking competent, confidential and professional treatment, with some redress to a professional body where necessary. Where professional bodies do not exist, or where individuals are not members of any organisation but are qualified in some way, details of individual therapists are given, along with their qualifications. Some organisations did not wish a list of their members to be published, and the organisations themselves can be contacted for the name of a therapist in your area. No responsibility will be accepted by the author or publisher for any form or instance of malpractice by practitioners listed in this book.

Author's Note on
the Seven Chakras
or Energy Centres

There are seven main energy centres in the human being. These are commonly referred to as chakras, and are described thus in the course of the text. The first centre occurs at the crown (the pineal gland), the second at the forehead (the pituitary gland), the third at the throat (the thyroid gland), the fourth at the heart (the thymus), the fifth at the solar plexus (the pancreas), the sixth at the abdomen (the adrenals), and the seventh at the base centre (the gonads). These energy centres are part of our *etheric* (energy) body. Besides these main centres, there are millions of other energy lines or meridians running through the etheric body, connected to our physical body.

These chakras are receivers and transmitters of energy or spiritual life force. Each chakra is tuned to a particular vibration or frequency, and vibrates with a particular colour of the spectrum. For example, the crown chakra is purple, the forehead is indigo, the throat is blue, the heart is green, the solar plexus is yellow, the abdomen is orange, and the base chakra is red. Kirlian photography can be used to photograph the state and colour of these chakras. Some people who are extra-sensitive can see these energy centres, individually or collectively, as an *aura* (meaning light).

When each chakra is in balance, we experience good health and a sense of well-being. When a chakra is damaged, or is not able to transmit or receive energy adequately, we experience dis-ease. Therapists and healers who work with spiritual energies, depending on the type of therapy being used, seek either to manipulate or to channel energies to the chakras, so that any blockages can be cleared and balance be restored.

Alternative and Complementary Medicine

Comment from the Department of Health

In a letter to the author, dated 14 November 1996, the position of the Department of Health regarding complementary and alternative therapies was stated thus:

Alternative Medicine and Complementary medicine are umbrella titles for acupuncture, osteopathy, herbalism, homoeopathy, aromatherapy, reflexology, psycho-therapy, massage, counselling, etc. The general position in regard to Complementary Medicine in Ireland is that it is not regulated and there are currently no proposals to regulate it. The reason for this is that practitioners of Alternative Medicine are not employed within the public health services and regulation should only be considered when practitioners in a particular field are employed in the health services.

Practitioners of Complementary Medicine are free to provide services to the public so long as they do not represent themselves as being registered medical practitioners. The legal position of practitioners of Complementary Medicine is that their dealings with their clients are regulated by civil law.

The Department of Health's approach to the provision of services in the area of Alternative and Complementary therapies is one of general encouragement to the various therapies in establishing their own regulatory structures and in developing mechanisms to inform the general public about the availability of services from reputable therapists.

A five year European Research Project on unconventional medicine was established in Brussels in June 1993 under European co-operation in the field of Scientific and Technical Research. In April 1994 the European Parliament issued an 'Own Initiative' draft report on the status of Complementary Medicine (Ref: A3-0291/94/PART B) calling on the Commission to take the measures required to harmonise the statutes of the various disciplines in Alternative Medicine. The Report also calls on the Council to enact legislation on the subject in order to guarantee patients free choice of treatment with all appropriate guarantees and to guarantee practitioners the right to establish in an effective manner. Finally the Report calls on the Council to forward a recommendation to Member States to include Alternative Medicine in their social security systems.

The Alexander Technique

When the natural subconscious mechanisms which control balance and posture are disturbed by injury or by constant misuse, the standard of our physical and mental functioning can be adversely affected. Most people unconsciously misuse their bodies by bending and twisting instead of keeping their backs poised and using their arms and legs naturally. They sit, walk and stand in a way that puts strain on certain areas of the body, especially the neck, the shoulders and the back. We cannot undo years of misuse by simply consciously telling ourselves to do so. It involves automatic reflex responses that appear to support the body almost effortlessly when they are functioning properly. By using the principles of the Alexander Technique and by learning to prevent interference with these complex mechanisms, pupils can begin to restore their effectiveness. Movement becomes freer and lighter and more enjoyable; breathing and speaking become easier.

The technique was developed by Frederick Matthias Alexander, a successful actor who suffered from recurrent hoarseness and breathing problems. When he rested he noticed that all symptoms disappeared, only to resume once he went back to work. He decided that the cause of his symptoms must be something he was doing while acting. He set up mirrors to observe himself at work and he found that he had a habit of stiffening his neck, pulling his head back, depressing his larynx and sucking in air with a gasp. Over several years he eliminated the old unconscious habits that had caused his difficulties and substituted new conscious movements which brought his body back into natural alignment.

What Happens During a Lesson Using the Alexander Technique?

You are asked to do many everyday things such as walking, sitting and standing. The practitioner observes your movements, and any areas of the body which are being put under strain by the various movements. Then the teacher will place his or her hands on certain parts of the body that need adjusting, and will show you how to move correctly, by keeping the hands held in that position. For example, when you are moving from a sitting to a standing position, the teacher may put one hand on the back of your neck, and the other under your chin, and then gently guide you forwards and upwards into a standing position, without putting any part of the body under strain. Then when you are standing, the teacher may guide you into a more correct standing position, by gently pressing the shoulders and diaphragm, easing the position of the head on the neck. Often those who experience standing in this way feel as though they are falling backwards, because for years they have tended to slouch forwards. You may also be asked to lie on a plinth, while limbs and shoulders are arranged to help you loosen up after many years of stiffness caused by misuse. After each lesson, you become more aware of your movement and posture in all sorts of areas of life. Gradually the movements come about naturally as your subconscious effortlessly controls the natural balancing reflexes of the body.

Benefits of Using the Alexander Technique

Many people can benefit from using the Alexander Technique. People who have physical problems caused by poor posture, or tense and tired muscles, may be amazed to discover that a lot of their problems are the result of constant misuse of their bodies on a day-to-day basis. Sports players and those who are health-conscious may wish to improve their co-ordination, performance and well-being. Performing artists may wish to add to their existing professional skills, by relearning how to move naturally, without strain or effort.

After as little as one lesson, many people report a feeling of lightness and well-being. As habits of a lifetime are gradually corrected, many report a definite improvement in the way they look, as well as in the way they feel. Back problems, neck and shoulder tightness and soreness, sciatica, and headaches are very common areas where there is a vast easing of symptoms. Other symptoms such as fluid retention, rheumatism, asthma, fatigue, menstrual problems, which may have been caused by poor posture and inhibited breathing, have also been reported to have lessened. It has also happened on occasions that tension, which had been trapped in the body because of emotional trauma, has been released. Many doctors have praised the healing and preventative aspects of the Alexander Technique. It may start by helping to ease backache but it can also lead to a transformation at the physical, emotional and psychological levels of the recipient, as old habits, attitudes and tensions are released from the system.

Practitioner: Frank Kennedy

Frank Kennedy first discovered the Alexander Technique when living in England in the 1960s. He studied for three years with the Society of Teachers for the Alexander Technique (STAT). Once qualified he returned to Ireland, and has been teaching the Alexander Technique in Dublin for over twenty years.

So many people misuse their bodies when moving, sitting, standing. Often people slouch or slump in chairs, hunch their shoulders and crinkle up their necks when working at their desks, hold the phone between their head and shoulders and write at the same time. This creates a state of strain and tension in the body. Poor posture can affect our breathing, our circulation and our digestion. I want to get people back to their natural height, and to their natural width. The back should be supporting itself. The head weighs in the region of a stone, and how we carry this affects everything else, including our balance and co-ordination. People need to become aware of how they are misusing their bodies, how it feels when they constantly put undue strain on certain parts of the body. They also need to feel the difference when their posture is corrected and they relearn to sit, to stand and to walk in a way that allows flexibility and less effort.

Our incorrect habits are second nature. We need to get in touch with first nature. As children, up to the age of about three or four, we knew exactly how to move and how to sit naturally without straining ourselves. As a race of people we have become largely desk-bound for many years of our lives, through studying in school and college, and later through working with computers, and in offices. This all takes its toll on the body. It takes time for people to relearn a natural way of moving and being. To change the habits of a lifetime which feel so familiar would be nearly impossible without assistance and practice. It would be like learning to swim or to drive without getting lessons. On average a person will attend for lessons at least once a week, for about twenty-five to thirty sessions. The Alexander Technique is both educational and therapeutic. It can bring about great relief to many people who have suffered for years with back pain, shoulder strain, stiffened muscles, sciatica, and other related complaints.

As well as being in private practice, Frank also teaches the Alexander Technique to the students in the College of Music, in Chatham Row, Dublin. He can be contacted at 35 Callary Road, Mount Merrion, Co. Dublin (tel: 01 288 2446).

Case Study: Emma

I decided to try the Alexander technique on the strong recommendation of other musicians who I respect, and when I realised that tension was present in my body. I also wanted to prevent any later damage and to check my current habits. I wanted to ensure that I would be able to play my instrument without pain for long periods of time. Initially I attended twice a week, then once a week and now about once a fortnight. At first I felt self-conscious and exposed. After the second visit I felt comfortable and relaxed, positive and focused. I always feel lighter after a session, restful and pleasant.

I'm much more conscious of my physical behaviour now. There is no more back and shoulder pain. I use less energy walking and running. I've begun to slow down a little. I think the Alexander Technique also encourages you to take yourself more seriously. My breathing has improved. I used to get chest pains, and a little wheezy, but now all that has changed.

Suggested Reading

Drake, J., *The Alexander Technique in Everyday Life*, London: Thorsons, 1996.

Hodgkinson, L., *The Alexander Technique and How It Can Help You*, London: Piatkus, 1996.

Leibowitz, J. and B. Cunnington, *The Alexander Technique*, London: Cedar, 1994.

MacDonald, G., *The Alexander Technique*, London: Hodder and Stoughton, 1994.

Aromatherapy

Aromatherapy (from aroma, sweet-smelling, and therapy, with intent to heal) is the practice of extracting oils from aromatic plants to enhance health and beauty, and bring about a sense of well-being. Essential oils are derived from the flowers, leaves, stems, roots and bark of plants and trees. Oils are extracted from a wide variety of plants and are very concentrated.

Properties of Aromatherapy Oils

Essential oils possess numerous properties which make them useful for treating many of the most common physical, mental and emotional problems. Smell has always been one of the most potent and instinctual of all our senses.

Each essential oil has its own unique properties. Some can be used as perfumes, air fresheners, aphrodisiacs and anti-depressants — for example, ylang-ylang, jasmine, and patch-ouli. Others have proven very beneficial in treating fear and anxiety — for example, geranium, bergamot and neroli. For centuries the oils of lemon, eucalyptus, clove, thyme and pine have been used to help fight infection. Lavender and rosemary are used for healing injuries, bruises, muscular aches, burns, and infections, and helping to quicken the natural healing process. Camomile is a soothing oil used to relieve itchy and dry skin and prevent allergies. Rose oil is helpful in the treatment of depression, eating disorders and trauma. At a physical level, lavender is used to help heal abscesses, acne, arthritis, cuts, headaches, hot flushes, nausea, sunburn and travel sickness. Psychologically it is used to aid insomnia, fear, hysteria, mood swings, panic attacks and anxiety.

It is very important, however, that we only ever use essential oils that appeal to our own unique sense of smell.

Uses of Aromatherapy Oils

The relaxing and soothing effect of aromatherapy is a deeply healing, sensual and enriching experience. Massage is probably the most important and useful way to use essential oils in aromatherapy. The essential oils used in massage can be diluted with a base oil such as wheat germ, grapeseed or sunflower. The oils work on the emotional as well as the physical plane. The inner relationship between mind and body in massage is one of the main keys to its importance. Aromatherapy massage combines the benefits of massage with the therapeutic properties of pure essential oils. The molecular structure of the essential oils is minute, so they penetrate the skin, and are taken into the blood and lymphatic system.

A few drops of a favourite essential oil, diluted with water and placed in an oil-burner, or placed on a log in an open fire, creates a real ambience in any home. Many oils are suitable for use in vaporisation. Oils can be put into baths to instil relaxation, to invigorate, to sedate, and to soothe tired or sore limbs and tense muscles. A compress or poultice can be applied to any area of the body to help burns, strains or skin problems to heal. This is a very simple way of using essential oils, especially when massage is contra-indicated. A poultice can bring relief to sprained or bruised areas, rheumatism, and menstrual cramps. Oils can also be placed in a bowl of boiling water, over which a person can then lean with a large towel, enclosing both head and bowl, and inhaled. Using this method and breathing through the mouth helps to soothe sore throats, while breathing through the nose is beneficial for sinusitis. Essential oils of lavender, eucalyptus, rosemary and marjoram are very useful as decongestants.

Aromatology

Aromatology enables the remarkable ability of essential oils to treat illness, to be applied to a far wider range of conditions. Having completed an additional three years of training and 200 clinical hours, aromatologists are the only practitioners qualified to prescribe essential oils internally and intensively. Training includes the study of aromatic medicine, which is used in France by many doctors as an alternative to pharmaceuticals. Over 150 essential oils are studied, as well as their uses internally, in the form of capsules, pessaries and suppositories, and their external uses in the form of aerosols, frictions and absorption creams. At present, Nicola Darrell is the only practitioner of aromatology in Ireland (see Directory).

Aromatherapy Practitioner: Kathryn Redmond

Kathryn Redmond works as an aromatherapist in Wexford. She studied aromatherapy and massage in the Natural Living Centre (NLC) in Raheny, in Dublin. Her qualifications include an ITEC diploma in anatomy, physiology and holistic massage, an ITEC diploma in aromatherapy and aromatherapy massage, and an NLC certificate in sports massage. Kathryn has successfully treated people who have had many and varied physical and emotional problems, including muscular aches and pains, insomnia, depression, PMT, menopausal syndrome, rheumatism, arthritis, skin conditions and migraine.

When a person comes for their first aromatherapy treatment, Kathryn conducts a thorough medical case history. It is important before using essential oils that the properties of each of the oils are known. Some of the oils can be harmful to use in certain conditions. Kathryn makes sure that the person likes the scent of the oils she has chosen. She makes up a special blend of the essential oils, mixed with grapeseed oil, which can be used in the bath between treatments.

In Kathryn's experience an accumulation of stress is a huge factor in the development of many illnesses.

Stress and stress-related illnesses are among the most prevalent health problems of 'civilisation', and certainly figure prominently among aromatherapists' case histories. Stress can be described as anything which disturbs the normal balance of mental and physical health. Stress from any source makes us less able to withstand further stress. When we are worried we may find that we have minor accidents, and we are much more prone to infections and illnesses when we are emotionally drained. External sources of stress are not in themselves the problem, but the way in which we react to them. After an initial reaction to a stressful experience, the body continues to function reasonably well, even though the source of stress is still present. This adaptation phase puts a certain degree of strain on the body, especially the adrenal glands. If the level of stress increases, the ability to adapt to it may break down. Then all kinds of symptoms, from allergies to muscular aches and pains, can manifest themselves.

Most people consulting with an aromatherapist are aware that they are stressed and have chosen this therapy for the deep relaxation that massage with essential oils can bring. A huge array of essential oils are at our disposal in coping with stress. All the sedative and anti-depressant oils induce relaxation, such as marjoram, lavender, camomile, clary, sage, bergamot, neroli, and rose. Oils which strengthen the action of the adrenal glands are geranium, rosemary and black pepper. Anybody who knows they are under stress can do a great deal to help themselves by having aromatherapy baths which instil deep relaxation. Obviously it makes sense to do whatever is possible to remove the source of stress. Sometimes I would refer people to see a professional counsellor, to help with deep emotional and psychological problems. Nutrition is also very important when the body is under stress, so taking some supplements, particularly of the B vitamin group, can be very helpful.

Kathryn also runs six-week courses in aromatherapy for home use. She can be contacted at the Beauty and Aromatherapy Salon, 28 Lower Henrietta Street, Wexford (tel: 053 22527).

Case Study: Ann

Ann presented with muscular aches and pains, mostly in her back and shoulders, and with tension headaches. A full consultation, including a medical history, was taken before commencing treatment. Ann had started her own hairdressing business about five months previously. She was married and had two children. She was feeling very stressed. She constantly tried to balance her time between looking after her family, doing household chores, and working in her business. She also found it difficult to sleep at night. The therapist chose two essential oils to use for aromatherapy back massage treatment. These were lavender, for its balancing effect on the emotions, and marjoram, which is used as a muscle relaxant, and for its sedative qualities. She explained to Ann the benefits of each of the oils. During the treatment, Ann's back and shoulders felt very tense and tight and had a build-up of lactic acid. This was probably the result of her work as a hairdresser, which demanded that she often kept her arms in one position, when holding hairdryers. Also there was a build-up of tension from stress and anxiety. Afterwards Ann said she enjoyed the treatment very much. The therapist advised her to have a treatment on her back and shoulders once a week, for about six to eight weeks. She also gave her a bath blend of the oils for use between treatments. Ann was advised to make time for her lunch, which she was inclined to skip.

When she returned the following week, the aches and pains in her back and shoulders had lessened quite a lot. She had used the bath blend every night. She was sleeping much better and felt more relaxed. She had also made sure to take the time for her lunch, and she had drunk less coffee and eaten less junk food. Ann's back and shoulders had slightly improved over the week. There was less tension, and less of a build-up of lactic acid. The therapist continued to work on Ann's neck and shoulders, and also worked on her lower back, where circulation and lymphatic drainage was poor. Ann was advised to go for walks and perhaps to join a gym, to tone up her muscles.

On the third visit Ann was looking more relaxed. There was less strain in her face. She said she was making more time for herself. She had even joined a gym. She was making sure to eat much better foods, and to have her aromatherapy bath every night, which helped her to have a good night's sleep. She said that she felt less stressed and much more able to cope with her busy life. She was eager to continue her aromatherapy treatment once every week, for a few more weeks.

Suggested Reading

Cochrane, A., *The Body Shop: Aromatherapy & Massage*, London: Futura Publications, 1985.

Davis, P., *Aromatherapy An A–Z*, Walden, Essex: C.W. Daniels, 1988.

Earle, L., *Vital Oils*, London: Ebury Press, 1991.

Price, S., *Aromatherapy for Common Ailments*, London: Gaia Books, 1991.

Ryman, D., *Aromatherapy: The Encyclopaedia of plants and oils and how they can help you*, London: Piatkus, 1996.

Tisserand, R., *The Art of Aromatherapy*, Walden, Essex: C.W. Daniels, 1996.

Tisserand, M., *Aromatherapy for Women*, London: Thorsons.

Valnet, J., *The Practice of Aromatherapy*, Walden, Essex: C.W. Daniels, 1993

Westwood, C., *Aromatherapy: A Guide for Home Use*, Dorset: Amberwood Publishing Ltd., 1991.

Art Therapy

Art therapy provides the opportunity for insight, self-expression and communication, within a safe, therapeutic relationship between client and therapist. It can take place in one-to-one settings, or in groups. It is often used in educational settings, in psychiatric wards, in art psychotherapy, in self-development groups, in nursing homes, in rehabilitation programmes, in prisons, and in many other settings. Art therapy can provide a fascinating pathway to your unconscious world. This world is a source of creativity, uniqueness and energy, but also of repressed emotions, impulses and conflicts.

What Happens During an Art Therapy Session?

The therapist usually provides a range of materials for you to use. These include paper, cardboard, paints, crayons, chalks, pens and pencils, clay, textiles, old magazines (for collage), wood, or any other type of medium which the therapist feels may interest and inspire you. You are either asked to create a picture or object with a specific theme in mind, or you are allowed to choose a theme. The therapist gently encourages you to experiment with different materials and themes during the therapy process.

It is important that clients feel in control of their work. The task of the art therapist is to help people find ways to relate to the images they have created, to make sense of their creation, and in so doing to apply any insights gained to their day-to-day lives. The meaning of the work is explored by discussing its atmosphere or mood — for example, whether it is peaceful, intense, or violent. The relationship between different elements in the work is also explored — for example, whether in conflict or in harmony. The colours chosen, and the size and thickness of brushstrokes, are also significant. Sometimes clients discharge a lot of emotion through their images — anger may be represented by fire, hurricanes or explosions, while control may be represented by a closed gate or a dammed-up river. It can also happen that clients may create only 'happy' pictures. This can be a form of either conscious or unconscious denial, a way of keeping their rage or sadness private, and of giving the impression to the outside world that everything is wonderful.

While much imagery has a universal significance, the images a person makes have a meaning that is personal. An interpretation made too readily by a therapist might well say more about the therapist's problem with transference, than about the client's work. For some, the process of creating the artwork is therapeutic enough and they may not need to discuss anything more, while for others the artwork may be just the beginning of the therapy process.

In a group situation, it can be interesting to see how members work together on shared art projects, such as a giant mural. The group process can provide a means of connecting with others, through having to share art materials, and space, and time. It can also be a fun and a healing experience to create a work of art with other people who have the same goal as yourself. It can create a feeling of camaraderie and togetherness.

Benefits of Art Therapy

Art therapy is a visual language, and a very effective mode of communication. For some people who find it difficult to talk about a traumatic experience (particularly in the case of sexual abuse), it can feel much safer to begin to put down their memories and feelings on paper, in their own time, and in their own way. It can enable adults and children who have speech difficulties, limited vocabulary or learning disabilities to communicate. Art therapy can also be effective for people who are highly articulate, who may tend to talk about feelings rather than experience them fully.

Art, like a diary, provides a tangible record of the therapeutic process. By putting images on paper, the feelings and thoughts behind them are made more concrete and real. The works can be viewed objectively, shared with others, or saved for later review. As a tool for self-exploration, it combines a deep journey into your psyche with a deep sense of fun and awe at your own inherent creativity and self-expression.

Practitioner: Liam Plant

Liam Plant trained as an artist, before studying art therapy at St Albans in England in the early 1980s. He has worked in Ireland as an art therapist since the mid-1980s, with people from all walks of life, in all kinds of therapeutic settings. He also gives weekend workshops in art therapy.

Liam sees art therapy as a means to a therapeutic end, rather than as a means of producing art. The usual relationship between the client and the therapist is central to therapy, but there is also a relationship between clients and their artwork.

Art for many can be a very powerful experience. Since human beings are innately creative, art can unlock a lot of forgotten feelings and experiences from childhood. Clay, which is a very tactile and elementary medium, can bring about very intense emotional reactions. This kind of emotional release can be cathartic and healing because it occurs spontaneously, in a safe environment.

Liam does not agree with forcing anyone to break down their boundaries or defences. These will only be relaxed when clients feel safe and able to trust the therapist, and gain insight into their own processes and behaviour. Liam can be contacted at 25 Windsor Road, Rathmines, Dublin 6 (tel: 01 497 9337).

Case Study: Jenny

A few years ago I attended a group art therapy class, for about ten weeks, one evening each week. Every evening was a new experience. I never knew what would come up for me, what kinds of emotions, or what kinds of insights I would get into my life. I never really liked communicating in groups before. This was different because we were communicating more through art than through words. I really enjoyed myself. At times I felt like a child, free and happy, sprawling with crayons on the floor. Other times I was amazed at the beauty of what I had created. Once I couldn't believe there was so much pain inside when it all came spilling out on the page.

The art therapist was really caring and helped us to explore ourselves, and our relationships to other members of the group, in a very safe way. There are a few exercises which really stand out in my mind. One was drawing my self-portrait. I drew myself by looking into a mirror. I was amazed at the result. It was an incredible likeness, and the other group members remarked on the feeling of calm and gentleness, especially in my eyes, which the picture evoked for them. I was delighted with this picture and hung it up on my wall. It was a very healing experience.

Another evening myself and Mary worked together. I had never worked with Mary before. We had one large sheet of paper between us and each of us had to try to communicate with the other through drawing. Mary began by stabbing the paper with black and red marks. I had the feeling there was a lot of anger and frustration going on inside of her. I drew big smiling red lips, then a kind of shiny yellow sun and a long healing river of purple and blue. The river was long because I really wanted to reach out to Mary, but I didn't want to touch her drawing in case she'd feel I was invading her space. Mary paused for a long time. Then she drew a green river between my drawing and hers. She allowed this to seep into my drawing, culminating in a blue heart. Mary smiled. I smiled too. I was delighted and amazed that such a deep level of communication had occurred between us, without either of us having spoken a word. Afterwards Mary said my drawings had really reassured her. I certainly learned a lot about communication from that exercise.

I did a clay model of my working environment on another evening. I had no liking or respect whatsoever for the management of this organisation. I made the bosses into little figures with big ties, and shoved them all to the back of my clay building. I put the large figure of myself at the entrance of the building. I was walking away from that despicable place, never to return. This was my big goal, to leave that job and find a much more fulfilling place. I revelled in making this model. I felt a release of anger as I dug my hands into the clay.

There were so many other things we did which really left a lasting impression on me. There was a group mural which really brought the whole group together. We were delighted with the wonderful vibrant forest we'd created. No one felt crowded or lacking in space. We each made our unique contribution. Then there was the night we all made a mask and a shield. This was the side that we showed to the world to protect ourselves and to keep our vulnerable sides hidden. On different evenings we worked with wood, plasticine, cardboard, textiles, magazines for collage, paint, crayons and clay. It was a really healing experience for me.

Suggested Reading

Case, C. and T. Dalley, *Handbook of Art Therapy*, London: Routledge, 1992.

Case, C. and T. Dalley, *Working with Children in Art Therapy*, London: Tavistock, 1990.

Dalley, T., C. Case, J. Schaverien, F. Weir, D. Halliday, P. Novell-Hall, and D. Waller, *Images of Art Therapy: New developments in theory and practice*, London: Routledge, 1994.

Dalley, T. (Ed.), *Art as Therapy*, London: Routledge, 1994.

Kramer, E., *Childhood and Art Therapy*, New York: Schocken, 1979.

Milner, M., *On Not Being Able to Paint*, London: Heinemann, 1977.

Schaverien, J., *The Revealing Image*, London: Routledge, 1991.

Thompson, M., *On Art and Therapy*, London: Virago, 1990.

Ulman, E. (Ed.), *Art Therapy in Theory and Practice*, New York: Schocken, 1975.

Aura Soma

Beginnings of Aura Soma

Aura soma, meaning 'light being', is the creation of Vicky Wall, the seventh child of a seventh child, who could see people's auras from childhood. When she lost her physical sight, her sixth sense became greatly sharpened. She was guided to make the first series of 'balance' or aura-soma bottles while in meditation, and at that time she was not aware of their later use. Subsequently she discovered that the crystal-clear oils, plant extracts and essences used in the contents of her aura-soma bottles were found to revitalise and rebalance the human aura.

What is Aura Soma?

Aura soma is a gentle holistic form of self-healing for body, mind and spirit. It is also a form of colour therapy. There are ninety-six bottles, the contents of each of which are divided into a top and bottom section. Each bottle is made up of two colours, one colour for each section, or of one colour. Each 'balance' bottle vibrates with a different energy frequency. It seeks to balance the chakras if any one of them is disturbed or weakened. There is a special balance bottle associated with each of the chakras, which is deemed to bring healing to the glands, organs and muscles linked to that chakra. If any of the chakras are damaged, problems can be felt at all levels.

What Happens During an Aura-Soma Reading?

You will be asked to choose four bottles to which you are drawn at a feeling or intuitive level. As each vibrates at a different frequency, it is assumed that the bottles chosen are the ones needed to indicate your current state of well-being, and the kind of chakra-healing needed. The order in which the bottles are chosen is also noted. The bottles indicate your unique life story. On a soul-level, each has a specific meaning.

The first represents the soul as far as your present consciousness can perceive it. It shows your potential, life purpose and the lessons that need to be learned. The colour at the bottom represents your true aura. The second bottle indicates problems you have experienced, which have had to be overcome to learn and develop — this shows your process of evolution. The third bottle indicates the here and now, the present state of the soul. The fourth bottle shows the present situation in relation to the energies moving towards the future.

The meaning of each bottle chosen is discussed with you. When you shake the bottle, sometimes it becomes bubbly, indicating that your energy field is vibrating with those of the bottle. A lack of harmony is indicated by the bottle becoming cloudy. Each bottle also has a special fragrance when opened. A few drops of the liquid can be put on the wrists and used to cleanse the aura when the hands are passed over the head and the main chakra areas. There are also aura-soma pomanders and quintessences which emit vapours and are used to cleanse the electromagnetic field, and protect the aura.

Case Study: Jacinta

I went for a reading when I was doing a colour course and I was curious to see what it would be like. At that time there were many changes going on in my life, and I wanted some kind of reassurance and direction. I was asked by the therapist to choose four bottles, and to place them on a table in the order in which I had chosen them. She said I should choose bottles I really felt drawn to. I chose: (1) Purple over Turquoise, (2) Turquoise, (3) Purple over Magenta, and (4) Blue.

The therapist explained the significance of each bottle. The first bottle chosen represents the person's soul path in life. The purple over turquoise indicates that I have a definite path of spiritual communication. Spiritual awareness at a very deep level was very important to me, she said. This is very true. I have always needed some form of spiritual meaning to feel at peace with myself. This is why I was really delighted some years ago to become involved in the spiritual and therapy areas. The colour at the bottom of the first bottle reveals the person's true aura. Turquoise is my true aura colour. I really love this colour. Both turquoise and purple are my favourite colours.

The second bottle represents the difficulties experienced, and gifts gained, from the past. The all-turquoise bottle is the bottle of heart-felt communication. This was again very true for me because deep and close connections have always been very important to me. This is also the ray of intuition, and of having a great affinity with the subconscious. Then the therapist said that I may have felt a lot of hurt, misunderstanding, and isolation as a child and I probably felt as though other children were on a different vibration from mine. I agreed with this 100 per cent! I had a very difficult childhood because I found it so hard to make friends. I was into poetry and art and song-writing, and all of those kinds of areas. As a result of this I was often laughed at by other kids. I suppose this is why I stuck with adults much of the time. Turquoise is also the colour of sensitivity, the therapist said, and this is something that I have developed as a result of past difficulties.

The third bottle represents who I am now. I chose purple over magenta. I had chosen a bottle which represented huge potential, the therapist said. She felt as though I had so many talents which could be used spiritually, and that I had vast and broad understanding of so many areas and so much to offer to others. Also she said I could link up the knowledge gained from studying and experiencing many different areas to reach new levels of understanding and awareness. Again communicating this knowledge, and intuition, which I would like to develop more, is very important for my self-expression.

The fourth bottle represents the future. I chose the all-blue bottle. This again represents communication at a very deep level, and is also the bottle of peace. The colour is very much richer, and stronger, than that of the past (turquoise), because in the future I will have learned to communicate my truth to others, and will, as a result, feel more comfortable with myself, and not as fragile as in the past. This is my mission, according to the therapist. I will probably be called upon in the future to talk to large groups of people and in that way I'll connect with many people. I had recently begun to facilitate a personal development group. This had been nerve-racking for me but I really did want to overcome my old problems with groups so I looked on this as an opportunity. Thus the reading gave me great hope for the future.

Suggested Reading

Wall, V., *The Miracle of Colour Healing: Aura-Soma therapy as the mirror of the soul*, London: Aquarian Press, 1993.

Bach Flower Remedies

Dr Edward Bach, a Harley Street physician, discovered his flower remedies having dedicated much of his life to researching and perfecting his approach to healing. His basic philosophy was that our emotional outlook and personality are ultimately responsible for our overall mental and physical well-being. His system of healing was intended to treat people at an emotional and personality level, and he believed in treating the cause rather than just the effect. His flower remedies are used to transform negative emotions (such as fear, bad temper, jealousy and worry) into positive emotions (such as calm, joy, hope and self-acceptance). The remedies are divided into seven categories which help to change feelings of (1) apprehension, (2) uncertainty and indecision, (3) loneliness, (4) insufficient interest in present circumstances, (5) over-sensitivity to ideas or influence, (6) despondency and despair, and (7) over-care for the welfare of others.

There are thirty-eight remedies in all, each one prepared from the flowers of wild plants, bushes and trees. Each remedy deals with a particular emotional state or aspect of personality. For example, olive is used to treat someone who suffers from tiredness, fatigue and exhaustion caused by excessive working, studying or concentration. Several remedies can be taken at a time, up to a maximum of six. The remedies in no way interfere with any other kind of medication being taken, and are entirely safe for use by adults, children, and even animals and plants. They are usually taken by putting a few drops of the chosen remedy into water. When a special remedy is being prepared a 30-ml bottle containing spring water and two drops of each remedy, or four drops of the rescue remedy (see below), is used. The flower remedies come in liquid form, preserved in brandy. They should be sipped or put on the tongue for a few seconds, before swallowing. Four drops of this remedy can then be taken four times a day. They may not be suitable for anyone who has a problem with alcohol, because of the brandy preservative.

The rescue remedy, which is a combination of Star of

Bethlehem, rock rose, clematis, cherry plum and impatiens, is used to treat shock, or in times of emergency such as following an accident. It is also helpful when someone is apprehensive of visiting the dentist, when a woman is anxious before childbirth, or in the case of trauma or bereavement. Rescue remedy can be applied to the skin to remove the shock and pain from an area that has been bruised or has suffered a minor burn. Rescue remedy cream can be used in treating lacerations, ulcers, scalds, burns, sprains and many other skin problems.

Bach flower remedies treat you as an individual, taking into account your feelings, temperament and personality. The remedies are not a direct treatment for physical complaints, but they can have a positive effect on our bodies. When we feel better emotionally, often any physical illnesses or ailments — which may have been originally caused by a suppression of our emotions or a depletion of our energy — can be cleared out of the system much more quickly and effectively.

Practitioner: Moira Griffith

Moira Griffith, author of *Flower Power*, has used Bach flower remedies for over forty years, as a way of helping to transform her own life, as well as aiding others on their own path to health and happiness. She works as a Bach flower consultant in Nature's Way in Tallaght, and from her home in Blessington. She also gives courses in the uses and benefits of the flower remedies. According to Moira:

The flower remedies contain the pure love, perfection and conscious-ness which emanate from the individual flowers. They are created by placing the flowers in a bowl of water and leaving them for a few hours in sunlight, so that their love and energy can be transmitted into the water. The water containing the flower's energy, which is the source of the flower remedy, is then used by the patient's higher self, to work through any negative traits which have developed in the per-sonality. These traits block us from accessing our higher selves, thus causing us untold problems and dis-ease in our lives.

The remedies help to open us to our higher selves, but they cannot permanently change us unless we work with them to bring about our own healing. We can only transform ourselves by willingly opening to

*life, to love and to the perfection of the universe, of which we are a
unique part. When we become ill we are much more likely to open
ourselves, and to consider change. The flowers help to free us from
feelings of self-doubt, fear, anger, intolerance, greed, resentment,
possessiveness, hopelessness and many other negative emotions, which
can be transformed into their opposite positive attributes.*

*My daughter-in-law had suffered from asthma for many years, and
had one dreadful attack of asthma in the middle of the night. Nothing
could calm her, until I gave her a few drops of flower remedy, containing rescue remedy, aspen and mimulus, to alleviate the feeling of
panic. Within twenty minutes she was breathing peacefully. Since that
night she has never had another attack of asthma.*

*I use a combination of knowledge, intuition and experience, to help
patients discover which flower remedies are most suitable for their
particular personality type. Often people have lost touch with the
essence of their true selves. Through pain, disappointment and trauma
they may have developed a shield of protection around themselves.
They may never admit their own failings, imagining themselves to be
different from how they really are. By bringing any negative traits to
consciousness there is always the possibility for healing and lasting
change. The flower remedies help to bring emotions to the surface. It
is, however, up to the patient to accept whatever truth is revealed and
to work, not just towards the alleviation of a symptom, but towards
total transformation. I combine the flower remedies with the use of
affirmations, to help people to bring the love and openness of the
flowers into their own lives. For this is who we really are, pure love,
and this is what we can recreate in our lives, with the help of the
flower remedies. The Bach flower remedies are available in most health
food shops, and in some chemists.*

Moira Griffith can be contacted at: Shroughan, Lacken, Blessington, Co. Wicklow (tel: 045 865 078) or at Nature's Way, Tallaght
(tel: 01 459 6268).

Case Study: John

*John was an epileptic, and had been confined to the house for over ten
years. He was constantly falling and breaking limbs, and he was on
heavy doses of medication. John suffered greatly from constipation,
which was a great source of worry for him. He had tried many long-*

standing remedies. Each type of laxative worked for a while but the effects were not lasting. The situation seemed particularly hopeless when he had been constipated for six weeks. The woman who was looking after him finally decided to try the flower remedies. The flower remedy counsellor she attended did her best to ascertain the personality of her patient, by asking the woman to give details of the patient's emotional state. The patient was reported to be fearful, anxious, reserved, not prepared to get emotionally involved with people, and constantly feeling hopeless as though he'd like to be dead. The counsellor made up a special bottle of the remedy containing aspen (to combat anxiety), mimulus (to help with fears and phobias), rescue remedy (to help with the emergency situation which was at hand), water violet (to help with feelings of being aloof and tending to withdraw from emotional involvement), and sweet chestnut (to alleviate feelings of deep anguish and wishes of death).

Four drops of the flower remedy were to be administered to the patient, four times each day. John was given four drops in the evening before his bedtime. In the morning he was given another four drops. That morning his six weeks of constipation ended. He never suffered from constipation again. He also began to go out of doors, to travel by bus, to live a full life for the first time in ten years.

Suggested Reading

Bach, E., *Heal Thy Self,* Walden, Essex: C.W. Daniels, 1994.

Bach, E., *The Twelve Healers,* Walden, Essex: C.W. Daniels, 1993.

Barnard, J. and M., *The Healing Herbs of Dr Edward Bach,* Bath: Ashgrove, 1995.

Chancellor, P.M., *Illustrated Handbook of Bach Flower Remedies,* Walden, Essex: C.W. Daniels, 1995.

Griffith, M., *Flower Power,* Kilkenny: Abundant Life Products, 1994.

Howard, J., *Bach Flower Remedies for Women,* Walden, Essex: C.W. Daniels, 1992.

Mansfield, P., *Flower Remedies,* London: Optima, 1995.

Bio-energy

Bio-energy is a form of energy healing that originated in China. It involves the re-channelling and balancing of all energies (cosmic and earth — biological — energies) contained both inside and outside the human body. When the energy field (the chakra system) is healthy, it is in complete balance, and the energy or chi is flowing in a harmonious way. When it becomes weaker or blocked, illness can manifest itself at a physical level. Bio-energy therapists seek to clear blockages and to replenish the energy field in areas that are depleted of energy, by allowing energy to flow through their own energy fields. They use their hands as sensors to diagnose what is wrong and then seek to rectify it. Both physical and emotional problems can be treated.

What Happens During a Bio-energy Session?

You can lie, sit or stand during the administering of treatment, depending on the presenting problem. The therapist begins by feeling the energy centres (chakras), and checking their condition. If any blockages are located, the therapist diagnoses whether their cause is physical or emotional. The therapist then applies certain learned techniques, which involve manipulating the energy and sometimes laying on of hands, to release blockages from the system. The energy can be felt by therapists in their hands and in their stomach (solar plexus) area.

A treatment can last from twenty or thirty minutes to an hour. Usually it is recommended that you attend for treatment on three consecutive days. Sometimes people will get results within that period, but depending on the chronic nature of the problem, it may take longer. People often experience heat, cold, tingling or tickling feelings during a session. Sometimes people are pulled backwards when the therapist is 'pulling' the energy.

Bio-energy Therapist: Michael Dalton

Michael Dalton holds a plexus diploma in bio-energy. He has been working with bio-energy for three years, and has had much success in using it to treat such physical problems as arthritis, lower back pain and stress. He also cites a recent case of a young child who visited him for three sessions with asthma, and was completely cured within that time.

I see bio-energy as a way for people to take control of their health. People create their own sickness. I believe that I attract people to my practice who are ready to be healed, and who can be helped by my experience and sensitivity to energies. The energies I channel have their source in the cosmos and the earth. Every chakra and colour vibrates with a different frequency, so I channel the energy of the combined colours from the full spectrum of light.

Michael runs eight-week introductory courses to give patients the opportunity to develop and learn techniques for themselves. He has also developed a year-long course, which he believes will teach people all they need to know about using universal energies to bring about healing in themselves and others. His course includes a section on the correct use of channelling energy so that the person's own energies will not be drained, as can happen if therapists seek to cure others from a power or ego basis instead of through the channelling energies.

Michael Dalton PBE Dip. can be contacted at The Natural Health Centre, 15 Wicklow Street, Dublin 2 (tel: 01 677 1021).

Case Study: Ann

I first went to the (bio-energy) clinic on the recommendation of a friend. I have to say I was unsure of what I was letting myself in for. However, after just one session, I felt immediate relief of back pain, and also my oesophagus inflammation seems to have eased considerably. After three sessions I also noticed an amazing occurrence. I have had an enlarged thyroid gland since I was very young, and both my husband and myself noticed that the usual swelling had been reduced a lot. I also feel generally in good spirits and have lost a lot of tension.

Suggested Reading

O'Doherty, M. and T. Griffin, *Bio-energy Healing*, Dublin: O'Brien Press, 1991.

Biofeedback

Biofeedback originated in America in the 1950s, and is a scientific method of measuring and monitoring a person's superficial and inner stress, by means of modern electronic equipment. It is often described as the teaching mirror because it reflects our state of health. An experienced biofeedback therapist can quickly measure the degree of stress and identify its cause. With this information the therapist makes clients aware of their stress levels, and teaches control. The great value of biofeedback therapy, for those who live a very busy and demanding life, is that stress can be self-controlled in almost any situation.

Everyone is subject to some degree of stress on a daily basis. It may not be obvious to us, however, exactly how much stress we are actually under. If not dealt with, stress may build up, and eventually become manifest through physical or emotional symptoms. Stress affects different people in different ways. Some manifest it outwards through physical aggression, while others suppress it, which often leads to pain or hypertension.

How Can Biofeedback Help Control Stress?

Bio- (from biological) feedback shows varying stress levels on a monitor. This is very helpful especially for those who are unaware that they are in any way stressed. There are several instruments used to measure stress levels. Electromyography (EMG) measures muscle tension. Small sensors are placed on the muscle, which measure electrical activity. Every movement requires muscle tension, but when muscles are at rest they should feel relaxed with no residual tension. When at rest, the EMG should register between 1 and 2 micro volts. Skin temperature is measured by attaching a thermister or thermometer bulb to the fatty part of the finger. This registers skin temperature on the monitor. Skin temperature indicates the level of inner stress. If we are relaxed, our blood vessels are dilated, and blood flow is increased so that the our hands are warm. When we are stressed, blood vessels are constricted, blood flow diminishes and our skin temperature is lowered.

With biofeedback therapy it is possible to raise skin temperature and in so doing to control the autonomic nervous system
which controls blood pressure, heart rate, etc. Low skin temperature is associated with migraine. By controlling skin
temperature, migraine headaches can be alleviated. Likewise
when patients suffer from panic attacks, biofeedback therapy
can teach them to control their breathing, which raises the skin's
temperature. This is important, as the basis of a panic attack is
the fear of losing control. The galvanic skin response device
monitors changes in the nervous system. This measures the
amount of electrical current that the skin allows to pass.

Benefits of Using Biofeedback Therapy

Biofeedback therapy can help in the successful treatment of
more than fifty major medical and psychological conditions
such as stress, anxiety, panic attacks and agoraphobia, migraine,
hypertension, peripheral vascular disease and irritable bowel
syndrome. Biofeedback teaches the patient to gain control.
Unlike other therapies, where the patient plays a passive role,
with biofeedback the patient is the therapist. The patient is
learning from the experience of past performance.

Practitioner: Ann Gallagher

Ann Gallagher works as a biofeedback therapist at Mount
Carmel Hospital in Dublin, and from her home in Terenure. Her
background is in nursing, midwifery, psychiatry and psychology. Ann sees biofeedback therapy as safe, holistic and non-
intrusive, often helping to reduce or replace medication.

*It is complementary to other therapies, but equally can be used suc-
cessfully on its own. During the initial consultation I take a detailed
case history, which includes details of the patient's lifestyle, exercise
and diet. As part of the biofeedback programme, I help the patient to
develop more effective ways of reducing stress. This may involve
taking more exercise, healthier eating, and breathing deeply at times of
crisis. The patient is also made more aware of the body's internal
warning signals, such as when the time has come to rest and recuperate, or when to release emotions of sadness, anger, or frustration in a*

safe and healthy way. It usually takes about six or seven sessions of therapy before the patient can learn to control stress levels successfully, but this of course varies between individuals.

Biofeedback is an effective way of showing patients the amount of stress that they are actually under. Once attached to the various monitoring machines it becomes obvious how stressed or relaxed the patient actually is. The amazing thing about these biofeedback machines is that stress levels can be changed consciously by a person's thoughts. For example, if you relax and think of a favourite setting, the readings will show increased relaxation, whereas if you begin to think of stressful situations in your life, the readings will visibly and immediately move to a more stressed level on the monitor.

I have seen great benefits using biofeedback therapy, especially with people who suffer with chronic stress, panic attacks, PTD (post traumatic disorder) and migraine. Biofeedback teaches many people to take back control of their bodies and their lives. Patients have learned to recognise alarm signals when these occur in the sympathetic nervous system, and to change their patterns of thinking and behaving to keep them balanced and calm. The benefits of learning to release stress are enormous physically. The heart, stomach, kidneys, bowel and circulatory system are all part of the sympathetic nervous system, so when levels of stress are no longer stored in these major organs, patients feel much fitter and healthier. Emotionally and psychologically patients learn how damaging it is to allow emotions to accumulate without expressing or releasing them appropriately. When this kind of emotional awareness is achieved the patient feels much more calm, clear and balanced.

Ann can be contacted for appointments at 20 Heathfield Road, Dublin 6 (tel: 01 490 5378).

Case Study: John

John is aged thirty-three years. He is a company director. He had his first panic attack at a board meeting. Suddenly and with no warning he started to hyperventilate. He got pins and needles in his arms and legs. He did not know what was happening and was terrified. These symptoms continued over a period of eighteen months. Each episode lasted three to four days, and occurred every few weeks. John had all the relevant medical investigations. During this time, his activities were limited and he lapsed into the 'sick role'.

John had experienced a classic case of panic attack, where the onset is sudden, there is no obvious cause, and there is a dread of losing control. Panic attacks are caused by a build-up of stress. They recognise no socioeconomic boundary and tend to occur in people who are outwardly controlled and perfectionist by nature. The symptoms in all panic attacks involve the autonomic nervous system, which is 'out of control'. With biofeedback therapy John learned to control this system. He could see the level of control on the biofeedback monitor. With practice and guidance from an experienced therapist, he not only felt much more in control, but was reassured by the visual evidence provided by the monitor.

Suggested Reading

Brown, B.B., *New Mind — New Body*, London and New York: Bantam, 1975.

Cade, C.M. and N. Coxhead, *The Awakened Mind — Biofeedback and the Development of Higher States of Awareness*, New York: Delacourt, Eleanor Friede, 1979.

Karlins, M. and L.M. Andrews, *Biofeedback — Turning on the Power of your Mind*, London: Abacus, 1975.

Schwartz, M.S. & Associates, *Biofeedback: A Practitioner's Guide*, New York: The Guilford Press, 1987.

Chiropractic

Chiropractic, born in the US in 1895, has become one of the largest drugless, non-medical healthcare professions in the world, helping millions to realise good health. Many aspects of chiropractic were a natural part of healthcare in many civilisations for thousands of years, but by the time Daniel David Palmer, the founder of chiropractic, treated his first patient, these arts had largely been forgotten by the Western world.

Chiropractic aims to improve the function of the individual, creating a healthier, stronger person, able to achieve more in life. The intensely complex expression of life that is the human individual has a master control system — the central nervous system — consisting of the brain and spinal cord. All communication between our bodies and our central nervous system is transmitted via our spinal nerves. The spinal cord and spinal nerves are intimately related to the bony spinal column. All vertebrae (spinal bones) are designed to move. The sum total of all this movement allows people to move and to carry out daily activities. When this movement becomes aberrated or abnormal, it can affect the spinal nerves as they exit from between the vertebrae. This causes an insult or interference to the nerves. This mechanism of aberrant spinal biomechanics (spinal movement), with the resultant nervous system impairment, is known as a 'vertebral subluxation'. It is often simplified by describing it as a spinal misalignment, or spinal nerve stress.

As these nerves are constantly carrying millions of signals between the central nervous system and the body, any interference will impair the transmission of these signals. The various body parts that are dependent on those nerve transmissions now do not function correctly. When left untreated, as is often the case, this leads to lowered health, vitality, and eventually overt symptomatology. Chiropractors are trained to locate and remove vertebral subluxations, assist patients in preventing the recurrence of these subluxations, and thereby help to improve the health and well-being of individuals.

What Happens During a Chiropractic Treatment?

On attending a chiropractor for the first time, you will usually be asked about your current and past health history, especially relating to injuries or accidents, even those that occurred some time ago. Then the chiropractor will conduct a physical examination which may include the use of a number of different tools including X-rays; thermographic and neurocalographic studies (the analysis of body temperature patterns); posture analysis; muscle testing; and muscle and motion analysis. The chiropractor may then decide that a patient is best served by referral to other medical or health-related agencies.

In correcting subluxations, chiropractors usually use their hands, but may avail of a variety of spinal adjusting instruments and specialist treatment tables. The spinal adjustment is a very specific type of manipulative thrust. It aims to restore normal function and spinal alignment rather than just improve mobility. Hence the use of the term 'adjustment'. The adjusting techniques are extremely safe and can be used to treat a range of people including pregnant women, babies, children, pensioners, athletes and people from all occupations.

Many chiropractors also recommend exercise programmes, give advice on posture and ergonomics (work postures), and may give simple diet and nutritional advice. There are at least forty spinal analysis and adjusting techniques designed to locate and correct vertebral subluxations. Most chiropractors use them selectively, depending on their patients' needs.

Conditions Treated

About half of all patients who consult a chiropractor do so for lower back pain. The next most common conditions treated are headaches and neck pain. Neural, muscular or skeletal conditions comprise almost all consultations with a chiropractor. However, many people first go because of a specific health problem.

How Does Chiropractic Work?

Because the subluxation interferes with the nerve supply to a particular area, it is thought that area does not function as well and will eventually show up as a symptom, such as pain, stiffness, ache, etc. The symptom is the body's alarm bell to say that there is a problem. By removing the subluxation, the chiropractor simply assists your body to repair itself by removing the nerve interference that has otherwise prevented it from happening earlier. Many patients find that other conditions that appear to have nothing to do with the back also resolve or improve under chiropractic care, because of the vast influence the nervous system has on the functioning of the body. Subluxations in one area of the spine may be influencing the function of another apparently unrelated region.

Before attending for treatment, you are urged to ensure that your chiropractor is a member of the Chiropractic Association of Ireland (CAI).

(Courtesy of Dr Christopher Barnett)

Case Study: Sophie

I had been experiencing severe pain in my back and hips for quite a while. The pain got worse when I did anything even remotely strenuous, such as dancing or lifting anything. I had recently begun a very stressful job, where I spent several hours a day working at a computer. The back problem really flared up when I moved jobs. Sometimes I felt a kind of numbness, or at other times pins and needles. I had been told about chiropractic by a friend who had gained a lot of relief from back pain.

Initially I was very nervous, especially when my spine was being examined. The practitioner asked me about my lifestyle, my diet and my job, and this helped me to relax. He used muscle testing, and palpation of the spine to check for irregularities. After the examination, he told me that I had a number of misalignments in my spine, which were causing the pain. This was a big relief, to know that it was nothing serious. I attended every week for about five weeks. Each time he did some work on the bones of my spine. The relief was good, and over the weeks I gradually felt better than I had in many years. I became aware of my poor posture when working at the computer. The chiropractor gave me some simple exercises to help this. I also started to take breaks at work, every forty-five minutes, to stretch my legs, and this helped a lot. I visited a nutritionist to advise me on a healthier diet, as I was in the habit of skipping meals. I now visit the chiropractor about once a month, for a check-up, to ensure that my spine is in good shape. Chiropractic has made a great difference to my life.

Suggested Reading

Moore, S., *Alternative Health — Chiropractic*, London: Optima, 1988.

Scofield, A.G., *Chiropractic — The Science of Specific Spinal Adjustment*, London: Thorsons, 1968.

Colour Therapy

Colour is a characteristic of the natural light energy of the universe. It occurs in the form of electromagnetic radiation, which emanates from the sun and stars. As a manifestation of energy, it affects us at all levels. Light and its component colours transmit in waves of energy which vibrate at different frequencies. Each colour has its own wavelength and frequency.

Properties and Healing Qualities of Colours of the Spectrum

Each colour of the spectrum — red, orange, yellow, green, turquoise, indigo, violet and magenta — is associated with one of the main organs and energy centres of the body. Each colour is beneficial in the treatment of specific emotional, physical and psychological conditions, when used in colour therapy.

Red, related to the base chakra or sexual energy centre, gives vitality to the physical body and is the colour of earthiness, stability, passion, creativity, and sexuality. It is especially effective in the treatment of anaemia, low blood pressure, chills and colds. It is also effective in helping us to recover our own power to think and act, and in the treatment of drug and alcohol abuse.

Orange, related to the abdomen, is the colour of health, vitality, activity, sociability, fun and freedom. It helps us to get in touch with our emotions, to overcome conditioning and to be ourselves. It is beneficial in the treatment of kidney and bladder problems, or for torn ligaments. It is also particularly good to use when we have just had a shock or a traumatic experience.

Yellow, related to the solar plexus, is the colour of detachment, of individuality and ideas. It is the colour of the sun, summer and natural light. This is the colour of the philosopher and the student. Yellow helps us to clear away old hurts and fears, to feel more secure in ourselves. It is also helpful in the treatment of digestive disorders.

Green, related to the heart, is the colour of unconditional love, harmony, healing, freedom, peace and group-consciousness. It is where the physical energies (red, orange and yellow) and the spiritual energies (turquoise, indigo and purple) are balanced. It is good to use if you need more space in your life, if you feel emotionally unbalanced or suffer from heart or circulatory problems. It can also help treat neuralgia, hay-fever, ulcers, flu, venereal disease and biliousness.

Turquoise, related to the throat, is the colour of communication, of peace, truth, gentleness, clarity, wisdom and trust. It is the colour of service to others, the colour of the sage, the counsellor and the writer. It can help with any kind of speech or communication problem, and is great for the immune system as it helps to ward off infections and has an antiseptic effect. It is also a soothing, rejuvenating and cooling colour, helping to heal sunstroke, sunburn or any inflammatory condition. It lowers high blood pressure, and can be used in the treatment of sciatica, backache and swollen glands.

Indigo, related to the forehead, is the colour of understanding, wisdom, intuition, awareness, truth and pure consciousness. It gives a feeling of calm and profound stillness. It is great for treating the skeletal system, varicose veins, any inflamed condition such as burns, bruises, eczema, arthritis and rheumatism. It is also helpful in stopping the flow of blood if haemorrhaging has occurred, and it is a great anaesthetic. It is a very healing colour; it protects the aura, helps combat insomnia, soothe fears and prevent nightmares.

Violet, related to the crown, purifies and cleanses the aura. It is the colour of self-sacrifice, nobility, power and dignity, artistic creativity and inspiration. It helps to normalise hormonal problems, and is used to treat emotional and personality disorders, nervous problems, and insomnia. It also helps to boost our self-esteem.

Magenta, situated above the crown chakra, is the colour of unconditional and universal love, of consideration and compassion, of co-operation, genuine caring and understanding. It helps to relieve headaches and head colds, lowers high blood pressure, and is beneficial in the treatment of nervous disorders and breakdowns, chronic tiredness, over-exertion and amnesia. It helps ease any situation where there is aggression or violence.

Each colour has a complementary colour which can be used to create harmony or if overuse of a colour has taken place. The complementary colour pairs are red and turquoise, yellow and violet, green and magenta, and indigo and orange.

How Can Colour Be Used as a Form of Therapy?

Colour can be absorbed into the human energy field through many different methods. A coloured silk, of whichever colour is indicated, can be placed over the part of the body that needs healing. Coloured lamps can also be used, as can visualisation of the colour flowing through the person's chakras. Coloured crystal pens are sometimes used to stimulate the reflex points, especially on the feet. Painting in the colour, wearing the colour, or drinking solarised water which has been stored in coloured bottles, are also methods which can be used in colour healing.

Most colour therapists will use a spine chart to find the colour with which you most need to work. The spine chart contains a diagram of the thirty-two vertebrae of the spine, divided into four sections. Each section contains eight vertebrae, and each vertebra is allocated a particular colour of the spectrum. You are asked to write your name on the back of the chart. The therapist then dowses or tunes into your energy, and reflects this on the chart by marking whether each vertebra has a strong, medium or weak reading of energy. When this is complete, the therapist can decipher which colour most needs to be worked on. The complementary colour is also worked on, to maintain harmony. Colour can be used to bring balance to the mental, emotional, metabolic or physical dimension of the person, depending on which is indicated by the spine chart. A full spectrum lamp can then be used, which contains two bulbs, one of the colour to be worked on, and the other of the complementary colour. Each of the bulbs is shone on you, in a predefined sequence, for 19.75 minutes.

Colour Therapist: Nuala Kiernan

Nuala Kiernan is a colour therapist and teacher, who gives individual treatments, introductory classes, and workshops for the Hygeia diploma course. She also works with colour reflexology, and as an aromatherapist, a reiki practitioner, a spiritual healer and an aura soma practitioner.

When we feel unwell, off-colour, it can affect all aspects of our being. So in my treatment I tend to look at whatever area of the person's being the problem is manifesting at, and take it from there. People often come to me when they are at a crossroads, when they want to make changes and need support, so emotional and spiritual healing is one of the areas I focus on. At the moment a young teenager is receiving colour treatment for bed-wetting, which occurred virtually every night. Since her third treatment, she has been 'dry' for six out of seven nights. Colour reflexology has cleared headaches that this particular person had suffered from almost constantly. In 1995, I myself had a bad fall where I tore ligaments from my shoulder, and chipped a bone. After a few colour treatments the ligaments healed and I was back working the following week!

Colour therapy works on an even more profound level emotionally, spiritually and mentally. It is the vibrational frequency of the particular rays that helps to clear the blockage or the cloud, so we can make the changes we need. When this happens we can be the truest expression of our own divine potential. We can shine in our truest colours.

Nuala can be contacted for appointments at 22 Treesdale, Stillorgan Road (tel: 01 283 5648).

Case Study: Eva

I originally went for colour healing because I had done an eight-week colour course and I could feel a lot of benefit from that. It was at a time when I was going through major changes in my relationship. Colour was a way of really pampering myself, and I loved doing the course. Consequently I went for colour therapy, about three times. Each session lasted about one and a half hours.

When I initially attended, the therapist had a chat with me and explained the different methods which could be used. The strongest kind of colour treatment is through a full spectrum lamp. The first time I went the therapist used coloured silks and hands-on healing, and a coloured crystal pen was used on the reflex points on my feet. For this session she used the lamp. I signed the back of the chart which she gave me, and she told me to relax and listen to the music while she worked out which colours I needed to work on. After a few minutes it emerged that yellow, the colour of detachment, was the colour I most needed treatment with, as well as its complementary colour, purple.

I needed yellow in all areas of my being: mental, emotional, metabolic and physical.

For about twenty minutes I sat and relaxed under the full spectrum lamp. The top bulb was yellow, and the bottom one was purple. I was advised between sessions to bring more yellow into my life. I bought some yellow flowers, balloons, candles, a scarf. I like yellow flowers, but it wouldn't have been a colour that I would ever have worn. I went back for a second session and again it emerged that I needed to work with yellow, but this time only at the physical level.

I certainly felt the benefit of going for colour therapy. Detachment was something I needed at that time. I needed to let go and clear out many aspects of my former life. I felt much clearer and lighter after the colour treatment.

Suggested Reading

Gimbel, T., *Colour Healing,* London: Gaia, 1994.

Gimbel, T., *The Colour Therapy Workbook: A guide to the use of colour for health and healing,* Shaftesbury, Dorset: Element, 1995.

Gimbel, T., *Form, Sound, Colour and Healing,* Walden, Essex: C.W. Daniels, 1995.

Gimbel, T., *Healing through Colour,* Walden, Essex: C.W. Daniels, 1995.

Graham, H., *Healing with Colour,* Dublin: Gill and Macmillan, 1996.

Sun, H. and D., *Colour Your Life,* London: Piatkus Books, 1992.

The Colour Therapy Workbook, Shaftesbury, Dorset: Element, 1993.

The Symbolism of Color, New York: Carol Publishing, 1989.

Counselling and Psychotherapy

Counselling is a special kind of relationship, where the client and the counsellor are committed to finding creative responses to the client's present difficulties and needs. It involves the giving of time, complete attention and respect to the client. Counselling provides an opportunity for clients to explore the roots of any traumatic or upsetting experiences they may have had in the past, or which they are experiencing in the present. They can then become conscious of the different options that are open to them to help resolve the problem.

Why Go for Counselling?

Many people find it difficult to open up and discuss their fears and past traumas, even with a close friend or partner. Often they may be having problems with the people to whom they are closest. Counsellors are trained to develop in themselves definite qualities and skills which are very beneficial in helping people to open up, to feel supported and cared for, to feel accepted, respected and understood. Counsellors do not offer advice: clients are encouraged to make their own decisions about situations.

The counsellor encourages you to grow in inner strength, self-understanding and self-esteem. Counselling can also be used for self-development. It can be a chance to explore with the help of a skilled and committed person many personal and philosophical questions. You may then discover hidden emotions and repressed thoughts, inner strengths and vulnerabilities, inner desires, dreams and goals for the future. The possibility of turning these dreams into reality based on your own unique potential can also be explored.

Some of the problems counsellors specialise in are bereavement, child abuse, rape and sexual abuse, AIDS, depression, stress, illness, anxiety, sexual problems and relationship problems. Counselling usually takes place in a one-to-one situation. Group therapy is also available and can be particularly effective in the areas of eating disorders and addictions.

Psychotherapy

Many counsellors are also psychotherapists — that is, they tend to go deeper, looking at past experiences and more deep-seated personal issues, seeking to bring about deeper changes, healing old traumas and hurts and helping clients to develop their unique creative potential. Some of the most commonly used approaches are briefly outlined below.

Behaviour Therapy

This therapy focuses on how a person is behaving when problems are encountered and needs are not being satisfactorily met. These behaviours are explored and discussed. New more appropriate behaviours are suggested when people are in distress. This is most effective with people suffering from phobias and fears, and compulsive-obsessive conditions.

Biodynamic Psychotherapy

This is a humanistic, body-oriented approach, which often uses methods such as biodynamic massage and expressive body-work, as well as verbal counselling and psychotherapy. It can be particularly useful when psychosomatic issues are presented at the beginning of therapy.

Bioenergetics

This emphasises the need to be grounded in the physical world. A variety of exercises that create stress in the body are used to bring repressed emotions to the surface. This also leads to an unblocking of energy previously trapped in the body.

Body-work

Body-work seeks to unblock and release energy trapped in the client's body owing to some trauma or painful experience which has disrupted the natural process. By working on these blockages through touch and gentle pressure, energy can be released and a sense of well-being experienced.

Client-Centred or Rogerian Counselling

In this type of counselling, the counsellor firstly explores the client's past and discusses any present problems, with a view to helping the client to understand the reasons why these problems exist, and over time to seek realistic solutions by developing an appropriate plan of action. Where a situation cannot be changed, for example when someone close has died, the client is helped to adjust to the new circumstances.

Co-counselling

This is where client and counsellor interchange roles. The emphasis is on encouragement, support and the balance of attention. Healing is believed to occur through the sharing of experiences and the discharge of emotions, which up until that time may never have been expressed. Co-counselling techniques are often taught and developed in group situations.

Emotional Release Work

The principle behind this is that memories are stored in the body. Working through these feelings physically, often by screaming, banging cushions and crying, can be a powerful way to encourage the client to release emotional pain while being supported by the therapist in a safe environment.

Inner Child Work

This is used mainly when a person has been abused or has undergone some very traumatic experience in childhood. The client is helped to recover the inner child, to feel exactly what it was like to be that child and, as an adult, to begin to nurture and care for that child. This is often achieved by using visualisation and self-expression through art and writing.

Psychoanalysis

In this approach the therapist relates current problems, anxieties and conflicts to childhood and adolescent experiences which were traumatic and subsequently repressed.

Relational-Emotive Therapy (RET)

This therapy aims to help the clients to rid themselves of 'irrational' ideas which are interfering with their enjoyment of life. It is believed that a more rational way of thinking will help the client to grow in self-esteem and to become happier and more able to cope with problems encountered in life.

Transactional Analysis (TA)

TA aims to help people become aware of the intent behind their communications with others, and to take responsibility for their behaviour by eliminating deceit and subterfuge from their ways of relating to others. Therapy takes place mainly in group settings where the interaction between group members is analysed in terms of the different parts of the personality which become prominent at any one time.

Counsellor in Practice: Eileen Boyle

I have been working as a counsellor for thirteen years. It has not been a straightforward journey. I became interested in counselling while working in administration in the World Health Organisation in Geneva. While working there I spent a lot of time listening to people's issues and problems. Somewhere along the line I realised that I did not have the skills to deal with some of the problems being presented. I returned to Ireland and studied at Trinity College. After obtaining my degree, the only counselling course available to me at the time was the guidance and counselling qualification. I completed this course and have worked in the education sector and as a freelance counsellor ever since.

It became apparent to me early on that I needed further counsellor training and I embarked on a varied route. I have taken courses in many areas of counselling. I was among the first group in Ireland to be certified in Reality Therapy. I am also qualified as a reflexologist and have a keen interest in alternative approaches to health and well-being. I have worked in schools and have enjoyed this very much. At present I work in a post-Leaving-Cert college. In this position I offer a counselling and guidance service to students. Recently there has been a new dimension added to my work with my involvement in the new one-year full-time counselling course at the Liberties College. I also have a private practice. I have been a tutor on the Maynooth counselling skills course for many years. In addition, I am involved in counsellor supervision. My interest and orientation is shifting towards archetypal psychology. I am exploring the areas of imagination and dreams, and am particularly drawn to soul work.

As a counsellor, people present with a wide variety of problems and difficult situations. Examples are loneliness, stress, confusion, relationship problems and many more. However, over the past two to three years I have found that there is a huge shift in people's awareness and in general I could say that clients are much less interested in problem solving and much more interested in their own personal development and growth. They tend to use the counselling sessions as a place where they can explore their own paths as well as looking at specific current problems and difficulties. With this in mind I use a varied approach encompassing parts of counselling models which will suit a particular client at a particular time. For me, however, the counselling relationship is all-important. I regard supervision as an essential part of my work and support system.

Eileen can be contacted for appointments at 57 Upper Grand Canal St, Dublin 4 (tel: 01 660 4574).

Case Study: Emma

Six years ago, at the age of thirty, I had a miscarriage. The circumstances around the pregnancy were difficult and it took time to come to terms with it. But I found that I began to get excited about the birth. Soon after, I had the miscarriage. I took it very hard as having a baby would have been one of my dreams in life. In the days that followed I began having flashbacks of child sexual abuse. I kept trying to push it away to the back of my mind. Eventually it faded into the background. Three years ago the memories surfaced again. I was in a job that was extremely challenging and stressful and my coping skills and confidence plummeted. I was waking up with thoughts of the abuse and I felt panicky. I finally contacted a counsellor.

I attended for counselling initially fortnightly for six months. Then I stopped attending for a while, but since I hadn't come to terms with the abuse I began attending again on a weekly basis. Initially I experienced only sadness. I talked a lot, trying to make connections with the past and my life as it was now. It took me a while to accept that it can be a slow process, especially because I was so used to censoring my feelings. It took time to trust. I have faced and worked through many difficult experiences with the help of the counsellor.

I am more able to understand my behaviours, some of them quite destructive, and my feelings. I have learned to be more accepting of myself and less critical. I feel as if I've experienced life in a richer way. There were times in the past when I'd go to bits and not want to wake up. I never think that way now. I have developed more respect for myself and more responsibility and control over my life. I am hopeful.

Suggested Reading

Kennedy, E., *On Becoming a Counsellor*, Dublin: Gill and Macmillan, 1977.

Murgatroyd, S., *Counselling and Helping*, London: Routledge, 1985.

Nelson-Jones, R., *Practical Counselling Skills*, Eastbourne: Holt, Rinehart and Winston, 1983.

O'Farrell, U., *First Steps in Counselling*, Dublin: Veritas, 1990.

Rogers, C., *On Becoming a Person*, London: Constable, 1990.

Creative Therapies

Creativity, when used therapeutically, can help any adult to explore and experience the joy and wonder of their own uniqueness. As children we were free to be creative, spontaneous, and imaginative — free to express ourselves through play and dance, colour and song, music and verse. But most of us lost this sense of our own creative essence when we were criticised and judged, or when we began to feel that we were 'too old' to splash paints across paper or to sing songs for the sheer fun of it.

Our creativity is part of our deepest selves. This creative energy can be expressed in all sorts of different ways, from singing, dancing, painting or drawing to writing, acting or gardening. Much pain comes from our fear of expressing this creativity. Without our ability to imagine and create, we risk becoming stuck and unfulfilled.

Listed in the Directory are people who run courses in creativity to help us reawaken and rediscover that inner dynamic, fun-loving self. (See also Art Therapy, Drama Therapy, Movement and Dance, and Music Therapy.)

Practitioner: Mary Roden

Mary Roden trained as an artist and in many other creative disciplines. Over the years she has worked in a variety of creative areas. During an illness she began to uncover her 'innate creativity' through painting, meditation, practical philosophy, and healing. Through these activities, she found great inspiration for her life and work. She has been working as a creativity therapist and giving creative counsel for a number of years now. Her work aspires to enabling people to express themselves creatively and in so doing to uncover their 'innate creativity'.

I believe that our 'creativeness', in all aspects of our lives, depends on our connection with our intuition: our inner guiding voice. Our intuition enables us to connect with an unlimited knowledge (spirit) and to experience our innate creativity. If we listen to our intuition we will always do what is best for ourselves and for all concerned. It releases us from our doubts, fears, anxieties and negativity. It gives us freedom to be ourselves, to grow in awareness and live an inspired life.

All creativity begins with an inspired thought, whether we want to arrange flowers, write a poem or design a garden. So to release our creativity we need to make a deeper connection with our intuition (unlimited knowledge) and allow ourselves to be creative in our thinking, thus eliminating all negative thoughts which prevent us from uncovering our innate creative potential.

The Arts Unlimited 'Creativity' process is a tool to uncover our innate creative potential. In an Arts Unlimited workshop you will experience an uncovering of your creativity and intuition. It is a process of learning to communicate with ourselves. To uncover our innate creative potential we use images (painting/drawing/collage/clay work), relaxation, guided meditation, dialogue and practical exercises. The format is always flexible to enable a 'person/group-centred' nurturing and growth.

Creating images can be energising, joyful, painful, sad, inspiring and freeing. It can give us insight and inspiration, and stimulate the senses. The colour and texture of the images, the creative process and the finished 'artwork' are all stages in the process of communication and healing.

Each person experiences the creativity session in their own individual way, uncovering what they need to, when they need to. People's growth in awareness during a 'creativity' programme is also reflected in their commitment to themselves and what they intend to gain by the experience.

Mary works with people on an individual basis and with groups in communities, universities (Trinity College Dublin) and the corporate sector. She is a reiki teacher/practitioner and artist. Mary also writes a regular column in the *Fitzwilliam Post*, Dublin. She can be contacted at Wicklow (tel: 0404 61248)s, or by writing to Arts Unlimited, 66 Lower Baggot Street, Dublin 2.

Crystal Healing

Crystals are concentrated forms of light energy which evolve in the earth over millions of years. They occur in certain areas that correspond to the earth's major chakras or energy centres. For example, crystal quartz is found mainly in Arkansas, in the US, and in parts of Brazil. Crystals are precious and semiprecious stones, which have been revered not only for their beauty and variety of shape and colour, but also for their ability to rebalance the chakras and so aid healing. Crystals most often used in healing are amethyst, ruby, sapphire, crystal and rose quartz, diamond, emerald, jade, tiger's eye, turquoise, lapis lazuli, malachite, peridot, opal, moonstone, citrine, calcite, aquamarine, amber, aventurine, agate, bloodstone, garnet, jasper, and pyrite.

Benefits of Using Crystals

The main reason for using crystals in healing is to help rebalance your own energy, which may be disturbed or depleted. An excessive amount of stress, or the suppression of emotions, can over time lead to problems on a physical, emotional, psychological and spiritual level. A release of any blockages in the main chakras or energy centres is aided by using the crystals' energy to amplify your own energy. Crystals can help ease depression, insomnia, stress-related problems, menstrual and ovarian problems, lower back pain and colitis.

The use of crystals, especially clear quartz, also helps to focus the mind and bring clarity, which can aid meditation. Rose quartz acts as an ioniser and helps to absorb any negativity which may have built up in a room. Crystals can be used to purify water, and to bring a plant back to blooming health if it has wilted or is not thriving in its environment.

What Happens During a Crystal Healing Session?

You are asked to select from a large range of crystals and gemstones seven crystals, to which you are attracted. A crystal reading is done by the healer based on your selection. Each crystal represents a certain aspect and chakra of the person (e.g. rose quartz and aventurine are heart stones and so represent emotions and need for love). The meaning of the crystals chosen is then discussed with you. Next, you are asked to lie on a plinth and the crystals are placed either next to or on you in an appropriate position (for example, rose quartz and aventurine stones would be placed over your heart area. If the crystals chosen were very large, they would be placed on the plinth as near as possible to your heart). This helps you to release stress or emotional or physical pain, without trauma, in a safe and gentle way. Healers may also use their own hands to channel energy.

A clear crystal quartz can be 'programmed' with positive thoughts, just as a blank tape can have a message recorded onto it which can be played back when required. This crystal can be carried by you, and acts as a reminder that old patterns of thinking need to be changed so that lasting healing can occur.

Crystal Healer in Practice: Terri Blanche

Terri Blanche works as a crystal healer, astrologer and holistic masseuse. She initially trained with the Faculty of Astrological Studies, and is also qualified in holistic massage (ITEC). She has attended many seminars and workshops in the Maitreya School of Healing in London, and in the Findhorn Community in Scotland. Terri first discovered the power of crystals around 1989. She realised that there were no workshops or courses being run in Ireland in the area of crystal healing, and, based on her own experience and intuition, began giving these courses some years ago.

When Terri works with a person using crystals she does not impose anything on the person's body. When the body realises it is safe, then it is free to relax. It allows the crystals to release the blockage, and restore a new and healthy pattern in the body, mind and spirit. A session usually takes about one and a half hours. Terri has also had much success in using crystals to bring about positive changes in people's lives. She recalls the man who chose five 'heart' crystals, including rose quartz, aventurine and sugalite, which greatly helped him to open his heart and to express long-suppressed emotions that needed to be released for healing to occur. And then there was the woman who chose orange calcite, which helped clear up her colitis overnight.

Terri very much feels that people are drawn to the beauty and healing power of crystals at this time because it is the Age of Aquarius, the dawning of a new concept and understanding of life and healing.

Many people are experiencing a new kind of energy vibration within themselves. The crystals help to hold and harness this energy while people are getting used to the change in vibration. They help us to remember that we are also repositories of energy. Listening to an enchanting piece of music can awaken us to the beautiful essence within us. Thus we can gain a greater clarity, of who we are, and where we are going. This helps us to integrate the new level of awareness into our day-to-day lives, so that real change and healing can take place.

Terri can be contacted for appointments and course details at 30 Sevenoaks, Frankfield, Douglas, Cork (tel: 021 891 527), or at Odyssey Healing Centre, 15 Wicklow Street, Dublin 2 (tel: 01 677 1021).

Case Study: Janet

Janet was a woman in her mid-thirties who attended for crystal healing. She spoke of feeling pressure in her head, and she had a problem with sleeping. She also felt a lack of job satisfaction and she worried a lot about money. She said she had no sexual feelings although she really wanted to have a relationship. During the first session she chose a large single quartz (a symbol of female and mother energy), a twin quartz (representing her desire to have a relationship), an amethyst (a symbol of her spiritual self), two rose quartz (which related to her heart and to her future), and two citrine crystals (which showed she was struggling with issues of personal autonomy).

This combination of stones, coupled with the healer's intuition, showed that Janet was intellectualising her feelings. Gentle work on the heart chakra, or energy centre, was indicated, which would help her to begin to feel her feelings. Janet was living very much in her head. She was not connected with her feelings or with the physical side of herself. This is probably why she found it so hard to sleep, with so many thoughts going around in her head. The amethyst was a great choice as it helped with her sleeping difficulties. The citrine helped her to become more in touch with her own personal power. It helped her validate herself, and overcome the effects of an authoritarian father who, she said, had always been very critical of her.

At the end of four sessions Janet was able to realise that her parents were just human like herself, and that it was up to her to make decisions to bring about change. She decided she would not enter into a relationship until she met a man who could really love her, and who she could also love. Previously she had kept her partners at arm's length by analysing them and not allowing them to get too close. A lot of anger which Janet had been holding in her system had dissipated and she was sleeping much better. The feeling of pressure in her head had also subsided.

Suggested Reading

Burgess, J., *Healing with Crystals*, Dublin: Gill and Macmillan, 1997.

Gardner, J., *Colour and Crystals: A Journey Through the Chakras*, Freedom, CA: The Crossing Press, 1988.

Holbeche, S., *The Power of Gems and Crystals*, London: Piatkus, 1995.

Irwin, N., *Understanding Crystals*, London: The Aquarian Press, 1991.

Raphael, K., *Crystal Healing*, Santa Fe, NM: Aurora Press, 1987.

Cutting the Ties

Cutting the ties is a form of psycho-spiritual therapy, which seeks to bring about a liberation from many sources of false security. There may be people on whom we depend for our emotional survival, and to whom we have given away our power, either at a conscious or a subconscious level. As children we are dependent on our parents or guardians. They provide for our physical, emotional, and psychological needs. When we become adults, however, it is time for us to fulfil our unique potential, as independent individuals.

In ancient cultures a ceremony was performed, when a child reached puberty, in which the ties of childhood and dependency on parents were cut. Since we no longer have these puberty rites, many people remain dependent on parents into adulthood. Their own needs are often sacrificed to fit in with the wishes of a dominant parent. A typical false escape from this dependent state is rebellion against all that parents stand for, and making further choices aimed at hurting, disappointing, and punishing them. In this case choices are still inversely influenced with reference to the parents, and control of the person's life is still external, not internal.

You may feel the need to cut the ties with one or both parents, with a sibling, with a lover or partner, with a child, or with anyone with whom you are over-emotionally and intensely involved. Ties may need to be cut when a relationship is holding you back from growing and moving forward in life. Ties can be cut with only one person at a time. If necessary, they can be cut with a deceased person. Those who cut the ties are set free to live their own lives without draining the energy of the person on whom they have been dependent. Often a much more mutual relationship will develop between both people when this has been accomplished.

What Happens During the Cutting of the Ties?

Both client and therapist work together to cut the emotional, psychological and spiritual ties, with the individual, through visualisation. It usually takes about three sessions. You sit with the therapist and visualise two circles touching (similar to a figure 8). You put yourself in one circle, and the person with whom the ties are being cut is placed in the second circle. You visualise a golden light flowing around both circles, and then a blue neon light is imagined, which magnetises each person into the centre of their circle. Tracing the figure 8 with golden and blue light is practised between sessions. A log of your dreams is kept, and these are discussed before each session. A complete list of the positive and negative qualities of the other person (with whom the ties are being cut) is written. The therapist then explores the extent to which you have been conditioned in the relationship. The therapist often makes a relaxing tape, to which you can listen each morning and evening between sessions to prepare for cutting the ties.

After tracing the figure 8, you usually lie down with your eyes closed and are covered with a blanket, to aid comfort and relaxation. Visualisation is used to relax each part of the body in turn. You visualise a golden light gently flowing from the feet, through the body, right up to the head and skull. You and the therapist are linked by a line of light — this line of light forms the base of a triangle, the sides of which are formed by the light flowing upwards from each person's spine until it reaches a point where you and the therapist connect with your higher selves. Your higher self is asked to guide you to visualise whatever is necessary to accomplish the cutting of the ties. The therapist asks you to visualise the ties binding both of you together. You are then asked what instrument will be best to sever the ties. When severed, they are destroyed in a manner visualised by you.

When the ties have been cut you are encouraged to thank the person with whom the ties have been cut, and to ask forgiveness, as well as granting forgiveness for past hurts. This is essential for taking back your own power and allowing the other person to do likewise. It is also often suggested to write a letter, which is not sent, to the person with whom you have cut the ties, stating that you are both free. The final visualisation usually involves you standing under a waterfall, which cleanses, heals and soothes the body, mind and soul. You are asked not to discuss what has happened for three days, so that the whole experience can be integrated into your psyche.

Benefits of Cutting the Ties

The greatest benefit is the feeling of emotional release, of freedom, of internal power and independence. During and immediately after the cutting of the ties the client experiences a release of old feelings and memories which need to be cleared away in order for healing to take place.

Practitioner of Cutting the Ties: Sarah Branagan

Sarah Branagan is a registered spiritual healer and has extensive experience as a facilitator for different meditation groups. She also holds a foundation certificate in hypnotherapy. Sarah is thus well acquainted with the use of visualisation and symbols for transforming lives and enabling people to regain their personal power. She also facilitates those who wish to do past-life regression. Sarah finds that spiritual healing provides an indispensable adjunct to cutting-the-ties therapy.

People can form attachments to almost anything: to having their own way, to their own opinion, or to strong emotions such as anger, jealousy, fear and pride. A person may become attached to appetites, such as food, alcohol, drugs, money, clothes, houses, cars, power and success. People can become so attached to their own life that they become terrified of death. Cutting the ties can bring about fundamental changes, accompanied by a new sense of freedom and contentment.

Sarah can be contacted for appointments at The Irish Spiritual Centre, 30/31 Wicklow St, Dublin 2 (tel: 01 670 7034).

Case Study: Linda

I decided to cut the ties with my mother because I felt I needed to gain more of my own power and self-esteem. I wanted to free up my creativity and to deal with my fear of childbirth. There had never been a lot of bonding with my mother. I first heard about this type of therapy when I went for a spiritual reading. It sounded like exactly what I needed.

The whole procedure took three sessions to complete. The therapist explained what was involved when I rang him, and then he sent me a tape which I was to play every day before the first session. I also had to make out a list of positive and negative traits, of my mother and father, and to record my dreams. He went through these with me at the beginning of the first session. I lay on the couch and closed my eyes. There was a female guide who I chose to work with during these sessions. I remember being brought back to when I was aged seven, and to the feelings I had at that time. Then I was brought back further to when I was a baby and my mother was washing me in the bath. I can't remember much more about this session, or the next one. There was really so much that I felt and experienced. Between sessions I had to trace out the figure eight, visualising myself in one circle, and my mother in another. I also had to listen to a tape of the first session every day until I returned for the second time.

The third session was when I actually did the cutting of the ties. I had a choice between staying in this life or reliving a karmic past-life experience. I felt it was the past life that I needed to deal with. I lay on the couch again, feeling my guide near me. I went back to a time when I was living in South America. I was living in a shack, in a very barren area. I was part of a large family. I then saw an incident in which I was having a baby. My parents didn't give me a lot of support. The baby was taken away from me soon after it was born and given to some other woman. I felt very upset. It was very traumatic. Then I was brought further on in time. Now I was married and I wasn't able to have a child. I was really afraid of giving birth and this was causing a lot of difficulty in my marriage. Then I returned to the present time. I could see myself overcoming my fear of childbirth. I could see myself in the future with a husband and three children.

The therapist then asked me if I was ready to cut the ties. I said I was. I could see my mother in her own circle and I was in mine. We were joined by lots of ties. One was the umbilical cord, another I remember was joined to each of us around the ankle. I cut some of these with a scissors. With one tie, I had to open the lock with a special key to free us. When all the ties were cut I visualised disposing of them by throwing them into a big fire. I got the gift of a lighting candle from my guide before I finished the session. I was asked not to talk about my experience for at least forty-eight hours. I was also asked to write a letter to my mother, which I wouldn't send to her, where I could say all the things to her that needed to be said.

I have really benefited in many ways from the cutting of the ties.

It is a very powerful experience. I have a better relationship with my mother now, and I don't give my power away to her anymore. I feel I can detach from her, which used to be a problem before. I also feel I have overcome my fear of childbirth which was a major obstacle for me. I really feel it has been worth doing. It has helped me gain confidence in myself. Many people have commented on the positive changes which have occurred in my life.

Suggested Reading

Krystal, P., *Cutting the Ties that Bind: Growing up and Moving on*, York Beach, ME: Weiser, 1993.

Krystal, P., *Cutting More Ties that Bind: Letting Go Fear, Anger, Guilt, and Jealousy so We Can Educate our Children and Change Ourselves*, York Beach, ME: Weiser, 1993.

Family Therapy

In the past thirty years in Ireland huge social changes have greatly affected family life and values. The changing roles of men and women have brought about much greater freedom for women in terms of choice of lifestyle. For many men, however, there have been feelings of anger, fear and confusion. Many women are now choosing to work outside the home, and child-rearing practices have consequently changed. There has also been a rapid increase in the number of one-parent families, of legal separations, and of partners choosing to live together without marrying. People want a better quality of life than ever before. This includes companionship and intimacy in relationships as well as personal space, fulfilment through career, and sexual satisfaction. Many feel under great financial pressure, because of high expectations in terms of housing and lifestyle. High levels of unemployment and the threat of redundancy have also taken their toll on the stability of the modern family.

Problems and Life Crises

As well as the above social changes, there are other problems that can affect every member of the family, when they occur. These include abuse, violence, alcoholism and drug abuse, gambling and other addictions, anorexia and bulimia, involvement in criminal activities, and extra-marital affairs. Great upheaval also follows from life crises such as bereavement, miscarriage, illness, children being bullied at school, children leaving home, retirement and parents needing to be nursed in old age.

What is Family Therapy?

In family therapy the therapist seeks to help the members of a family to resolve their current difficulties. The aim is to help the family as a unit, as well as the individual members, to learn to communicate with each other. Intimate and honest communication is important not only at times of great stress but in everyday life. Many families first come to therapy when a serious crisis strikes. This may be the family's presenting problem. Often, however, when one person is experiencing difficulties, all the family may need to look at their internal coping mechanisms and their patterns of communication and behaviour, both as a family unit, and as individuals within that unit. The main approaches of family therapists are briefly outlined below.

Nathan Ackermann

Ackermann is called the father of family therapy. His emphasis was on the influence of social class or ethnic group on individual psychological development within the family.

Murray Bowen

Bowen is considered to be one of the pioneers of family therapy. His name is linked with the origin of the theory of multigenerational transmission of mental illness, and the development of genograms (or family trees), which are used to show the pattern of relationships, health, education, etc. in a family over several generations. He also believed in the significance of social origins.

Bowen developed the concept of triangulation. When there are problems between two members of a family, a third person is often drawn in or 'triangulated' to create a scapegoat who redirects the point of conflict. For example, one parent may persuade a child to side with him or her against the other parent. Greater differentiation from a person's family of origin is encouraged, but not a complete cut-off.

Virginia Satir

The mother of family therapy, Satir, whose background is in social work, is recognised as having made a large contribution to early family therapy. Her belief is that children's symptoms are related to marital difficulties in which they have become triangulated. In this way the depressed or withdrawn child within the family expresses the family's internal pain.

Satir talks of the importance of 'nurturance', care, trust and affection in the psychotherapeutic situation. She believes that a therapist must become involved and show deep caring for family members in order for healing to take place.

Salvador Minuchin

Minuchin's therapeutic method is to create enactments to help family members redefine their plight in a way that illuminates every member's role in it.

Milton Erickson

Erickson is hailed as the mentor of strategic therapists. Strategic family therapists believe in helping families to solve their pre-senting problems with the minimum interference possible from the therapist. The emphasis is on helping the family to com-municate, and encouraging them to try new ways of improving their lives together.

Carl Whitaker

Whitaker invites the family to develop a caring and probing relationship with him. He believes that the real problems faced by a family are birth, growing up, separation, marriage, illness and death. Using a type of psychoanalysis, he sensitises the family to its own subconscious life. He usually will not begin a therapy session unless all family members are present, as he believes any person absent is symbolic of the whole family's reluctance to be in therapy.

Milan Systemic Therapy

This was developed by Maria Selvini Palazolli and some of her colleagues in Milan, originally to treat families with a schizo-phrenic member. Their method places a great emphasis on the work of the team. One mixed-sex pair of therapists works with the family, and another pair operates as the observing team behind a one-way mirror. Information is gathered from the family by means of 'circular questioning', a method which examines how the symptoms of the person with the presenting problem affect other family members.

Practitioners of Family Therapy

Freda Roche, Linda Fulton, Gail Grossman Freyne and Vivienne Shields are registered family therapists with the Family Therapy and Counselling Centre. Freda's background is in occupational therapy and health education. She is also trained in trager massage and in zero balancing, and has a particular interest in combining body-work with psychotherapy. Linda's background is in social work. She studied integrative psychotherapy and body-work with Patrick and Inger Nolan. Gail trained as a mediator and has a special interest in personal development and couples therapy. Vivienne's background is in education and law, and she is also a trained mediator.

The centre mainly uses the systemic and strategic approach. This ensures the least possible amount of interference from the therapist. Family members are encouraged to continue doing what they usually do, and the role of the therapist is to observe and to help the family to see how a seemingly small change may bring about a tremendous effect in solving the problems. Each member of the family is asked their opinion on the nature of the problem, and how they are affected by it. Families can come with any kind of problem, from sexual abuse to anorexia, from drug abuse to unresolved grief. They are encouraged to communicate more honestly, to help to prevent a build-up of stress and strain in the family in future.

Perhaps the greatest benefit of the process is to create a safe space for individual family members to explore their feelings, the reasons for their conflicts, and their needs. Many parents behave to each other and to their children in ways that they have learned from their own family of origin. By helping them to draw up a genogram, much insight can be gained as to the reasons why current problems are being experienced.

Information can be obtained from The Family Therapy and Counselling Centre, 46 Elmwood Avenue Lower, Ranelagh, Dublin 6 (tel: 01 497 1188/497 1722).

Case Study: Siobhán

At ten years of age I suffered from anorexia. I went to many doctors and hospitals for two years before I was correctly diagnosed. A child psychologist recommended to my parents that we all should go for family therapy. Overall we attended therapy for six months. I was a full-time resident in a treatment centre for six months and a part-time resident for two months. I had huge feelings of anger and victimisation. At first the family therapy sessions were very tedious. I was very apprehensive of everybody in the family being together. I felt very unsettled in the group sessions, and once I had a hysterical tantrum because I felt so angry and frustrated. In the end I was cured of anorexia. All the members of my family were forced to confront problems within the home, which had been highlighted by my illness. My father realised that making money wasn't the only requirement or responsibility of being a father or a husband. I learned not to bottle my emotions and thoughts, but to voice them and to share my problems. After many years of harbouring anger it began to diminish slowly. I am still in contact with my family, though I have now moved away from home. Watching how other families behave towards each other has always been extremely important to me since. I suppose it's a way of learning how different people relate to each other.

Suggested Reading

Lerner, H.G., *The Dance of Intimacy*, London: Pandora, 1992.

Minuchin, S., *Families and Family Therapy*, London: Routledge, 1996.

Skynner, R. and J. Cleese, *Families and How to Survive Them*, London: Cedar, 1996.

Gestalt

Gestalt arose out of the humanistic movement in the height of the 1960s' anti-war campaign and flower-power counter-culture. The humanistic approach was a reaction to two world wars, to authority and to rigid ways of doing things. The basic philosophy of gestalt is existentialist — human beings are free to choose to take responsibility for their destiny. The word 'gestalt', which is German in origin, has no literal translation. The closest meaning is 'a whole made up of parts'. As a therapy, gestalt focuses on the here and now. It emphasises the importance of experiencing feelings in a counselling session rather than just talking about them, and the need for the client to become more aware of their interaction with, and relationship to, the environment. Gestalt is probably most identified with Fritz Perls, who was one of its leading exponents.

Those who come for therapy are usually 'stuck' or 'frozen' in some aspect of their past, and searching for a way of integrating these past experiences into present life. In gestalt therapy every word gives an indication as to what you are thinking and feeling at that moment. By emphasising the importance of being in the present, it helps you to see how you actually relate to the environment, and the extent of the role played by past conditioning in your present life.

Approaches Used in Gestalt Therapy

The gestalt therapist helps clients to focus on the here and now, on their breathing, and on any feelings that pass through their body and mind. When you become anxious, you cut off your breathing. When this happens the therapist encourages you to breathe through your feelings, really to feel them and then let them go. You can then become aware of when you're avoiding a feeling or a situation, or when you're playing a role that belongs to a time in your past.

Gestalt encourages you to keep connected to the moment. If you are introduced to someone for the first time and are instantly attracted to them, is it because there is an immediate connection between you? Or does that person remind you of a family member, or a past lover, or one of your parents? If you find it hard to trust and confide in a friend, do you have reason to doubt that person or is it that you have never been able to trust anyone in your life, since your mother neglected you?

The gestalt therapist's job is to help sharpen awareness, so that clients recognise their own process — what it is, and how they interrupt it. Gestalt is all about learning to feel and express your feelings honestly, and to relate to others in a genuine non-clichéd way.

Gestalt Therapy in Action

People attend gestalt therapy for a variety of reasons. Some present with feelings of low self-esteem, others have a lot of stored-up anger that they find very difficult to express. A lot of people present with issues of abuse: sexual, emotional, neglect, and physical violence. Some are dealing with loss, relationship problems, alcoholism or life crises. Others feel a lot of guilt or are very inhibited about their sexuality. Many feel a sense of confusion because of the changing roles of the sexes, and the frequent breakdown of intimate relationships. Others feel a huge gap between the generations, which causes difficulties between children, parents and grandparents.

It is vital for the therapist to remain in contact with the client, to listen intently, to observe, to give feedback, and to keep gently guiding the client back to the present and to feelings. An important part of the therapy is to guide people to an awareness of their own uniqueness, to what feels right for them, so that they can actually own their own feelings. The therapist gently challenges the client, to assist in exploring the roots of feelings. Gestalt is a very powerful therapy for anyone who has difficulty facing their feelings, who tends to intellectualise or over-analyse, and always needs to be in control.

Group Gestalt

Gestalt work can be done in one-to-one situations or in groups. If working with a group, the facilitator takes the participants through a series of exercises, all designed to help them explore their reactions to their environment, and to connect with each other through their shared experiences. Individual members are encouraged to disclose how the exercise felt for them. Feedback is then given to that person by group members, as to how they perceived the person's body, voice, words etc. Group members are also encouraged to challenge each other, to become aware of defensive barriers by facing other group members with their perceptions and feelings about each other. This will either expose their own tendency to project feelings and experiences onto others, or will lead to others gaining valuable insights into their behaviours, fears and conditioning, which will lead to increased self-awareness.

Case Study: Cathy

Cathy is thirty-five. She originally attended gestalt therapy because she felt a lack of confidence, a fear of speaking out, and a fear of confrontation. She also felt that she had unfinished business in relation to her family of origin. In her first session she was asked about her relationship with her parents and her brothers and sisters, and whether there had been any deaths in the family. Cathy's family history revealed that she had a violent alcoholic bully of a father, and a depressed cold mother, who died when Cathy was in her teens. Cathy was the eldest of four children. She had become burdened with practical and emotional problems at an inappropriate age, and had experienced and witnessed violence and conflict within the home.

Through therapy Cathy began to realise how she had turned her feelings of aggression and anger over the years, which should have been directed towards her parents, towards herself, out of a fear of violence. She had also suppressed her need for love and care by becoming the family fixer and rescuer, in a desperate attempt to make everything seem okay. Her grief and loss around her mother's death was 'frozen' as she very quickly became her father's surrogate spouse and emotional cushion. Cathy was eventually able to 'defrost' her emotions by working through her fears and finally expressing her anger with her father, and then freeing up the sense of loss (for her childhood) and her grief.

Cathy's feelings about her relationship with her husband began to emerge when she had released her feelings for her parents. A flood of repressed needs and anger surfaced around her marriage as she recognised how she still tried to rescue and take responsibility for her husband. This is something that Cathy is still working on. She has already felt an increase in her confidence and a release of energy, and she has become more in touch with her creativity and potential. She has also released a lot of grief, which she had carried for years after the death of her mother. At times during therapy Cathy looked to her therapist to be a 'nice mother figure' to her, because the therapist was someone who listened, supported and didn't judge her. Sometimes Cathy's real mother had not been 'nice'. So on some occasions the therapist challenged Cathy, and she was able to get angry at the therapist, and finally at her mother. Then she expressed a lot of anger and hurt that had been previously repressed. When Cathy's marriage difficulties have been resolved, she will finish therapy.

Suggested Reading

Houston, G., *Red Book of Gestalt*, London: Airlift, 1990.

O'Leary, E., *Gestalt Therapy*, London: Chapman and Hall, 1993.

Schiffman, M., *Gestalt Self Therapy*, Berkeley, CA: Wingbow Press, 1990.

Schiffman, M., *Self Therapy*, Berkeley, CA: Wingbow Press.

Herbalism

Animals instinctively turn to plants to gain relief in times of illness. So too, our ancestors, by trial and error, found the most effective local plants to heal and soothe the mind, the body and the spirit. Now, with the advancement of science, which enables the chemical constituents of these plants to be identified, we can better understand their healing powers.

In traditional herbal medicine the whole plant is used for healing. The leaves, flowers, stem and root may act in different ways, but all are important and are used. The region where the patient usually resides is also the best place for the herbalist to gather the herbs, as this is the home environment to which this particular person's body is accustomed. Herbs are natural substances whose molecular make-up is easily assimilated by the human digestive system and so cause few or no side-effects when correctly administered.

Plants with a particular affinity for certain organs or systems of the body are used to nourish and restore to health those parts that have become weakened.

Diagnosis and Prescription

Medical herbalists are trained in the same diagnostic skills as orthodox doctors but they take a more holistic approach to illness. The underlying cause of the problem is sought and, once identified, it is this that is treated rather than just the symptoms. Herbalists use their remedies to restore balance to the body, thus enabling it to mobilise its own healing powers.

The initial consultation with a patient usually takes about one hour. The diagnosis involves assessing your medical history and current state of health from a medical and holistic perspective. If the herbalist feels that more detailed tests are necessary, a visit to your doctor is advised. Likewise, if you disclose a long-standing emotional problem, referral to a counsellor may be suggested. Treatment may include advice about diet and lifestyle as well as herbal medicine.

Herbs can be prescribed in several forms, the most common being tinctures, ointments and teas. Some herbs are very powerful and should be prescribed only by a qualified herbalist. When prescribed by a professional herbalist, herbs are very safe and effective, and are complementary to any other form of therapy.

The second consultation usually takes place two weeks later, though if your condition is acute it may take place after an interval of one week. It lasts between twenty and thirty minutes. About 60 per cent of people report that they are feeling better after just a few weeks of taking the herbs. About 20 per cent have not noticed much initial improvement, while the remainder may report a worsening of the symptoms which is usually temporary, and may be accounted for by a clearing out of the system. Another examination may be carried out, and sometimes a new prescription is given. Further consultations take place at about one-month intervals. After taking the herbs for six months the patient often reports a full recovery. Sometimes people who have been on long-term medication are able to dispense with it. At this stage the herbalist may recommend a check-up, and some preventative remedies, about every six months.

Benefits of Herbal Medicine

Herbal medicine can treat almost any condition that patients might take to their doctor. Common complaints seen by herbalists include skin problems such as psoriasis, acne and eczema, digestive disorders such as peptic ulcers, colitis, irritable bowel syndrome and indigestion. Problems involving the heart and circulation like angina, high blood pressure, varicose veins and varicose ulcers can also be treated successfully, as can gynaecological disorders like pre-menstrual syndrome and menopausal problems. Conditions such as arthritis, insomnia, stress, migraine and headaches, tonsillitis, influenza and allergic responses like hay fever and asthma can also be effectively treated. Herbs can be used to help former drug addicts during their initial withdrawal from drugs to aid pain relief and sleep, and to help the body recuperate and the organs to be strengthened and nourished. People who are HIV positive can also be sympto-matically treated with herbs that have anti-viral properties and that have fewer side effects than many medically prescribed drugs.

Practitioner: Helen McCormack

Helen McCormack is a member of the National Institute of Medical Herbalists, and president of the Irish Association of Medical Herbalists. She did the four-year course with the National Institute in England. Helen has worked as a medical herbalist for several years in her own clinic in Dublin, and she spends one day a week working in the Walmer House clinic in Raheny. She also runs a six-week course in herbal medicine. As a medical herbalist, Helen combines her medical and scientific training with her knowledge and experience of the properties and healing abilities of plants. In her practice she uses about 200 plants. Some of these she grows and picks herself, while others she obtains in tincture and ointment form, prepared using traditional remedies.

The healing ability of herbs and nature is magical. Going back thou-sands of years, people had a much deeper connection with nature. The appearance of a plant, the colour, texture, and shape, as well as the area it grew in, gave people an idea of what conditions the plant could best be used for treating. There are thousands of plants which grow in the wild which have marvellous healing powers, and there are probably many more whose medicinal qualities we are as yet unaware of.

Treating the whole person and not just the presenting problem is a very important part of my work. Helping people to see the links between their lifestyles, their diets, their emotions and their health is vital to aid a patient's treatment. It is also a way of helping to em-power a person, because when we have a better understanding of the reasons for the manifestation of illness, we feel more able to prevent illness. We therefore feel more in control of our health and our lives.

Helen has seen many successes in treating her patients with herbs, especially in the areas of skin problems, asthma and chest problems, and digestive disorders. She can be contacted at 186 Philipsburgh Avenue, Marino, Dublin 3 (tel: 01 836 8965), or at

The Natural Living Centre, Walmer House, Station Road, Raheny, Dublin 5 (tel: 01 832 7859).

Case Study: Geraldine

Geraldine is a forty-two-year-old married woman with one child. She has suffered from recurring infections for most of her life. She contracted pneumonia in the first few weeks of life and has been prone to bouts of bronchitis, especially in the wintertime. There is a family history of asthma, and her condition necessitated the use of an inhaler twice a day with additional medication. She complained of increased difficulty in breathing and lack of energy. She had been on three separate courses of antibiotics over a period of eight weeks and was still feeling unwell. She had been on sick leave from her job for two weeks when she first visited the medical herbalist. She eats healthily and takes exercise when she feels energetic enough. In recent years too, she has been suffering from sinusitis and had a permanent 'blocked-up' feeling. She also complained about the dual pressures of work and home. While she enjoys her work very much, it is a busy job with much responsibility.

The treatment prescribed for Geraldine by the herbalist was to supplement her diet with vitamin C and garlic, which was the first step towards building up immunity to infections. Inhalations using camomile and eucalyptus to clear the airways of congestion were also recommended. The herbal remedy consisted of: Inula helenium (elecampane), which is a stimulating expectorant with excellent anti-bacterial action; thymus vulgaris (common thyme), which loosens phlegm and eases spasmodic bouts of coughing; echinacea angustifolia, which is an immuno-stimulant and has important anti-viral proper-ties; plantago lanceolata (plantain), which encourages expectorant of phlegm while also soothing inflamed and sore mucous membranes; zingiber officinale (ginger), which is a warming herb that is stimulat-ing to the circulation and encourages lung function.

Geraldine's second visit was two weeks later and she reported less congestion. She was taking less of her prescribed medication and her symptoms of breathlessness and tightness in the chest were reduced. She felt she had more energy, and she was back at work. She was instructed to continue with the herbal remedy as prescribed.

On her third visit four weeks later, Geraldine reported some recurrence of the asthmatic symptoms. The wheeze had been worse of late. She was also having broken sleep most nights as her young son was waking up a lot during the night, probably because of a head cold, which was making him restless. She still felt that her health had improved overall and that she had more energy. Her chest was still clear on examination and her blood pressure was normal. The herbalist suggested that Geraldine cut out cheese (of which she was very fond) or switch to goat's or sheep's cheese for a while to see if that improved the wheeziness. Certain breathing exercises were also recommended as an aid to relaxation and to help with the functioning of her lungs. The prescription was slightly changed to include euphorbia piluifera and ephedra sinica in very small doses to relax any spasm of the bronchial airways and to loosen the accumulation of sticky phlegm.

On her fourth visit, Geraldine was feeling very relaxed and much improved. She had reduced the use of her inhaler to a significant degree. She has had no recurrence of any chest infection to date and is on a maintenance level dosage of herbal medicine, which is altered from time to time, depending on her needs.

Suggested Reading

Brooke, E., *Herbal Therapy for Women*, London: Thorsons, 1992.

Buning, F. and P. Hambly, *Herbalism*, London: Hodder and Stoughton, 1993.

Griggs, B., *The Green Pharmacy*, London: Pan.

Griggs, B., *The Home Herbal*, London: Pan, 1995.

Hoad, J., *Healing with Herbs*, Dublin: Gill and Macmillan, 1996.

Hoffmann, D., *The Holistic Herbal*, Shaftesbury, Dorset: Element, 1966.

Mabey, R., *The Complete Herbal*, London: Penguin, 1991.

Scallan, C., *Irish Herbal Cures*, Dublin: Gill and Macmillan, 1994.

Holotropic

The name 'holotropic' literally means 'aiming for totality' or 'moving towards wholeness' (from the Greek, 'holos', meaning whole, and 'trepein', meaning moving in the direction of).

In the late 1970s, Stanislav and Christina Grof developed a simple but powerful and safe method for inducing non-ordinary states of consciousness, called holotropic breathwork. It has been known for centuries that it is possible to induce profound changes of consciousness by techniques that involve breathing. In a typical breathing session the tensions and blockages in the body will be manifested and amplified. Continued breathing tends to bring them to a culminating point of release and resolution. Like breathing, music and other forms of sound technology have been used as powerful consciousness-altering tools. The continuous flow of music creates a carrying wave which helps you to surrender and let go, overcoming psychological defences, and moving through difficult impasses and experiences. The last component of holotropic breathwork is focused body-work. This is used only when the breathing and music did not bring a complete resolution of the experience.

A basic assumption of holotropic breathwork is that we, in our culture, operate in a way that is far below our real potential and capacity. This impoverishment is caused by the fact that we identify with only one aspect of our being, namely the ego. This leads to an inauthentic, unhealthy and unfulfilled way of life, and contributes to the development of emotional and somatic disorders of psychological origin. Holotropic breathwork has brought about remarkable changes in the understanding of emotional and psychosomatic disorders that clearly have no organic cause. When we start experiencing symptoms of a disorder that is emotional rather than organic, it is important to realise that this is not the beginning of a 'disease'. It is the emergence into our consciousness of the material that was previously buried in our unconscious. Thus the emergence of symptoms is not necessarily the onset of disease, but the beginning of its resolution.

The Inner Healer

The key to the holotropic perspective in general is: 'the healer is within'. The subject — in this case, the breather — is the expert. If something happens that could be referred to as healing, it is the result of that mysterious inner healing capacity, which might even be known in more mystic circles as grace.

Holotropic Breathwork Workshops

Holotropic breathwork is usually done in a group setting, although everyone's process is individual. Often weekends are residential, offering participants the time and space to enter into the experience fully. Much time is given to preparation and integration before and after the sessions. At a workshop every participant in the group chooses a partner with whom to work. In the sessions, participants function alternately as 'breather' and 'sitter', with the facilitators overseeing the whole workshop. It is not unusual for the experience of being a sitter to have a deep and significant impact on the person involved.

The Healing Potential of Holotropic Breathwork

Holotropic breathwork is not an easy, quick-solve process, and should not be entered into lightly. It can involve expressing emotional suffering and difficult physical experiences, over time. If worked through thoroughly, the benefits can be immense. It offers a very effective adjunct to conventional verbal psychotherapy, and can be used to work with various forms of psychopathology that do not respond so well to traditional psychology. It can help you to realise and experience unfulfilling, self-defeating or even self-destructive patterns that are preventing you from living up to your full human potential. It can help you to find a more satisfying approach to life and a new way of being. Finally, holotropic breathwork can be an important tool in the spiritual and philosophical quest. It can mediate the connection between the transpersonal domain of our being and of existence.

When evaluating the results of holotropic breathwork we have to realise that it is quite different from verbal therapy, although it works best as an adjunct to it. Major changes can occur within a short period of time. There is often release of general muscular tensions and opening of energy blockages in the sinuses, throat, chest, stomach, intestines, pelvis, uterus and rectum. In some instances such energy unblocking has been followed by clearing of chronic infections in these areas, such as sinusitis, bronchitis, and cystitis. Often people have had dramatic relief from anxiety states and phobias, and a clearing of depression. There can sometimes be a disappearance of headaches, migraine, menstrual cramps and a wide variety of psychosomatic pains.

Holotropic Centres

These centres (see Directory) run one-day and weekend holotropic workshops. Workshops are suitable for qualified and trainee psychotherapists who wish to broaden their therapeutic skills, and also for those who need to search more deeply within for personal healing. Using group work, relaxation, meditation, art, music, guided imagery, focused body-work, and breathing, participants will be enabled to move through deeper states of consciousness and to work through struggles and difficulties that are currently inhibiting well-being and personal growth. These centres also run professional counselling and psychotherapy courses, which include training in holotropic therapy.

(*Courtesy of Elis Clare Lynd O'Connor*)

Case Study: Karmel

My reason for attending holotropic therapy was to clear myself of childhood sexual abuse. I had reached a point where I knew I had to look at my past closely. I was thirty years old, in a co-dependent relationship. I had two children, one of whom had disclosed to me incidences of sexual abuse when he was three years old. Physically I was always tired, yet restless, and I suffered many kidney infections, colds and backache. Mentally I was highly strung, prone to paranoia and severe depression. Emotionally I was unstable and not really available to others. Spiritually, I was listless and in need of nurturing this side of myself. I heard about holotropic therapy from my sister, who had also undergone childhood abuse. I began attending Professor Ivor Brown, who ran holotropic workshops, fortnightly, for several months.

The room consisted of several mats and beanbags. Beside each mat was an empty basin and a box of tissues. Each person going through the process had a sitter with them. The sitters had previously gone through this process themselves, and most of them had medical experience. The sitters' job was to be there for the person without imposing. My sitter wiped away my tears, of which there were many, held my hand and encouraged me to stay in my body. All memory is stored in the body, so I had to go into the physical sensations to relieve the blocked memories.

Each session lasted three hours. I was taught how to use controlled breathing and relaxation, while soothing, rhythmic music filled the room. I began to deep breathe down into my body. As I quickened my breath, under instruction, I began to feel numbness in parts of my body. I'd feel a lump rise in my throat. This lump came out as a childlike cry, a whining. I tried to control its sound. I was encouraged by my sitter to let it out. I was safe. It was okay. I let it out, crying, sobbing, then rage, anger. I kicked and screamed. I bashed the beanbags. I was livid. The background music got fainter. For the first time in my life I could express all the anger, the pain, the terror, the fear, the trembling, the loss, the guilt, the shame, and the immense sadness I had felt as a child. For the most part, it was feelings I released during therapy, but there were flashbacks too. These must have been similar to what a war veteran might experience, like those who fought in Vietnam: post-traumatic stress disorder. Though it was traumatic to live through the experiences, I felt relieved after each session. I had gone into my inner cave, where I'd found a strong, yet frightened, little girl, an innocent angel. I nurtured her, and we walked away from the past, together.

During one of my last sessions, I went through a labour and birth. I thought then that I was reliving one of the births of my two children. Yet I was adamant during the process that there was no baby. Several months after therapy, I began to have memories of babies. At the time my sister was also having flashbacks of seeing a baby being buried in the garden. I knew it was mine. I was terrified. I didn't want to face it, but I went back to therapy and had recall of being pregnant at the age of twelve. The baby was taken from me before it was full-term. I remember thinking, at that time, that my 'sin' was being taken away. The revelation was the hardest to deal with, but suddenly all the pieces fitted: the reasons why I had never respected myself, my difficulty in my relations with men, especially in trusting them, and with women.

The benefits of knowing the truth of my life far outweigh the losses. I'd rather live in light and awareness than slowly die in darkness. Now I feel free to be me. I have nothing to hide, no more hidden skeletons in the closet. I know there may be times I'll have more memories, but at least I know I can and will handle it. All the answers are inside us, if we want to know.

Suggested Reading

Grof, C., *The Thirst for Wholeness: Attachment, Addictions, and the Spiritual Path*, London: Harper Collins, 1994.

Grof, C. and S. Stanislav, *The Stormy Search for the Self: Understanding and Living with Spiritual Emergence*, London: Thorsons, 1995.

Grof, C. and S. Stanislav, *The Holotropic Mind*, London: Harper Collins, 1993.

Grof, C. and S. Stanislav, *Realms of the Human Unconscious: Observations from LSD Research*, London: Souvenir Press, 1996.

Home Birth

Home birth is where women choose to have their babies born at home with a midwife or general practitioner in attendance. Childbirth is a natural function of a woman's body, and many women do not see themselves as patients, or wish to undergo a medical procedure in a hospital in order to give birth. Most women choosing home birth have previously had unsatisfactory experiences of giving birth in hospitals, which seemed impersonal and greatly lacking in choice. Others may have talked with friends or family members who have given birth at home and who have spoken highly of the experience.

What About the Safety Aspects of Home Birth?

Studies in Britain and the Netherlands suggest that home birth can be safer for mother and baby than birth in hospital. Researchers concluded that when 'low-risk' women gave birth in a consultant unit in hospitals geared for 'high-risk' women, they too were treated as 'high risk', and so were offered interventions which led to complications. There is also a reduced risk of infection for both mother and baby in the home setting. The two risks that cause most anxiety — post-partum haemorrhage (PPH) in the mother and the failure of the baby to breathe — rarely happen in home-birth situations where there is no intervention during the birth. Rare circumstances of retained placenta or haemorrhage can be dealt with at home, and if needed the woman can be transferred to hospital. When women are less stressed themselves, distressed babies are a rarity. If any of these situations should happen, however, the midwife is well trained and equipped to follow a definite procedure to ensure the safety of both mother and baby at home, and will transfer to hospital only if necessary.

Midwives are practitioners in their own right and are qualified to practise independently in providing all services to pregnant women, including home birth. They are experts in normal maternity care while the obstetrician's skill is only necessary in the case of abnormal pregnancy and labour.

Midwives will not deliver at home if there is the slightest risk of danger to either mother or baby. A few doctors are willing to co-operate with midwives during home births so that the woman can have an enthusiastic GP and a skilled midwife. (A list of supportive doctors can be obtained from the Home Birth Centre, or the regional contacts — see Directory.)

Benefits of Home Birth

Many women who give birth in the comfort and privacy of their own home feel it to be a deeply satisfying experience. The chance of forming a close bond of trust and rapport with your chosen midwife is also very reassuring. Ante-natal visits are usually in the comfort of your own home, at a time convenient to you. The midwife will also individualise your care according to your needs. The father-to-be, and other children, can be involved in your care in pregnancy, and be present at the birth.

At birth, you are in familiar surroundings and are uninhibited in labour, allowing for ease of progress towards the birth. The midwife is completely devoted to the welfare of you and the baby, and so gives you undivided attention. The birth is not 'managed' in any way. You are not coerced into giving birth within a set time limit. You have complete freedom to move around, to squat, to walk in the garden, to use massage, aromatherapy oils, or any other complementary therapy you please, to help with pain relief. Medical procedures such as amniotomy (breaking of the waters), electronic foetal monitoring during labour, intramuscular injections of syntometrine (to speed delivery of placenta), and episiotomies (cuts made in the birth canal to speed delivery) are rarely used. If, however, a procedure is vital to the delivery, it will be performed after your informed consent has been given. There is also more successful breastfeeding with continuity of midwifery care at home.

After the birth, the mother, the father and other members of the family will be able to stay together with the baby. If there are other small children there will be no need for them to be separated from their mother. If the mother wishes to breastfeed the baby she will be given information and support by her midwife. All post-natal visits are done in the privacy of the woman's home, for up to six weeks after the birth. Usually women are visited six to ten times post-natally, depending on their needs.

Midwife in Practice: Bridget Cummings

Having my second son at home led me to become a midwife, in 1987. In 1989 I decided that truly to practise as a midwife, I wanted to see each woman through the birth and post-natally, and so became an independent midwife with my own case-load practice. Home birth is midwifery as it used to be, but with easy transfer to obstetric care, if needed. Women contact me at home and we discuss birth options. A booking for a home birth is done in the woman's home and all the usual ante-natal visits follow either in my clinic or in her home. Once the pregnancy reaches thirty-seven weeks I am 'on call' for the birth, and attend the mother-to-be when she goes into labour, giving continuous one-to-one care.

After a natural birth there is usually a natural delivery of the placenta. I stay for about two hours after the birth, longer if needed, where I enjoy the special atmosphere and ensure the comfort of all involved. Breastfeeding is encouraged as early as possible. When all the work is completed and the family have eaten well and tucked themselves up in bed to rest after the labour, whilst admiring the new arrival, I leave for home. I return later on and continue intermittent post-natal support for six to ten visits, over a six-week period.

Women book my services for planned home birth because they want to see the same midwife, build up a relationship of trust and know who will attend them in labour and afterwards. They want to avoid conflicting advice and be given information to help them make informed decisions in all aspects of their care and their baby's. Breastfeeding support is given priority, as well as the role of family and friends. Ante-natal classes and post-natal support groups are arranged so that the father-to-be can be involved. Women learn best from other mothers and my role is to facilitate the empowerment of women to birth their babies as best they can. I offer research based on evidence for effective care in pregnancy and childbirth.

Women are well designed to give birth, and can do so with dignity, beauty, and smooth recovery post-natally. Home birth is a safe option to consider for many women where there is continuity of care. As a professional, I provide a safety net where parents can experience birth and child-rearing as a positive, healing and enjoyable period of their lives. I see my work as supporting the most important job in the world: parenting. By offering informed choice I empower parents to meet their individual needs for pregnancy, birth and parenting. I prepare women for pregnancy and birth so that their confidence is enhanced. My priorities are to promote all that is natural and safe, avoiding unnecessary interference with birth, the new baby and nurturing.

Having undertaken a four-year part-time course in homoeopathy, I am able to combine both professions successfully, and work as an independent midwife with a homoeopathic clinic for mothers and babies. The natural and non-toxic aspect of homoeopathy, with its gentle action, makes it attractive to many pregnant women. It gives women more choice and can be used as a safe effective therapeutic tool to promote a normal straightforward birth. I have found that homoeo-pathy relieves trauma, aids the healing process and reduces the feeling of vulnerability of both mother and baby.

Bridget can be contacted for midwifery and homoeopathic services at Calva, Ballybawn, Enniskerry, Co. Wicklow (tel: 01 286 3501). She also holds clinics at the Donnybrook Medical Centre, and at the Homoeopathic Women's Clinic, in the Dublin Well Woman Centre (tel: 01 661 0083/661 0086).

Case Study: Claire

Claire decided to have her third baby at home. She went into labour after having had the flu. The midwife, whom she had built up a great rapport with over the preceding months, attended at the birth. Claire felt exhausted and found the contractions too forceful to bear. The midwife offered her a homoeopathic remedy of camomile to help her cope better with the contractions. The labour seemed long for a third baby and Claire was losing energy fast, despite a light diet which had been prepared for her by the midwife. Kali-phos was recommended by the midwife every twenty minutes. Claire said that she clearly felt a 'huge surge of energy'. Soon after, she gave birth to a seven pounds, twelve ounces baby girl, surrounded by her family, in the comfort of her own home.

Suggested Reading

Balaskas, J., *The New Active Birth*, London: Thorsons, 1991.

Balaskas, J. and Y. Gordon, *Water Birth*, London: Thorsons, 1991.

Castro, M., *Homoeopathy For Mother and Baby*, New York: Macmillan, 1992.

Flint, C., *Sensitive Midwifery*, Oxford: Heinemann, 1986.

Gaskin, I.M., *Spiritual Midwifery*, Summertown, GA: The Book Publishing Company, 1977.

Junor, V. and M. Monaco, *The Homebirth Handbook*, London: Souvenir Press, 1984.

Kitzinger, S., *Home Birth and other Alternatives to Hospital*, London: Dorling Kindersley, 1991.

Kitzinger, S., *The Midwife Challenge*, London: Pandora, 1988.

MacFarlane, C., *Where to be Born?*, Oxford: National Perinatal Epidemiology Unit, 1987.

Moskowitz, R., *Homoeopathic Medicines for Pregnancy and Childbirth*, Berkeley, CA: North Atlantic Books, 1992.

O'Connor, M., *Birth Tides*, London: Pandora, 1995.

Savage, W., *A Savage Enquiry — Who Controls Childbirth*, London: Virago Press, 1986.

Tew, M., *Safer Childbirth: A Critical History of Maternity Care*, London: Chapman and Hall, 1994.

Tiran, M., *Complementary Therapies for Pregnancy and Childbirth*, London: Bailliere Tindall, 1995.

Homoeopathy

Homoeopathy is derived from the Greek words 'homo', meaning 'similar', and 'pathos', meaning 'suffering'. Homoeopathy is one of the safest and most effective forms of medicine that has ever been discovered. In 1786 Dr Samuel Hahnemann discovered that the result of taking a small dose of the cinchona bark, which had been used by contemporary doctors to treat malaria, caused him, a healthy person, to exhibit the symptoms of malaria. Testing out many other natural substances, he discovered that people suffering from particular diseases or ailments could be treated effectively by taking minute doses of substances that caused the same symptoms. Thus he formed the foremost principle of homoeopathy, the law of similars: 'let like be cured by like'.

By using this method, the body's self-healing system seemed to be galvanised into action; the body responded, when invaded by a similar disease to the one it already had, by throwing off both the original and the artificially-added disease. Therefore, whatever the illness, the cure for it lies in finding the substance that is capable of producing effects similar to the symptoms of the diseased person. In giving even a tiny molecule of the substance to someone, their immune system will be activated and strengthened — the self-healing powers of the body will be brought to the fore. All cure comes from within the patient: it is not the substance that cures but this natural healing energy inherent in all life.

Homoeopathic remedies are made from very tiny and highly diluted amounts of the substances after which they are named. The substance to be used is first mixed with lactose. It is then diluted with water and alcohol, and shaken, to strengthen the potency of the remedy. It can be diluted and shaken further depending on the potency required. Dilution can be by multiples of tens (denoted by X on the bottle) or hundreds (denoted by C). The higher the amount of times a substance has been diluted, the more potent it is. Some substances have been diluted so much that scientific analysis will no longer be able to detect any molecules of the original substance. No one knows exactly how this is so, but it has been suggested that water molecules can hold or 'memorise' the healing energy of the original substance. This homoeopathic remedy will still be extremely potent as it is the vital life force of the plant or mineral that is being used to boost your immune system and set your own healing process into action.

Homoeopathic remedies are very safe, using vegetable and mineral substances, with a few derivatives from animal, prepared in such a way that they are powerful without being toxic. If a child were to swallow a whole bottle of homoeopathic tablets, there would be no ill effects. All kinds of illnesses, from minor health problems — emotional as well as physical — to serious conditions, can be effectively and quickly cured by homoeopathy. There are over 3,000 substances available for use by homoeopaths.

Diagnosis in Homoeopathy

In the initial consultation, the practitioner spends quite a lot of time ascertaining your medical history, family medical history, and the type, severity and pattern of any symptoms. Each person is unique so the remedy is chosen by taking the whole person into consideration, including emotions, physical condition, age and lifestyle.

The homoeopath decides which symptoms are most important and unique in each case and then consults books (the *Repertory* and various *Materia Medicas*) to find the most appropriate and similar meaning. Sometimes a remedy will be suggested after a quick consultation of the *Repertory*, or if the case is complicated, the remedy can be posted to the person within the week.

The potency of the remedy prescribed for you, and the number of times to be taken, also depends on the individual. Most remedies come in either tablet or drop form, and are taken orally, well apart from meals. Usually there is a follow-up consultation after one month to see how you are progressing. Like all therapies, during the treatment some people may experience a healing crisis. This may be necessary in order to clear toxins out of the system, or to readjust in some way so that healing can occur. It may take the form of a runny nose, a rash or some other mild symptoms. Some people do not feel any of these symptoms but experience a period of exceptional well-being and optimism.

Benefits of Homoeopathy

Homoeopathic remedies can be used to treat any physical or emotional problems, including pains and aches, insomnia, depression, constipation, bed-wetting, acne, circulation problems, bowel disorders, mental fatigue, stress, menopausal problems, shingles, migraine and headaches. They are suitable for all age groups from new-born to elderly. Many expectant mothers turn to homoeopathy for common pregnancy-related problems, because of its excellent safety record. Remedies can also be used during labour, to help with pain relief, tiredness, excessive bleeding and bruising, and in the post-partum period, to aid healing and to help with breastfeeding. Babies and children respond especially quickly to homoeopathy for childhood complaints such as teething, colic, and fevers. Some homoeo-pathic treatments are available for home use and can be purchased in healthfood shops and some chemists. These can be used to treat many complaints, and can be especially beneficial to include in a first-aid kit.

The Art and Science of Homoeopathy

Homoeopathy is a blend of art and science. Art, because it requires practitioners to be very much people-centred as well as having a certain amount of intuition to steer them towards the correct diagnosis and remedy. Science, because of the knowledge and understanding of the patient's body, mind and spirit, as well as the exact uses of each remedy, which homoeopathy requires to treat the patient successfully.

There is no limit to the possibilities of healing using the remedies, because of the holistic nature of homoeopathy. It is your own energy which uses the remedies to bring about healing in whatever way it is needed. This has nothing to do with your belief system, as many benefits have been recorded when remedies have been given to babies, animals and plants, who cannot be affected by the 'placebo' response. The greatest benefit is the degree of long-term healing which can occur without suffering any unnatural side-effects as is so often the case with drugs.

Case Study: Lisa

Lisa was in her mid-twenties, and was seven weeks pregnant with her fourth baby. She presented with 'morning sickness'. In each pregnancy she had suffered from this complaint up to about eighteen weeks and was anxious that it might happen again. The nausea was much worse when she was hungry. When she ate, she felt fine for about half an hour. She coughed, retched, and vomited occasionally, but she felt no better after vomiting. Lisa was very sensitive to smells, especially of soup, but she craved pickles, onions and spicy foods. She sometimes felt a bit dizzy if she hurried or was going up or down stairs. In past pregnancies Lisa had also felt very irritable, finding the children and everyday chores too much.

The two remedies considered by the homoeopath in this case were SEPIA (inky juice of cuttlefish) and COLCHICUM (meadow saffron). COLCHICUM did not fit the totality of the case as well as SEPIA, which was preferred because of the strong keynote symptom of nausea, ameliorated by eating and food, and desiring pickles, both of which are very distinctive pregnancy-related symptoms. While this was an acute prescription, the remedy also helped with the constitutional effects of having had several children in quick succession, as Lisa's three children were under six years of age. The prescription was SEPIA 6C, with one tablet to be sucked every two to four hours until improvement. After three days Lisa was much better and reduced the frequency of the dose. All symptoms disappeared after one week.

Suggested Reading

Aubin, M. and P. Picard, *Homoeopathy: A Different Way of Treating Common Ailments*, Bath: Ashgrove Press, 1989.

British Homoeopathy Association, *Homoeopathy: The Family Handbook*, London: Thorsons, 1992.

Castro, M., *The Complete Homoeopathy Handbook*, New York: Macmillan, 1990.

Chappell, P. and D. Andrews, *Healing with Homoeopathy*, Dublin: Gill and Macmillan, 1996.

Chappell, P., *Emotional Healing with Homoeopathy*, Shaftesbury, Dorset: Element, 1996.

Handley, R., *Homoeopathy for Women*, London: Thorsons, 1993.

Vithoulkas, G., *Homoeopathy: Medicine for the New Man*, London: Thorsons, 1985.

Hypnotherapy

Hypnotherapy is a very effective and speedy technique of psychotherapy. It utilises the natural phenomenon of hypnosis to gain access to the roots of many kinds of physical, emotional and psychological problems, which are deeply embedded in our subconscious. It cuts through our built-in habits, strategies and inhibitions, to release those deeply-buried memories for evaluation, enlightenment and assimilation. Using hypnosis, with its calming and relaxing effect, positive suggestions can be planted in the subconscious by a therapist to alter negative habits that have led to difficulties for a presenting client.

What is Hypnosis?

Hypnosis has been used for thousands of years. Modern-day hypnosis has been used successfully in pain relief and in psychoanalysis. It has been subjected to much research and experimental testing, by such people as James Esdaile (the Scottish surgeon who performed over 300 painless operations using hypnosis in India in the 1840s), Émile Coué, Pavlov, Sigmund Freud and Milton Erickson.

Hypnosis is a deep state of relaxation, and an altered, though absolutely natural, state of consciousness. It is also a heightened state of suggestibility. It is only possible if there is complete consent and co-operation between a hypnotherapist, who uses acquired knowledge and techniques, and a client, who uses imagination and creativity.

During hypnosis you become sufficiently relaxed, mentally and physically, for the subconscious mind to become much more accessible than is ordinarily the case. The suggestions of the therapist are absorbed by the subconscious mind, without interference from your conscious mind. The subconscious mind is also the storehouse of our total experiences. During hypnosis long-forgotten incidents which are still affecting you can be brought back into consciousness, allowing the presenting symptom to disappear.

Self-Hypnosis

Self-hypnosis is the induction of hypnosis without the presence of the hypnotherapist. The simplest way of attaining this ability is to be hypnotised and have the hypnotherapist make a suggestion to the effect that whenever you say a certain phrase you will go into a deep hypnotic trance, which of course you can terminate at will. In the state of self-hypnosis you can give yourself whatever beneficial suggestions you may wish. For example, you may use self-hypnosis to become more confident in a particular situation, to enhance concentration, or to increase your learning abilities.

What is Hypno-analysis?

Hypno-analysis or analytical hypnotherapy is the combination of hypnosis and psychoanalysis. It usually requires approximately eight sessions of therapy. The success rate is very high. It can bring about a surprising feeling of liberation, enlightenment, and self-insight.

What Does it Feel Like to be Hypnotised?

Unlike many misconceptions surrounding the subject of hypnosis, the reality is that people who are hypnotised are in complete control of what they are doing. Although the word 'hypnosis' comes from the Greek word, 'hypnos', meaning 'sleep', being hypnotised is in fact a state of heightened awareness. At any time during hypnosis you can bring yourself out of the trance.

The induction of hypnosis can take many and varied forms, but in a clinical setting the method generally used involves you relaxing in a chair or on a couch. The hypnotherapist talks in a monotonous, but soothing, tone. In some cases you may be asked to gaze at a bright object or rotating disc, whilst the hypnotherapist talks. Drugs are never used.

During hypnosis, people usually feel deeply relaxed, lethargic, and very peaceful. There are many physical signs of hypnosis which can be observed by the therapist, including regular deep breathing, rapid eye movement, eyelids fluttering, facial flush, and limbs limp and relaxed.

How Does Hypnosis Work?

In good-quality hypnosis the conscious mind is in neutral gear and so the subconscious mind comes to the fore. It is only when we access the subconscious mind directly (through hypnosis) that it will respond and co-operate to bring about desired changes. Hypnosis is not a treatment in itself but is used as an aid to therapy.

Benefits of Hypnotherapy and Hypno-analysis

Medically it has been stated that up to 80 per cent of all patients visiting their GP with a host of varied symptoms are suffering from psychosomatic disorders — illnesses that have their origins in the mind. The hypnotherapist can locate the exact cause of the presenting symptoms instead of treating the symptoms themselves. The problems successfully dealt with include excessive drinking, nail-biting, some skin disorders, allergies, nervous tension and anxiety, phobias, fears and compulsions, nightmares, insomnia, sexual problems, fetishes, enuresis, shyness and blushing, nervousness, inability to make decisions, lack of confidence, and migraine.

An ethical hypnotherapist will seek to alleviate pain only when the client has been examined by a medical doctor who has certified that the cause of pain is not physical. Hypnosis has been used by obstetricians as the sole analgesia (painkiller) for normal childbirth. Sports performance can be greatly enhanced using hypnotherapy, as can students' performance and concentration during study and examinations.

Hypnotherapy Practitioner: Dr Joe Keaney

Dr Joe Keaney works as a hypnotherapist, psychoanalyst, and psychotherapist at his Cork clinic. He holds a Bachelor's degree in Clinical Hypnotherapy from the American Institute of Hypnotherapy (AIH). He is principal of the Irish School of Ethical and Analytical Hypnotherapy, and he lectures in hypnotherapy in Dublin and in Cork.

Hypnosis is a widely used method for helping people make changes. It involves entering a trance state and then making good use of it. The subconscious mind causes symptoms, therefore it is only logical to suggest that only the subconscious mind has the ability to correct them. The mind is like an iceberg, we are not even aware of its full capabilities because nine-tenths are submerged below the surface. It is also like a heat-seeking missile. Programmed correctly it will work towards its target, dealing with all obstacles. If you programme the computer of your mind correctly using hypnosis, what you expect to happen will materialise. Unfortunately, 95 per cent of people flit through their lives like bats without radar, disappointed and hurt when they keep bumping into brick walls. The only lasting way to bring about change is to access the subconscious.

Transformation of the deep-seated characteristics is achieved by gaining access to the deeper mind and informing it directly. Hypnosis can help us alter our negative programming in order to achieve beneficial changes in ourselves. The therapy enriches the mind and instructs it on its own self-improvement. Imagination is a very powerful force and children exhibit far greater powers of imagination than do the majority of adults. Hypnosis is the recovery of those powers of imagination, and hypnotherapy is the training of the client in the constructive use of them.

Joe can be contacted for appointments or course information at the Cork Hypnotherapy Clinic, Therapy House, 6 Tuckey St, Cork (tel: 021 273 575).

Case Study: Maria

Maria was a married woman of thirty-five who presented with symptoms of insomnia and migraine. She had suffered from migraine since her early teens and the insomnia had developed only in the previous two years. Other forms of treatment had failed to alleviate both problems. During hypno-analysis she released many childhood repressions of sexual abuse by an older brother, and one in which he actually hit her on the head (origin of migraine). However, she went on to release a lot of repressed guilt about an extra-marital affair which she had started two years before, and also her reasons for not wanting any children, which was always an area of conflict in her marriage. By the end of the eighth session of hypnotherapy, Maria was sleeping and was free of headaches, although she still had a lot of work to do in her personal relationships.

Case Study: John

John was a thirteen-year-old boy who was failing in school and who had a blinking tic in his eyelids for three years. The constant blinking was accompanied by severe conjunctivitis. He had been treated unsuccessfully by psychotherapy. His father was a physician and wanted John to follow in his footsteps. However, John was more interested in mechanical hobbies, such as radio and electronic devices. It was apparent that the frustrated father was attempting to live out his life through his son. Under hypnosis, he was asked, 'Would you mind twitching the forefinger of your right hand several times a minute? This will take the tension off your lids.' Four sessions were required for reinforcement of this suggestion under self-hypnosis before the blinking tic of the lids was transferred to a finger-twitch. During the next six sessions, the finger-twitch was reduced in frequency until it too subsided. The father's faulty attitudes were discussed, and he decided not to push John.

Suggested Reading

Gibson, J., *The Life and Times of an Irish Hypnotherapist*, Cork: Mercier Press, 1989.

Ousby, W.J., *The Theory and Practice of Hypnotism*, London: Thorsons, 1990.

Shone, R., *Autohypnosis: A Step-by-step Guide to Self-Hypnosis*, Wellingborough, Northants: Thorsons, 1982.

Yapko, M.D., *Essentials of Hypnosis*, New York: Brunner/Mazel, 1995.

Yapko, M.D., *Trancework: An Introduction to the Practice of Clinical Hypnosis*, New York: Brunner/Mazel, 1989.

Kinesiology

Kinesiology is the study of muscle testing in relation to the movement and functioning of the body. The word 'kinesiology' comes from the Greek word *kinesis*, meaning 'motion'. Kinesiologists use muscle testing to discover energy imbalances that may be effecting your health. They draw on the theories of acupuncture to understand how these energies can be balanced. Applied Kinesiology was the name given by its inventor, Dr George Goodheart, to the system of applying muscle testing diagnostically and therapeutically to different aspects of healthcare. Today the name Applied Kinesiology (AK) refers only to the original system, which has its roots in chiropractic.

Kinesiology is used by doctors, dentists, physiotherapists, chiropractors, osteopaths, nutritionists, counsellors, naturopaths, and other healthcare professionals, as well as people from other disciplines. A major development was the formulation of a system of training called 'Touch for Health' which made it possible for members of the public to learn the basics. It is now the most widely used system of kinesiology in the world.

Basis of Kinesiology

In a computer system, the circuit is either open or closed, on or off. In the human being, if the energy is switched on, the muscle and the meridian governing the functioning of that muscle are in good order. If the energy is switched off, there is an imbalance or a blockage in that muscle. This may be caused by problems occurring in any of the following areas: chemical (e.g. allergic reactions, nutritional deficiencies, hormonal imbalances), structural (e.g. muscle or bone weakness, joint or spine problems, poor posture), emotional (e.g. beliefs, feelings, thoughts, past traumas) or electromagnetic (i.e. energy circuits in the body, affecting organ and gland functioning).

Kinesiology Techniques

There are many techniques used by kinesiologists to correct energy imbalances. Manipulation is used by kinesiologists who are also chiropractors and osteopaths. Neuro-lymphatic massage stimulates points on the body to increase elimination. Lightly holding neuro-vascular reflex points, which are located mainly around the head, restores strength to muscles. Meridian tracing stimulates the flow of energy. Holding acupressure points for a few seconds has a balancing effect on the muscles, organs and glands. Muscle reprogramming stimulates the muscle to increase energy flow. The kinesiologist will also advise you on aspects of diet, exercise, and lifestyle.

Benefits of Kinesiology

Kinesiology does not focus on specific symptoms but tests for, and corrects, imbalances throughout the whole body and mind. Many kinesiology treatments bring about instant results. Other deep-rooted problems, however, may take much longer to treat. Some of the problems that can be helped through kinesiology are: accident trauma, addictions, allergies, anxiety, asthma, backache, bed-wetting in children, bladder and bowel problems, breast soreness, candida albicans, chronic fatigue syndrome (ME), constipation and diarrhoea, depression, digestive problems, eating disorders, emotional upsets, fatigue, eczema, food intolerance, headaches, indecisiveness, injuries not requiring surgery, insomnia, irritable bowel syndrome, joint pain, learning difficulties, low self-esteem, migraine, mood swings, menstrual disorders, muscle strain and pains, nausea, neckache and stiffness, nervous problems, neuralgia, phobias, post-operative pain, restlessness, sciatica, sinusitis, skin disorders, sports injuries, stress, tinnitus, and weight problems.

Uses of Kinesiology

Teachers and health professionals who are trained in kinesiology use muscle testing, special exercises, movements and energy corrections as part of their work. They help children who have difficulties in learning to read. They also teach children how to obtain states of alertness for peak performance and concentration. Some nutritionists use kinesiology to test for food and other sensitivities in their patients. Counsellors and psychotherapists can use muscle testing as an indicator of how negative patterns of thinking, feeling and behaving have affected their client's health and day-to-day functioning.

Case Study: Jack

I attended a therapist who was both a nutritionist and a kinesiologist as I was feeling bloated and lethargic after eating. I was also contracting a lot of colds and flu. I heard about this therapist from a friend who had benefited from her treatment. It took just two visits for me to feel a big improvement in my energy levels and my overall health. I was made to feel very comfortable and relaxed by the therapist's informal approach, and her method of getting information to make a diagnosis. This was in contrast to how I felt many times when visiting doctors, to try to get solutions to these problems.

The therapist asked me to lie on a couch, and proceeded to put certain substances on my stomach. She then tested my arm muscles with downward pressure, for my ability to resist or succumb to that pressure. Most times I resisted. On a few occasions my arm could not resist her pressure. When this happened the therapist noted which substances she had placed on my stomach at that time. These were the substances I was having trouble with: coffee, tea, and alcohol. I was also found to be sensitive to electricity. This had the potential to affect me a lot as I work directly with electricity. Also she discerned that my energy was quite low in several parts of my body. She recommended that I take iron tablets and desiccated liver to build up my immune system, and to boost my energy levels. She also recommended that I eat more vegetables, and try to eat a more balanced diet.

I can honestly say that, yes, I did benefit from the treatment. However, these benefits showed only over a long period. What was recommended to me involved not only a change in diet, but also changes in my day-to-day life, to compensate for the negative effects of my working environment.

Suggested Reading

Thie, J.F., *Touch For Health*, Marina del Rey, CA: De Vorss & Co., 1973.

La Tourelle, M., *Thorson's Introductory Guide to Kinesiology: Touch For Health*, London: Thorsons, 1992.

Valentine, T. and C., *Applied Kinesiology*, London: Thorsons, 1985.

Massage

Massage, the art of touch, has always existed. Touch is essential for our physical and emotional development, for optimum health, and for a feeling of connection and love. It is a natural instinctive reaction to rub any part of the body that is injured, tired or sore. In all ancient cultures and civilisations worldwide, massage has been used either as a healing therapy or as a general healthful recreation.

Principles of Massage

Massage uses the medium of touch to bring about a feeling of deep relaxation and healing at the physical, mental, emotional and spiritual levels of a person. In massage therapy, the main strokes used are effleurage (light stroking), petrisage (kneading) and tapotement (tapping). There are many different types of massage, and most practitioners will use a variety of strokes from each type. Some of the most common forms of massage are Swedish, ki, holistic, Chinese, aromatherapy, remedial, and deep-tissue. Ki and Chinese massage therapists, like those of shiatsu and acupuncture, seek to bring healing and harmony to all levels of the person. These therapists use massage to help restore the flow of energy (ki or qi) in the person's system, which may have become blocked through the stresses and strains of life. This can have tremendous benefits for the patient at a physical and emotional level.

Benefits of Massage

Used as a holistic therapy, treating a person at the physical, mental, emotional and spiritual levels, massage can help to alleviate fatigue, to instil deep relaxation, and to encourage the body's organs and systems to function at their full potential. Massage can speed up the healing of damaged tissue, as well as eliminating fatigue and stress to create a deep sense of well-being. One of the primary functions of massage is to unlock deep-seated muscle tension by working around the knots of tension and releasing it. This means relief from aches and pains, especially back pain, and an improvement in posture. Massage acts as a mechanical cleanser of tissue and muscle, removing overloads of toxins, such as by-products of heavy exercise or the after-effects of illness. Having a massage is a way of increasing energy levels that have decreased through stress, worry and day-to-day living. Massage relaxes you, and in this way your natural energy and vitality will be restored. It is a safe and effective method of releasing stored stress without side effects.

Massage can also be used in conjunction with counselling and psychotherapy to help to express and release repressed emotions. It can greatly help survivors of any form of abuse or a person with a negative body image to reconnect with the power and beauty of their own unique body.

What Happens During a Massage?

In a full body massage, a base oil, blended with an essential oil, is generally used. This creates a powerful and relaxing effect. It also enables the therapist's hands to glide easily over your body's surface and to promote a much deeper, more comfortable massage. You usually lie face downwards on a plinth (a special type of couch), and are covered with towels to help you to feel comfortable and warm. The usual routine for a full body massage is to begin by massaging the back of the legs, the thighs, and then the back, shoulders and neck. Then the practitioner asks you to turn over and begins massaging the stomach area, then the front of the legs, the feet and finally the face. A full body massage usually takes about one hour.

Practitioner: Noreen Farrell

Noreen Farrell, and her team of professional masseurs at the Tony Quinn centre in Grafton Street, practise ki massage therapy. Ki massage is one of the safest and most effective therapies available, and has the largest membership of all complementary therapies in the country. It relaxes away stress and tension, and allows the natural ki or life force of the patient to heal body, mind and spirit. Many people who come for a ki massage treatment experience a change, not only in how they feel, but in their whole attitude towards themselves and their world view. Ki massage helps to awaken people to their own potential and creativity. People who benefit from ki massage therapy come from all walks of life.

Tony Quinn designed the ki massage course of training himself, along with his development of yoga and nutrition. His purpose was to make available to the Irish public a holistic therapy which affected them positively at the physical, mental and spiritual levels of their being, and which helped them become more aware of their unique potential. The difference between ki massage and other massage therapies is the understanding of what brings about transformation in a person's life. This kind of change is greatly helped by the state of the therapist, the amount of life force that comes from and through the therapist. Therapists must keep working on themselves: healing and wholeness are not the destination but are part of an ongoing journey of growth and renewal. Noreen and her team can be contacted at 10/11 Grafton Street, Dublin 2 (tel: 01 671 2788).

Case Study: Jacinta

Massage has become a part of my life since I had my first massage back in 1989. I have gone for all kinds of different massage treatments: aromatherapy, holistic, ki, oriental, and deep tissue. A few of the physical complaints which I have had over the years and which have been greatly helped by massage were tense neck and shoulders, sciatica, severe lower back pain which went into spasms when I walked, and over-tiredness from mental exertion (around exam times). At emotionally difficult times I found massage a great balm for my tired mind and soul, a way of being recharged. Gentle, soothing touch by a warm and caring therapist I have found to be deeply healing, especially when I felt so respected and special during the entire treatment. I especially remember a time when I had just split up with my boyfriend, after quite a traumatic and emotional scene. The next day I was in bits. I knew the most healing thing for me was to go for a massage. I was worn out physically and emotionally by the strain of the difficult relationship. I found it hard to sleep or eat, and I felt sick inside. The massage I received from a very sensitive and understanding therapist gave me a kind of peace of mind. It restored my confidence in my own ability to find fulfilment and happiness, without being completely dependent for this on anyone else. That night I had a really great sleep, and I felt that life was still there to be lived, fully.

Suggested Reading

Cassar, M.P., *Massage Made Easy*, London: Wardlock, 1996.

Hudson, C.M., *The Complete Book of Massage*, London: Dorling Kindersley, 1995.

Jackson, A.J., *Massage Therapy*, London: Vermilion, 1993.

Shen, P., *Massage for Pain Relief*, London: Gaia Books, 1996.

Thomas, S., *Massage for Common Ailments*, London: Sidgwick & Jackson, 1989.

Movement and Dance Therapy

Moving and dancing to music, chants and drum rhythms have been a part of human expression since time began. Tribes and societies throughout the world still gather together to dance, as a way of celebrating special events and connecting with other members of their group. Movement and dance not only stimulate us at a physical level, but also deeply affect us emotionally, psychologically and spiritually.

The importance of relearning how to express ourselves through our bodies is vital to the development of self-esteem and the regaining of personal power. In using the full range of the body's natural capacity to move, we express our authenticity, and our zest for life. Movement and dance help to free us from inhibitions, from past hurts which are still stored in the body, from feelings of inferiority and lack of love for our selves and our bodies. Through moving, swaying, stretching, running, rocking, jumping, and being truly in our bodies, and not stuck in our minds, we can experience the full pleasure and enjoyment that our bodies can give us.

Movement and Dance as Therapy

Movement and dance are used by therapists to help people connect with their bodies, to rediscover sensations and feelings and to learn to express the self through the body. This can lead to a reawakening of the love and joy that are a natural and spontaneous part of life for a happy child. Many of us have become disconnected from these feelings because of conditioning, criticism, abuse, self-hatred and a feeling of being in some way unacceptable. Dance is an elixir of positive emotions, attitudes and actions.

When we are fully aware of, and alive in, our bodies there is a deep feeling of harmony, freedom and integration. We possess an inner confidence, a sense of vitality and a responsiveness to the world around us, which is the essence of true sensuality and wholeness. Learning to free our bodies, however, is not easy. Our inhibitions and defences have become ingrained in our ways of being and living, so that dissolving our conditioning takes a lot of exploration and commitment. Yet the journey to regain our own unique way of expressing ourselves and our bodies is truly liberating, and the rewards of re-connecting with the essence of the self are always deeply healing.

Practitioner: Joan Davis

Joan Davis has been working in the field of movement, sound and the healing arts for over twenty years. She is a certified Body Mind Centring Practitioner and has extended her body-work practice with cranio-sacral massage, somato-emotional release and visceral manipulation techniques. Joan works with both individuals and groups.

My work is about the experience of being in motion. It is about how much we can be present in this moving and transient moment that we live in, in order to experience it to its fullest potential.

The personal benefits to those who participate regularly in dance and movement workshops can be immense. We become skilled in our own individuality — in other words, we learn to know our patterns and preferences. We can then learn to differentiate between that which is our own inherent creativity and potential, and that which is conditioned and approval-seeking. To explore this we work through the media of movement, dance, voice and sound, music and song, colour and art, touch and relaxation; the elements of earth, air, fire and water; meditation and examining themes such as boundaries, paradox, transitions, freedom of choice and other relevant day-to-day issues. But the most important medium of all is the sense of spontaneity, fun and freedom. If this reawakens the body, mind and soul to ancient forms and original ways of moving and sounding, then that could be considered a goal of the work.

'Theatre of the Unconscious' is a moving experience, facilitated by Joan over eight weekends. It is a reawakening and a bringing together of the body, the mind and the soul, the conscious, the subconscious and the unconscious. It is an exploration of the uniqueness of the self, but also explores our relationships with others. As well as dance and movement, other media used for self-expression and communication include art and colour, voice and sound, hill-walking, meditation and storytelling. These weekends are held at special times of celebration: the Autumn Equinox, Samhain, the Winter Solstice, St Brigid's Day, the Spring Equinox, May Day, the Summer Solstice and Lunasa. 'Theatre of the Unconscious' also takes place over longer periods at Christmas, Easter and in summertime.

Joan can be contacted at 'The Studio', Rere 330 Harold's Cross Road, Dublin 6 (tel: 01 287 6986).

Case Study: Amy

A few years ago I tried some movement and dance workshops. I wanted to give more focus and attention to my body. I had gone for counselling previously but now I really didn't need to talk any more. I needed to move and to free myself from painful experiences which were still lodged in my body from the past. I can remember vividly sitting in a circle with six other people including our facilitator, breathing deeply and focusing on the moment, on my feelings. We warmed up by lying down on the floor alternating between curling up into a foetal position and spreading ourselves out to take up as much space as possible. I felt like a tiny child, playing on the floor, living in my body, feeling every sensation as the surface of the carpet brushed against the skin on my hands, my feet and my face. Next we were given a big huge bouncy ball. I sat on it and lay across it, rolled it on the floor and then rolled it along my body. Then we found a partner and placed the ball between our stomachs while we tried to manoeuvre across the room without letting the ball fall. This was great fun. I felt connected with the other person but I was aware of the safety in having the ball as a barrier between us.

Next we changed partners and did another exercise where we took turns at supporting and being supported. I volunteered to be the supporter. This was easy, as I used my back and my hands and arms to support my partner. It was when it came to my turn to be physically supported that I felt so untrusting of my partner. I found it so difficult to trust — this was a real struggle. I was surprised how much this 'dance' had mirrored my usual way of behaving in relationships, of being the supporter while often not being supported, and usually not daring to trust. Myself and my partner talked together after this exercise and I found it really helpful to explore these issues and the feelings that had surfaced during the exercise.

The authentic movement work we did was my favourite of all. We could move and dance in any way we wanted to. The music was wild, rhythmic, ancient and tribal. We each began to move in our own way. I began swaying and rocking from side to side. I felt stiff and awkward at first, but no one was watching me. Everyone was doing their own thing, and anyway I didn't feel that I'd be judged in any way. After a few minutes I began to warm up, and I raised my hands in waves above my head. I felt like a beautiful golden goddess, free and perfect, connected to the whole of nature and to people everywhere. I danced across the room, moving from my own place, aware of the others around me who were moving around in their own way, doing what they needed to do. I danced on, becoming more and more absorbed in the rhythmic beat of the music, flowing, gliding, twirling, twisting. Then the music was gently turned down, until it grew very faint and died away. I just needed to lie down, to curl up and to feel safe and nurtured like a tiny child. I felt happy and content. I heard one woman crying softly at the other side of the room; another man was lying on the floor, laughing. This was their stuff — I just felt calm, centred and connected. Afterwards we each talked with a member of the group about our unique experiences. That night I felt I'd released a lot of tension from my body. I felt grounded and full of energy.

To end the evening we all came back into the circle. We each shared what we'd gained from the evening. We also did some singing and voice work. We held hands and did a short meditation. I floated out of the studio, feeling refreshed and excited that I had discovered a new place where I could explore all aspects of myself in a safe and healing way. I learned many things about myself through attending these workshops. I gained an insight into the way I've been conditioned through socialisation so that my own unique style of being has so often been hidden for other safer options, but also I have learned the importance of being authentic, of expressing my own truth. It is okay for me to be who I am and to feel and express what I feel.

Suggested Reading

Payne, H. (Ed.), *Dance Movement Therapy: Theory and Practice*, London: Routledge, 1992.

Jones, K.S., *Introduction to Dance Movement Therapy in Psychiatry*, London: Routledge, 1992.

Siegel, E., *Dance Movement Therapy: The Mirror of Ourselves. A Psycho-analytic Approach*, New York: Human Sciences Press, 1984.

Stenton, C., *Dance Movement Therapy in Psychiatry*, London: Routledge, 1992.

Journals

American Dance Therapy Journal, Suite 230, 2000 Century Plaza, Columbia, Maryland 21044, USA.

The Arts in Psychotherapy, 20 Ridgecrest East, Scarsdale, New York 10583, USA.

Neuro Linguistic Programming (NLP)

Neuro linguistic programming (NLP) began in the 1970s when Richard Bandler, then a mathematician, and John Grinder, then an associate professor of linguistics, set out to study the work of three of the world's leading therapists — Fritz Perls, Virginia Satir and Milton Erickson. Their studies revealed that all three were using the same underlying processes in their work. To make sense of all the information they gathered when building their model of subjective experience, Bandler and Grinder drew on several disciplines, including neurology, psychology, linguistics, and systems theory (computer programming). The synthesis of many components from these diverse fields led to the development of NLP.

NLP is based on a curiosity about people, and an approach to others that considers each experience as a rare and unprecedented opportunity to learn. It is a way of thinking about and studying people and the process of communication. It has a range of specific techniques that allow therapists to organise perceptions and behaviour to get extraordinary and well-defined results. NLP is about having the awareness and the skills to know what motivates and influences people. This knowledge can then be used to good effect in any form of communication.

'Modelling' in NLP

The process Bandler and Grinder used was modelling — they relied not on what the three therapists thought they were doing, but on the patterns of language and behaviour they actually used. They devised a structure to teach others how to build rapport when communicating in any human relationship. A most important element of this structure was mirroring, where a person was taught to mirror, or reflect back, the other person's posture, breathing patterns, body movements, and language patterns. When two people are naturally in rapport, their body posture and gestures become almost identical, because they are so much in tune with each other. NLP takes what is natural and often unconscious, and devises a series of techniques to achieve the same results consciously. Once rapport has been achieved, the therapist can 'lead' the client into a more relaxed frame of mind, by sitting back and breathing deeply.

Sensory Modes

NLP sees a tendency in people to respond in predominantly one or two sensory modes. The various sensory modes that we use are sound, vision, touch, or occasionally smell and taste. By careful observation of the kinds of verbs, adverbs, and adjectives used by people in their everyday speech, it is possible to discover which is their primary sensory mode. John might say: 'it sounds okay to me', and 'yes, I hear what you're saying', so his primary sensory mode is auditory. Jenny constantly uses phrases such as 'I see very clearly what you mean'. Her primary sensory mode is visual. Mary says something like 'that feels right for me, but I'll have to smooth out the rough edges'. Mary's primary sensory mode is kinaesthetic (feeling).

Your predominant sensory mode can be determined by observing not only your words, but also the way your eyes move when you are asked certain questions. If you are asked a question that requires some piece of information to be retrieved from memory, and you look upwards, then your predominant sensory mode is visual. If you look straight in front, then your main sensory mode is auditory, and looking downwards shows your main sensory mode to be kinaesthetic. In a therapy situation, if a therapist can detect the main sensory drive of the client, and begins to use this mode, rapport will be quickly established.

Benefits of NLP

Not only is NLP an effective communication tool, it is becoming more widely used by psychotherapists, dentists, doctors, educationalists and complementary therapists to aid their clients in bringing about desired changes in their lives. The best-known therapeutic application of NLP is the treatment of phobias. This technique involves seeing yourself experiencing the phobia in a detached state, so that you are distanced from the usual feelings of fear and distress.

Practitioner of NLP: Aidan Maloney

Aidan Maloney is an NLP practitioner, psychotherapist and hypnotherapist (member of the Council for Hypnotic Psychotherapy and Counselling) with the Centre for Creative Change, in Dublin. He studied NLP with John Grinder and gained his certification in the US. According to Aidan:

'Neuro' refers to the pathways that develop in our brains when we think. 'Linguistic' refers to language and the pictures, sounds and feelings that we store in our minds to represent our experiences. 'Programming' refers to the patterns of behaviour that emerge from our experiences. NLP is a way of detecting the steps that people use unconsciously, to achieve successful results.

Aidan has successfully used NLP to treat problems including redundancy, unemployment, phobias, addiction, over-eating and under-eating, career, relationship, stress, sexual problems, bereavement, depression, abuse, pain control, cancer, and performance peaks. Aidan works with individuals, groups and couples. He was originally involved in the training, development and research area, and he still uses his training skills when giving his fourteen-week course in NLP techniques. Aidan can be contacted for appointments and workshop information at the Centre for Creative Change, 14 Upper Clanbrassil Street, Dublin 8 (tel: 01 453 8356).

Case Study: Rita

Rita was a successful professional who was moving up the career ladder. She had considerable motivation and was very good at her job. Her problem was that she stammered. She stammered only when she was talking to a group of between three and approximately seven people. She didn't stammer when speaking one-to-one or addressing large groups.

In an NLP consultation the therapist wants to find out as early as possible what positive outcome the client wants. Rita wanted to get rid of her stammer but that is a negative outcome — to get rid of something.

I went through a process with Rita, helping her to specify an achievable outcome. She wanted to have as much control, and to feel as relaxed, when dealing with the small group as she felt when addressing a large group. The essence of the procedure is to elicit the outcome in a positive format, to help the client to see, hear and feel what it will be like to achieve the desired goal. An important element is to find out if the goal is ecological — are the changes that will occur as a result of getting the desired outcome compatible with the person's values?

I was conscious that when Rita was describing her desirable experience it was primarily an auditory and kinaesthetic one. I anchored the positive experience by associating it with a consistent tone in my voice when I mentioned it.

I then asked Rita to recall a stammering experience. I told her I wanted her to be able to experience the uncomfortable feelings, because they represented the best clue we had to the origin of her response when speaking to small groups. I coached her on how to dissociate from the feelings if they became too intense. I told her to look at herself in the small group situation as if she were watching a film, rather than experiencing it as if she was the centre of attention.

I asked her to hold the feeling and let her mind go back in time and to headline any experiences that came to mind, by mentioning some aspect by which we could identify them later. Rita recalled about six experiences and then she arrived at one where she was in primary school. This was the first instance of stammering she could remember.

Rita had been the best reader for her age in the school. The teacher had instructed her to take a small group of students, who had reading and stammering difficulties, and to teach them how to read. Because of the pressure of the situation, instead of Rita teaching her peers to read as well as she did, Rita learned to stammer. I pointed out to her how incredibly fast she learned how to stammer.

I asked Rita to give her younger self whatever she needed to cope with the situation. She chose self-confidence and detachment. I told her to watch her younger self deal with the situation with these new qualities, and when the outcome was to her satisfaction she could step into the situation and experience it.

As I observed Rita's expression I saw the non-verbal signals to confirm that the altered experience coincided with what she wanted.

*I then asked her to go through all the other experiences she had re-
membered, and see herself dealing with them in this new way. As she
was doing this I told her a story. I said she could listen with unconscious attention.*

*I talked about the development of sound recording technology. Ini-
tially there were records, and once the soundtrack was laid down it
was impossible to change the recording. When tapes were invented it
became possible to erase the original and record a new song. Another
tremendous benefit of this technology is that once a great performance
is recorded it can be listened to again and again in any context we like,
at home, in the car, out walking, anywhere. I asked Rita to imagine
how she was going to behave in the future when speaking to a small
group of people.*

*Rita came for three sessions and she was happy to report in the
third session that she had addressed a small meeting without stammering. When she experienced any anxiety she would quickly recall the
image of herself with confidence and detachment, and imaginatively
step into this image.*

(Courtesy of Aidan Maloney)

Suggested Reading

Bandler, R., *Magic in Action*, CA: Meta Publications, 1992

Bandler, R. and J. Grinder, *Frogs into Princes*, Enfield, Middlesex: Eden
Grove, 1990.

James, T. and W. Woodsmall, *Time-line Therapy and the Basics of Personality*, CA: Meta Publications, 1988.

Lewis, B. and F. Pucelik, *The Magic of NLP Demystified*, Portland, OR:
Metamorphous Press, 1993 .

Seymore, J. and J. O'Connor, *Introducing NLP*, London: Thorsons, 1995.

Nutrition

Our basic health depends on whether we are getting enough nutrients from our diet. When people attend other holistic therapists, the initial diagnosis includes a section relating to the client's diet. To remain fit and healthy, it is important to eat regularly, and to eat a well-balanced diet, containing as wide a variety of whole foods as possible. Three good meals a day should be sufficient to nourish and replenish the body. In our often fast and furious world many people find it difficult to take enough time to eat these three basic meals. Having an occasional day like this won't really matter. However, if it becomes a way of life, it can lead to serious health problems. Poor nutrition can be the cause of constant pains and aches; poor teeth, hair and nail quality; liver and kidney problems, digestive and intestinal disorders; rashes and infections; constipation; diarrhoea; fatigue and lack of energy; and constant colds and flu.

Eating a Well-Balanced Diet

To maintain our maximum health we need to consume a sufficient amount of the following: proteins, fats, carbohydrates, vitamins, minerals and water. Proteins are found in most vegetables — especially in beans, peas, and lentils — in nuts, and in meat. Fats are our most easily converted source of energy. They can be saturated — usually animal fats such as those found in meat and dairy products; or unsaturated — usually found in vegetables and olive oil. Unsaturated fats can help in reducing cholesterol. Carbohydrates include potatoes, rice, pasta, flour, cereals and vegetables. Vitamins and minerals are found in most fruit and vegetables. If care is not taken while cooking, vitamins C and B may need to be supplemented, as they are water-soluble and are often lost in food preparation. Vitamin D can be absorbed from the sun, which also shows the importance of taking in fresh air and sunlight. It is advisable to consume foods daily which have a high vitamin content, as some vitamins cannot be stored or produced by the body. All vegetables and cereals contain fibre, which is beneficial to the elimination system, and can prevent diseases such as colon cancer and diverticular disease. When there are problems with elimination, the body seeks other avenues to rid itself of toxins, such as through the skin. Drinking plenty of pure, fresh water is also important for flushing toxins out of the system.

What Happens During a Nutritional Consultation?

When you attend for a consultation, the nutritionist will look at your current symptoms and past medical history. Often the system is sluggish and overtaxed as a result of the lack of nutrition and a build-up of toxins. The nutritionist might recommend that you go on an elimination diet for a while, to help boost your immune system and clear out toxins. This consists of cutting down on saturated fats and refined carbohydrates, eating more fruit and vegetables, and drinking more water. This is just one option as each person's diet is a very individual thing. If your digestive system is particularly weak, it is better to eat cooked foods, as raw foods might be too hard to digest until the digestive system has been strengthened. The nutritionist will discuss different methods of cooking food, to ensure that most nutrients remain in the food until it is consumed.

Clients are encouraged to develop a balanced and healthy lifestyle, as well as a healthy diet. Many people give their power to others, where their health is concerned, instead of taking control of it themselves. Often people need to be educated that there are definite links between certain diseases and their diet. The importance of obtaining sufficient amounts of sleep, recreation, exercise and fresh air are also emphasised. The consultation usually takes one hour. There is usually a follow-up session a few weeks later, to see how the client is progressing. This lasts about thirty minutes.

Practitioner: Catherine Brady

Catherine Brady works as a diet consultant in the Natural Health Clinic, in Rathmines. She obtained her Bachelor's degree in food science in Aberdeen. Catherine also runs courses on food nutrition, and gives cookery demonstrations, at Old Bawn Community School, in Tallaght. Most people who attend

Catherine for a nutritional consultation have been referred by other therapists who feel that the client's ailments will clear up much quicker if their diet is improved. Catherine estimates that about 80 per cent of people's health problems can be linked to poor diet. There may be some tell-tale signs in the person's ailments — for example sports injuries that won't heal because the body needs more nourishment, or constant colds and flu caused by a poor immune system, which is a result of a build-up of toxins in the system.

Many people have got into the habit of taking vitamin supplements instead of developing a good well-balanced diet which suits their individual needs. If you are very run down or have not been eating properly, supplements can be a boost until you get yourself back into a routine of sensible and nourishing eating. Also some people spend their lives dieting. This can lead to food and calorie-counting obsessions and a constant craving for food as the body goes into starvation mode, literally eating up muscle tissue to feed itself. This is not healthy eating — if you are overweight, you can reduce the amount of fat in your diet, and increase the amount of fruit and vegetables you eat and the amount of exercise you take. To become aware of the feeling of being full is always a natural indicator that enough food for the body's needs has been consumed. This indicator can, however, be lost through constant overeating.

Food can also affect us emotionally. A build-up of toxins has been linked with PMT in women, depression, and mood swings. Also the physical symptoms which can develop through poor eating habits — for example, rashes, colds, pains and aches — certainly will not induce us to feel full of the joys of living. An excess of any food or substance can lead to a sensitivity or an allergy developing in the system. Some people can become allergic to drinking tea and coffee. The consumption of large quantities of alcohol on a regular basis may lead to poor blood quality and liver problems, as alcohol affects our ability to absorb nutrients. If you are very healthy, all kinds of foods will probably agree with you. It is particularly when we've let our system become weak through a lack of nutrition that we may develop allergies and sensitivities. When we begin to clear out the system and eat more healthily, we may find that we no longer have problems with these foods. It is important, however, to become aware of which foods agree with us, and which do not. It may be a good idea to keep a food diary, and if you find that, for example, your skin flares up every time you eat chocolate, take it as a fair indication that chocolate is causing the skin problem.

Catherine can be contacted for consultations at the Natural Health Clinic, The Mews, 154 Leinster Road, Rathmines, Dublin 6 (tel: 01 496 1316).

Case Study: Niamh

Niamh is in her late twenties. When she attended for a nutritional consultation she was slightly overweight, and she smoked fifteen cigarettes per day. Niamh had a leg injury that hadn't healed after several months. She had attended four sessions of acupuncture and the acupuncturist advised her to consult with a nutritionist. Niamh's blood quality was poor because of her lack of nutrition. She was taking a lot of supplements, such as multi-vitamins, and iron. Her diet was very poor: she ate a lot of meat and very little fruit and vegetables. She also drank about twenty bottles of alcohol per week. Alcohol affects the body's ability to absorb nutrients, and was felt to be the direct cause in this case of poor blood quality. Niamh ate quite regularly but she consumed a lot of take-away foods. Her hair had disimproved over the previous few months, her nails split easily and she had a constant bad taste in her mouth. On examination, it was found that her tongue was coated. There were signs of acne around her chin and nose. She complained of tiredness and a bloated feeling, as well as PMT. She was also prone to mouth ulcers and sinus problems.

The nutritionist advised Niamh to go on an elimination diet to improve her blood quality and the body's elimination functioning. She was also advised to reduce her alcohol intake greatly. Niamh said that she could cut down to four bottles per week. She was asked to increase her intake of fruit and vegetables, and to reduce the amount of meat and take-away foods that she ate. She was also coached on the best ways to prepare food to retain the highest amount of nutrients. Niamh agreed to try the diet and to become more aware of her overall lifestyle. When asked whether she did any exercise, she said that she didn't at the moment but that she'd take up swimming because this wouldn't put much of a strain on her sore leg. She also agreed to cut out citrus foods and drinks as these could be very hard on the digestion, and to

reduce temporarily the amount of bread she ate.
Niamh began to draw up a list of nourishing food items each week
and then to go shopping. *She began to take an interest in cooking, and
even invited some of her friends around for nutritious meals. Her leg
injury healed rapidly. It took only a further two sessions of acupuncture for her leg to be back to full health. At the follow-up session with
the nutritionist, Niamh reported a much greater feeling of well-being,
and a noticeable improvement in her former symptoms.*

Suggested Reading

Charles, R., *Food For Healing: How to Prevent and Cure Common Ailments
with Nutritional Therapy*, London: Cedar, 1996.

Davis, G.H., *Overcoming Food Allergies*, Bath: Ashgrove, 1996.

Daniel, R., *Healing Foods: How to Nurture Yourself and Fight Illness*,
London: Thorsons, 1996.

Greer, R., *Recipes For Health: Wheat, Milk and Egg-Free*, London: Thorsons, 1995.

Kenton, L., *High Juice*, London: Ebony Press, 1996.

Kenton, L., *Lean Revolution*, London: Ebony Press, 1996.

Kenton, L., *Raw Energy Food Combining Diet*, London: Ebony Press,
1996.

Lazarides, L., *Nutritional Therapy*, London: Thorsons, 1996.

Terrass, S., *Nutritional Health Series: How Your Diet Can Help: Allergies*,
London: Thorsons, 1996 (also in the same series: Arthritis, Candida
Albicans, Eczema and Psoriasis, Irritable Bowel Syndrome, Menopause, Stress, Weight Control).

Ursell, A., *Eat to Beat Indigestion*, London: Thorsons, 1996.

Osteopathy

Osteopathy (from the Greek 'osteo', meaning 'bone', and 'pathos', meaning 'disease') deals with disorders of the structural and mechanical balance of the body — the bones, joints, nerves, ligaments, tendons, muscles and general connective tissues, and their relationship to one another. Dr Andrew Still, the founder of osteopathy, believed that the human body was self-healing, and that an uninterrupted nerve and blood supply to all the tissues was necessary for the body to function properly. If any kind of structural problems occurred — for example, spinal/pelvic disorders, muscle spasm/strain/trauma or pregnancy — the self-healing power of the person was interfered with and disease would result. He developed a system of manipulation/adjustment, intended to re-align any structural deviation or abnormalities, and to treat their symptoms, such as pain, or loss of movement or power. Hippocrates described techniques for treating the spine about 2,000 years ago, but Dr Still applied manipulation/adjustment not only in the case of back problems, but to a whole host of other conditions where impaired structure affected the body's proper functioning.

The 'working' relationship between the spine, pelvis and cranium (head), and their attendant articular/muscular/neural and circulatory systems, is essential to the maintenance of health, as it envelops the spinal cord, and brain. As the brain controls all functions of the body, any interference to the nerve and circulatory pathways to and from the brain, via the spinal cord, must affect the normal functioning of the tissues to which those nerves/vessels pass, or from which they arise.

What Happens During an Osteopathic Session?

Before the osteopath embarks on a course of treatment, a detailed background and medical history is obtained, followed by a physical examination, in which your posture and movement will be examined, and any restriction or exaggeration of movement in any area, and any pain or weakness on use, will be observed. A detailed examination of your postural structures —

pelvis, hips, spine, cranium etc. — and appropriate joints and muscle groups, and nerve conduction will be tested to see whether there is any irritation, displacement or disturbance, or loss of mobility or power. The osteopath may recommend X-rays, blood or urine tests to aid an accurate diagnosis. Following examination and diagnosis, treatment, if indicated, can begin.

The purpose of treatment is to balance the spine/pelvic ratio, and any tension around it, as well as balancing stress in any other structures — hips, knees, shoulders, ribs, etc. Osteopathy will normalise the movement of all structures of the body and reduce any irritation of the nervous system, disturbances of circulation, and swelling. Many practitioners use 'soft-tissue' techniques, such as massage, stretching, electrical and neuro-muscular techniques to treat muscles and ligaments, as well as, or instead of, manipulation/mobilisation.

The first session usually takes up to an hour, and subsequent sessions take up to thirty minutes. Relief from pain usually takes from one to four visits, though this depends on the individual's response and the nature of the condition being treated. You are also advised on preventative and rehabilitative strategies such as flexibility, exercise, correct seating, work habits, and weight, which have a direct bearing on the type and degree of physical stresses. Following rehabilitation, an occasional check-up should be sufficient to ensure a pain-free existence.

What is the Difference Between Osteopaths and Chiropractors?

Although chiropractic evolved from osteopathy originally, and though they often treat similar problems, the type and application of treatment administered is different. Both use manipulation, but the osteopathic manipulation/adjustment is somewhat gentler as it uses 'minimum force'. The osteopath will also precede manipulation with treatment of the muscles and other 'soft tissue' around the injured joint. This relieves soft tissue or muscle disturbance, which contributes to much of the pain to start with. Thus, you are more relaxed for the manipulation/adjustment, and any post-treatment tenderness is much reduced. Besides the spine and pelvis, the osteopath treats problems in the joints and soft tissue of the limbs and cranium (head), whereas the chiropractor tends to treat the spine only.

What Type of Problems Does Osteopathy Treat?

Most people first consult an osteopath complaining of back trouble, or less often, of pain and discomfort in other regions, such as limbs and pelvis. It is not unusual to find that after treatment for their chief complaint, patients also report improvement in other conditions from which they may have been suffering, which they did not consider to bring to the osteopath's attention. For example, a patient suffering from neck and shoulder stiffness and pain may find that adjustment/manipulation of the neck has also relieved ringing in the ears, dizziness, or headaches. Adjustment of the structures such as the spine or pelvis and cranium, therefore, can be shown to be of value in the treatment of many conditions, including migraine, asthma, constipation, heart disease, digestive disorders and pregnancy (ante and post-natal), and loss of mobility or power, not to mention chronic or acute pain.

Osteopathy does not, however, consider the spine and pelvis to be the only factor in the onset of disease. It cannot deny that genetic, developmental, dietary, environmental, psychological, viral and bacteriological factors can cause disease; nor does it claim to be able to cure disease brought about by these factors.

Is Osteopathy Recognised by the Medical Profession?

Although osteopathy is even older than 'orthodox' medicine, the medical establishment has been slow to recognise its vast potential in the relief of pain and restoring movement. Many countries, including the US, Australia, South Africa and Britain, use osteopaths in hospitals, schools, the armed services and sporting establishments. The UK government recently gave full legal recognition to the profession through the Osteopaths Bill, 1993. A growing number of doctors recognise its value and refer patients who have found little or no relief with previous treatments, for chronic or acute neuro/musculo/skeletal pain disorders. Many doctors themselves attend osteopaths.

BUPA Ireland and Hospital Savings Association give their members refunds for osteopathic treatment (see Directory of Helplines and Useful Addresses, p. 301).

Osteopath in Practice: James Doyle

Some years ago, Sarah, a young lady of nineteen years, attended with her parents, complaining primarily of pain between the shoulder blades. Consultation revealed further pain on both sides of the rib cage, the left side of the chest, lower back, left shoulder, neck and head. It was also noted that she had chronic breathing difficulties, and frequently required an inhaler, as the range of movement in her lungs had been severely restricted. Bronchial pneumonia as a child didn't help matters. At the time, she was attending physiotherapy twice a week, which, she stated, 'makes no difference'. She had been given an outline diagnosis of scoliosis. If one observes the body from behind, the spine should run in a straight line from the tail to the back of the skull. A scoliosis is a lateral (or sideways) deviation of the spine, which may lead to compensatory mechanisms, leaving the spine in an S-shape. Not surprisingly, the ribs are often displaced from their attachments at the spinal column. In turn, this can lead to severe deformities of the rib-cage — an extreme example would be the posture of Quasimodo. Eventually, the thorax, containing the heart and lungs, undergoes changes in pressure and the mechanics of simple breathing may be severely compromised, as in Sarah's case. Spinal surgery was indicated as the next step.

As suspected, her examination revealed a chronic 'pelvic torsion' with consequential changes in tone/elasticity and power of all muscle groups associated with the lower back and pelvis. There was a severe rotation fixation of the right pelvic bone, upon the sacrum, with secondary fixation at the Lumbar 4-5/Lumbar 5-Sacral 1 joints. The consequential scoliosis deformity was almost beyond a simple description. The rib cage was so deformed it looked as though someone had set about it with a large lump hammer. The neck and head were fixed in compensatory side bending, with the head bent towards the left shoulder. This, I assessed, was in keeping with the upper body symptoms she had described.

I asked the parents how this had not been noticed in school in the early days of this insidious deformity. They shrugged their shoulders and looked sheepishly at each other. I could hardly control my anger and told them that, in my opinion, this was a case of 'criminal' negligence, and the condition should have been noticed years ago, before it had a chance to develop into the deformity it was now.

I began treatment with a gentle loosening and balancing of the sacral joints. Afterwards I told Sarah I would like to continue treatment as soon as possible and asked her how she felt. She said the pain, at least, had reduced considerably. She was weeping when I told her I should at least be able to make her existence more comfortable, less painful and at least 'arrest' the condition even if we didn't 'straighten her up' completely. This was a young woman whose life had been totally ruined — a normal social life was impossible because of her condition, never mind any romance. I think I felt more sad than she did when she left after the first visit.

I never saw her again. I heard later that her parents had followed the surgeon's advice. Metal rods were placed alongside her spine, to 'straighten the back'. I could have told them that it would not work in this case, and sure enough I later heard that the rods had started to protrude through the shoulder. The sadness is made worse by the fact that it was all preventable in the first place.

James Doyle DO MIOA can be contacted for appointments at 17 Windsor Terrace, Portobello, Dublin 8 (tel: 01 473 0828).

Case Study: John

John presented with mild lower back ache, and left calf pain. A keen sportsman, he was eager to recover from this 'injury' which had sidelined him. After examination and three treatments of his lower back, the lower back had improved but there was no change in his calf pain. The osteopath decided to examine the calf area closer. Weakness of the left calf muscles was accompanied by acute tenderness at the muscles' junction with their (Achilles) tendon. This is a common injury in racquet sports. John remembered a 'calf strain' some years back, playing squash. With rest it had cleared up, though he did not return to squash. Specific 'soft-tissue' treatment to this area cleared up the residual injury and weakness, and with subsequent rehabilitation exercises he was able to resume all sports.

Suggested Reading

Sandler, S., *A Guide to Osteopathy (New Ways to Health)*, London: Hamlyn, 1989.

Sneddon, P. and P. Coseschi, *Healing with Osteopathy*, Dublin: Gill and Macmillan, 1996.

Psychodrama

What is Psychodrama?

Psychodrama is an active and holistic method of psychotherapy that encompasses the body, mind and spirit. It integrates emotion, intellect and imagination, through the development of spontaneity and creativity. It uses enactment and group process to help clients explore their inner worlds, and relate to the world about them. Some practitioners have adapted it for use with individual clients. In psychodrama people have the opportunity to re-enact what happens in their daily lives, to heal wounds from their past, and discover how past coping mechanisms may still be operating to their detriment in the present. Features of the work include the development of insight, the safe and supported expression of feelings, and formulation and rehearsal of strategies for the future.

The Background to Psychodrama

Viennese psychiatrist, Jacob Levi Moreno (1889–1974), is the founder and creator of psychodrama, sociodrama and sociometry. He observed how much children at play learned about life through assuming different roles, and the importance of this in their self-healing. This work was confirmed and expanded when he later worked with actors. He incorporated insights he gained about the dynamics of groups from his experience of group work with Viennese prostitutes and community work with refugees.

Moreno's approach pioneered the treatment of individuals in groups and the use of action methods within psychotherapy. He had evolved the method of psychodrama by 1921.

Spontaneity and Creativity: Core Concepts in Psychodrama

Spontaneity and creativity are twin concepts central to the theory and practice of psychodrama. Moreno defined spontaneity as a new response to an old situation or an adequate response to a new situation. It is seen as the catalyst for creativity. Not to be confused with impulsiveness, it is seen as intentional and can be just as present in actions that are still, as actions that are flamboyant. It is characterised by openness, freshness of approach and a synthesis of intuitive, rational, emotional and spiritual functions. When we have a basic respect, an openness and a curiosity for the unconscious, we can develop more of our spontaneity and creativity.

What Happens in a Typical Psychodrama Group?

Each psychodrama session moves through three distinct phases: warm-up, action and sharing. Having established the ground rules and boundaries of confidentiality and respect, the director (therapist) uses a variety of exercises and games to build trust within the group. This is the warm-up phase.

The focus then moves to the group members and what they want from the group. The depth of work will be determined by the individuals in the group, and the group as a whole. Usually a theme will emerge or a group member will present an issue to explore. The issue chosen will represent the major group concern. The exploration is guided by the director (therapist) with the help of the group. The 'protagonist' (client) presents their story through enactment, structured with the help of the director. Various relevant scenes are enacted, with the protagonist and auxiliaries (group members) taking a variety of roles. The audience (group members not directly involved in the action) is actively empathic during the protagonist's exploration. They move through the protagonist's journey with them, and are at the same time aware of resources within their own life experience. When part of your own story unfolds on the psychodrama stage, through the work of another, you can feel less alone. Through this connection you can venture to acknowledge some of your own vulnerability. When the protagonist's journey is complete, group members share the resonance the work has triggered for them.

This is helpful both to the protagonist and the group members. The protagonist feels less alone and the group members have an opportunity to process their own material. Psychodrama uses drama and enactments, as opposed to words alone, to help people share their story with others. In conventional therapy, the therapist might help track what is happening with a client, by summarising what is going on in the session. This is automatically done in psychodrama through enactment or symbolic representation. We hear and see and feel what happens in the client's day-to-day life, and maybe what gives rise to this from the past. All of us operate in the present through memory filters of our early experiences. The beliefs we hold about ourselves need to be explored and challenged at source. We do this in psychodrama by recreating their original context. When we can acknowledge the connection between past events and current situations, and deal with the problem at source, we can heal and come to terms with past hurts. We are then free to deal more directly with what confronts us in the present. Psychodrama allows us to try out things differently without fear of making a mistake or getting it wrong, and learn how to turn a mistake into a re-take, experimenting with different approaches for the future.

This does not mean that you need to be good at drama. We use enactment for the purpose of exploration and rehearsal for living, not for performance. Enactment is less akin to acting than it is to children's play, which we have all experienced, embodying the essence of experimentation, and rehearsal for living. However, one of the things much loved about psychodrama is the wonderfully aesthetic moments that happen so naturally, as the end result of people daring to be more essentially themselves, and trusting themselves and one another to co-create together. The group will laugh, cry, sing or dance, be playful, triumphant, or celebratory. It is not without just cause that Moreno's epitaph reads 'Here lies the man who brought joy and laughter back into psychiatry'.

(*Courtesy of Catherine Murray, Doneraile, tel: 022 24117*)

Case Study: Teresa

My first experience of psychodrama was in Chrysalis on a co-dependency week. This is run primarily for people who have lived with, and experienced, the negative effects of a dysfunctional family.

I had the opportunity to act out a scenario with the help of the group. I found it a very powerful tool in confronting a very significant issue. The psychodrama tool used was that of sculpting. It involved selecting three individuals from the group, one as my father, one as my mother, and the other as myself. Once selected, I was encouraged to arrange the three, in postures that I identified them with. Then I had to place myself in relation to my parents. With the help of the therapist I gained an understanding and an insight into my relationship with my parents. I was encouraged to say what I felt I needed to say to them, in a way that I needed to say it. The experience helped to move me from a very stuck position with my parents and allowed me to express feelings that I had suppressed for many years. It was very powerful and freeing.

I subsequently attended an eight-week psychodrama course. Through the group work, I faced and acknowledged some well-buried feelings, through acting out some of my own experiences and by participating in other group members' scenarios. I found that psychodrama helped me to identify and face feelings that I was previously unaware of, and the negative effect of suppressing them. A very freeing experience.

Suggested Reading

The following books, and many others on psychodrama, may be ordered from: The British Psychodrama Association, 8 Rahere Road, Crowley, Oxford OX4 3QG (tel: 0044 1865 715055).

Fox, J. (Ed.), *The Essential Moreno*, New York: Springer, 1987.

Goldman, E. and D. Morrison, *Psychodrama, Experience and Process*, Dubuque, IA: Ilendall-Hunt, 1984.

Holmers, P. and M. Karp (Eds.), *Psychodrama Inspiration and Technique*, London: Routledge, 1990.

Kellerman, P.F., *Focus on Psychodrama*, London: Jessica Kingsley, 1992.

Psychosynthesis

Psychosynthesis can be practised as an aid to healing, to education and to living. It was developed by Roberto Assagioli as a way of looking at the mystery of the human being, of a person's inner life, behaviour and psyche. It is concerned with the individual's journey towards personal growth and self-awareness. As a therapy, psychosynthesis can be practised in either group or one-to-one situations.

Psychosynthesis seeks to bring the many parts of a person together, thereby creating a synthesis, so that no part of the psyche is excluded. It shows us the value of nurturing and acknowledging all of our parts: the physical and sexual, the psychological and emotional, the spiritual, our multiple personalities, the experiences of the past which have shaped us, the relationships and situations which form our present, and the potential we each have to create a more fulfilling future.

The Psyche

The various parts of the psyche which are analysed and gradually integrated during psychosynthesis are (1) the lower unconscious, (2) the middle unconscious, (3) the super or higher conscious, (4) the field of awareness or consciousness, (5) the personal self, (6) the transpersonal self, and (7) the collective unconscious. These are represented in the diagram (p. 136). The lines are broken to show that there is a constant interchange between the conscious and unconscious parts of the self, and between the different parts of the unconscious. The oval divided into three parts represents the unconscious with its lower, middle and higher sections. The uneven shape in the middle of the diagram represents our field of consciousness, which is constantly changing. The central point of psychosynthesis is represented by the line drawn between the dot (the personal self) and the star (the transpersonal or spiritual self): I am at one and the same time an individual, connected to all other living beings.

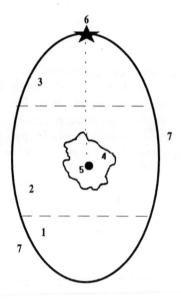

The lower unconscious (1) includes repressed complexes, memories of past experiences, instincts and physical functions, and our primitive urges. Repressed memories can often be expressed in the form of unconscious controls such as phobias, obsessions, and compulsions. The middle unconscious (2) is all that we have an awareness of, all the information that we can call into our mind when it is necessary to do so. We may suppress memories or knowledge not relevant to our current field of awareness (4). The super or higher conscious (3) is the region from which we receive all our inspiration and illumination. It is the source of our inner genius and wisdom.

The personal self (5) is the part of us that experiences itself as having sensations, emotions and thoughts. Often this self is not experienced in a very clear way. It may become identified with one or more of our personalities. Through psychosynthesis we can learn to become more aware of this personal self, in all its many guises — the different personalities we show to the world, or the many roles we play in our life. We can learn to choose which roles and personalities we want to identify with and show to the world, and those that we would rather express in a more appropriate and creative way. In psychosynthesis we also gain an understanding that the personal self is but a unique aspect of the transpersonal or spiritual self (6). The transpersonal self is both universal and individual. The collective unconscious (7) is common to all living beings. We are not isolated individuals, but part of a collective field of consciousness in which all beings play a part.

When we become self-conscious we lose an awareness of our connection with all other people and life forms. When we interact in relationships we often feel pain and a sense of rejection if we cannot open the self to others, or others cannot open themselves to us. Psychosynthesis can help us to become more aware of the many feelings, thoughts, and sensations that flow through our consciousness each second of our lives. It can teach us to observe that we are not our thoughts, our feelings or our sensations, although we can often become identified with them.

Psychosynthesis can help us to experience the inner dance of all of our parts, while not losing sight of the whole. This can bring about a deep feeling of liberation and peace, and an awakening of creativity and joy in living.

What Techniques are Used in Psychosynthesis?

Meditation is used to help you become internally focused and fully present to the self. The three types of meditation used are reflective, receptive and creative. Reflective meditation is probably best described as directed thinking. Receptive meditation is tuning into the unconscious and intuitive part of the self. Creative meditation looks at the insights gained from both the reflective and receptive meditations.

Art is used as a medium for expressing any symbols or images that have come up for you during meditation. This will make the experience more concrete, and may lead to further insights being gained at a conscious level.

Case Study: Carla

I attended several workshops in psychosynthesis at a time when I was doing a lot of soul-searching. The facilitator would pose a question to the group, often while we were in meditation, such as 'Who have been the most important people in your life?', 'What have been the most important experiences in your life?'. I found these very helpful, especially since we meditated on each one, and I was sometimes surprised by the answers and images that came into my mind. Afterwards we'd write what had come up for us, and we'd also draw pictures of the symbols that we had seen. Then we could discuss anything that had come up for us with another member of the group.

One meditation I remember very clearly. I went on a journey through a forest, until I came to a big old house. In this house there were two people who I was to meet. The first welcomed me at the door of the house. He was a wise old wizard, dressed in a flowing robe with a long beard. He was very tall and he had very loving eyes. I knew I could really trust him. I felt that he'd help me to solve any difficulties I'd ever have in my life. This was the outer part of myself which I show to the world, the capable, caring, 'in control' person who others come to for guidance. When I went into the house a tiny naked child ran over to me and hid her beautiful face in my coat. She needed my protection, acceptance and love because she felt so vulnerable and fragile out in the world. This was the inner part of myself which I keep hidden, and share with very few people. This meditation helped me to see so clearly the two main personalities which are a part of me. I realised how important it was to nurture, and to risk sharing more of my inner child to bring a greater balance into my life between strength and vulnerability.

Suggested Reading

Assagioli, R., *Psychosynthesis: A Manual of Principles and Techniques*, London: Aquarian, 1993.

Assagioli, R., *Transpersonal Development: The Dimension beyond Psychosynthesis*, London: Aquarian, 1993.

Parfitt, W., *The Elements of Psychosynthesis*, Shaftesbury, Dorset: Element Books, 1990.

Reality Therapy

Reality therapy was devised by William Glasser, an American psychiatrist in the mid-1960s, and was brought to Ireland by the Irish Institute of Guidance Counsellors in 1985. It is becoming firmly established in many institutions in Ireland, especially in the treatment of addictions.

As well as our physiological survival needs, human beings also have basic psychological needs — belonging and love, power and self-worth, freedom and fun. Although we all have the same needs, the intensity of these needs varies between individuals. Reality therapy aims at helping people find better ways of meeting their needs and taking responsibility for their lives whilst respecting the needs of others.

Throughout our lives we each store pictures in our minds of special people, events and activities which fulfil our basic needs. This is our quality world. Each person's quality world is unique. The more pictures that match from two people's quality worlds, the more they will have in common, and the easier it will be for them to get along with each other.

Often behaviours which we may have chosen as children to try to have our wants met are no longer effective as adults. Reality therapy is mainly concerned with our present behaviour — what we are doing, or choosing, that is leading to problems and lack of fulfilment in life.

The Theoretical Basis of Reality Therapy

Control Theory explains behaviour as a totality of doing, thinking, feeling and physiology. Behaviour is our way of meeting our needs and it is controlled from within. Reality therapy can help us become more aware of our choices, and help us choose better ways of meeting our needs.

Reality Therapy and Counselling

In counselling, reality therapy is used to bring about change, in manageable stages, in people's lives. Therapy usually takes place between a counsellor and an individual client, but it can also work well with a couple, or in a group situation. It is very important for the counsellor to show involvement, acceptance and respect for the client during each stage of therapy.

Reality Therapy and Lead Management

Reality therapy is also used as a system for lead management. When workers are treated with fairness and respect, they are more likely to put the workplace and their boss into their quality world. When they see work as a need-satisfying experience, quality work is produced. This method of lead management was practised by W. Edwards Deming who applied his skill and experience to the Japanese workforce in the 1950s.

Reality Therapy and Education

In the educational setting, teachers can benefit from learning reality therapy. When students feel involved, respected and liked, in a non-critical environment, they are much more likely to place their teacher, their school, and learning into their quality world so that the quality of their schoolwork greatly improves. This has been tried in several schools, including school reformatories for problem children in the US, where there has been much success.

Practitioner: Lucy Costigan

When I completed my diploma course in counselling skills I wanted to specialise in a form of therapy which I felt would be even more beneficial to clients with whom I was working. The appeal of reality therapy, when I first discovered its existence, was its emphasis on taking responsibility in the here and now, no matter what kind of past we had come from and no matter what kind of difficult problems we faced in the present. The expression of emotion is a vital part of our health and our healing process, but we mustn't become trapped in, and by, our emotions. It is important to pull ourselves back into the reality of today, to admit that what happened yesterday may affect us today, but that we still have control over what we choose to do with our lives today. This is the essence of taking responsibility for our lives, our present and our future. The reality therapist can help a client to become aware of patterns in their behaviours which are causing difficulties. *Change is chosen by the client when there is involvement and encouragement given by the therapist in a non-critical environment. Change is also facilitated by exploring the client's wants, needs, and goals for the future, and by providing support in planning realistic ways of making these changes in a gradual realistic time-frame.*

I have worked with people who were depressed and suicidal. Some had been bereaved many years previously and were still stuck in their pain and felt they could not move on. Others had suffered abuse and found it impossible to pick up the pieces and recreate a much better life for themselves. Reality therapy has proven to be very useful for people on their own path of self-discovery, who wish to explore their individual needs and their habitual patterns of behaviours in relationships, or for those who wish to grow in self-esteem, goal-setting and decision-making. Unlike many other forms of therapy, reality therapy can help bring visible changes in a person's life in a comparatively short space of time — even during the first session clients are encouraged to think of even one small concrete thing they could do before the next session to help improve life in some way.

Reality therapy has been used successfully, in conjunction with such groups as AA and Narcotics Anonymous, in helping people who have been addicted to substances or activities. It has also been used with those who had been involved in criminal or anti-social behaviour. Clients have learned to change their self-destructive behaviours and to become immersed in a more beneficial and satisfying activity. The changes in behaviour which may initially occur in people's lives may seem quite simple and insignificant, but for many this is the key to gaining the confidence to make bigger changes when the time is right. The rewards of changing and growing and learning to take responsibility for our own destinies can be remarkable. There is often the dawning of a whole new sense of our own beauty, a realisation of our worth as human beings, an appreciation of our courage, and an awareness of our ability to create new possibilities for our lives.

Case Study: Paddy

Paddy was in his early forties. He had been seriously depressed and suicidal for three years, since his father had died suddenly. He had never been a person to socialise. Most of his life had been spent in the family home with his parents and one sister. *He was never really close to his sister who had married quite young and gone to make her own life, so that he would see her only very occasionally. His mother had died about seven years before. He had always been closest to his father, so felt completely bereft when he died. Paddy had never worked in his life. His family was well off and he had never had any money worries. His father had left him the family home and all of his possessions.*

Before attending for reality therapy Paddy had been seeing a psychiatrist. He felt unbearably alone, empty inside and isolated. He tried to hang himself once, and he made several attempts to take an overdose of sleeping tablets. At the time of attending a reality therapist he was on medication. He said he had no hobbies and no friends. He lay in bed most of the day, wishing he could die. He rarely went outside. The first thing the therapist did was to ask Paddy to choose to sign a contract stating that he wouldn't commit suicide or harm himself in any way as long as he was in therapy, and for six months after he'd attended the last therapy session. Paddy reluctantly chose to sign.

The therapist chatted with Paddy about things he enjoyed doing in his life, although he said he couldn't enjoy anything, and exploring hobbies that he had enjoyed in the past. He was very familiar with the emotional part of himself. He believed that once he felt a certain way, this prevented him from doing anything. The therapist asked Paddy what kind of a life he'd like to be living. He answered that he would like to feel happy. The therapist then asked Paddy to describe what he was doing in his present life. He said that he spent his days lying in bed crying and feeling depressed. The therapist then asked whether what he was doing at the moment — lying in bed feeling depressed — was helping him in any way to achieve his goal of being happy. Paddy wasn't used to being questioned as to what he was doing. He was much more at home with how he was feeling. He answered, after pausing to think for quite a while, that lying in bed wasn't helping him to feel happy. And so the therapist asked whether there was even the slightest thing that he could do to make himself even a tiny bit happier. Paddy thought for a long time again before answering that he could go for a walk sometimes in the evenings, because he used to like doing this as a young boy. On which evening would he go for a walk? Paddy said that he would go on Wednesday evening. And what if it was raining on Wednesday evening? — the therapist wanted to try to cover all eventualities so that Paddy would not think up excuses.

Paddy said that he would go on the next fine evening. The therapist said that Paddy could use it as an experiment to see whether what he chose to do had any effect on what he felt, and then they could discuss the results at the next session.

After this initial session Paddy began to explore his quality world with the therapist. This took a lot of time and patience as Paddy would sometimes relapse into his feelings of despair. Then he would refuse to take responsibility for any aspect of his life. There were a few things he liked doing, which he had forgotten about, like reading, watching television, talking with Jack, an old friend of his father, doing a bit of gardening, going for walks in parks, and he really liked dogs but he had never owned one. So gradually over several weeks he began to bring a few more activities into his life. He renewed contact with Jack and called to visit him at least once a week. He started to take an interest in his big back garden, and even got Jack to help him on a few occasions with digging the soil and sowing plants. He visited his sister on one occasion, and met his six-month-old nephew for the first time. Paddy was surprised that his sister asked him to call back again soon, and he said that he would. He finally decided that he'd take the responsibility of looking after a dog. Thus Paddy's needs for belonging, for fun and for self-esteem, which had been completely neglected after his father's death, were at least beginning to be met again.

Suggested Reading

Glasser, N. (Ed.), *What are you doing?*, New York: Harper & Row, 1980.

Glasser, N. (Ed.), *Control Theory in the Practice of Reality Therapy*, New York: Harper & Row, 1988.

Glasser, W., *Reality Therapy*, New York: Harper & Row, 1965.

Glasser, W., *Schools without Failure*, New York: Harper & Row, 1969.

Glasser, W., *Positive Addiction*, New York: Harper & Row, 1976.

Glasser, W., *Control Theory*, New York: Harper & Row, 1984.

Glasser, W., *Control Theory in the Classroom*, New York: Harper & Row, 1986.

Glasser, W., *The Quality School*, New York: Harper & Row, 1990.

Rebirthing

Rebirthing is a safe and powerful tool for coming to terms with any limitations that may result from birth and early childhood traumas. Using a technique known as conscious connected breathing, rebirthing can bring about a new awareness of the self, healing at a very deep level, and a major transformation in your life. The roots of rebirthing can be traced to the ancient esoteric yogic traditions of the East. In its present form, rebirthing has been taught and practised in the West since the 1970s. The aim is gently to let go of physical, mental and emotional blocks which may have developed as a result of early traumas.

Breathing is one of the main sources of healing available to us. When we stop breathing, even for a few minutes, we cut off our life force. Often when we are in a state of trauma, shock or distress, we hold our breath to try to suppress our emotions, and sometimes to try to deny that the experience is happening. These trapped emotions can exert a huge influence over us at a physical, emotional and spiritual level. They can affect our energy level, our sense of well-being and our capacity to enjoy life. Events from birth and early infancy exert a strong conditioning on many people, especially overwhelming feelings of fear, pain, struggle, and separation from the source of love and security. Many problems, such as phobias, neuroses and difficulties in relationships, can be caused later in life by the suppression of these feelings in the subconscious.

Benefits of Rebirthing

Rebirthing, or conscious connected breathing, when practised in the presence of a rebirther, can free the breathing mechanism trapped since birth, allowing you to breathe fully, deeply and freely. When we become conscious of the need to breathe fully, no matter what we are experiencing, the feelings just flow through the body and cleanse the whole system. The natural energy of the body and mind can then be released, integrating these early experiences gently into consciousness, to bring about transformation. In this way moving backwards through the core events of the past, the actual circumstances of birth can be re-experienced, and such birth-related tensions can be finally let go in a safe environment.

A Rebirthing Session

The first time you visit a rebirther, some details of the circumstances of your birth, childhood, family, school, etc. are noted to give the rebirther a better understanding of where you are in life. The first session can last up to three hours, and subsequent sessions can take up to two hours. It is recommended that you take ten sessions with the same rebirther, after which time you can rebirth yourself.

The rebirther demonstrates the breathing technique, breathing in and out through the mouth without pausing between inhaling and exhaling. You usually lie on a mattress during the session. While you are breathing in this way, the rebirther sits at the side of the mattress, supporting, encouraging and helping you to remain conscious of your breathing at all times. Breathing in this way often reawakens buried feelings which occurred at the time of birth, or early childhood. Feelings and memories spring up during rebirthing. The task is to keep breathing into the feelings in a conscious way, surrendering to the experience without suppressing or pushing away that feeling. People can have amazing insights during a rebirthing session, where the reason for previously unconscious patterns of thinking and behaving become crystal clear. This can bring a feeling of deep release and empowerment, leading to major change occurring in your choice of thoughts and behaviours in the future.

Practitioner: Brenda Doherty

Brenda Doherty works as a rebirther, and a body harmony practitioner, in the Odyssey Healing Centre. She first trained in the area of rebirthing in 1989, with the LRT (Loving Relationships Training) form of rebirthing. She is now a member of the ARTI (Association of Rebirther Trainers International) and the AIR (Association of Irish Rebirthers).

Rebirthing is a gentle and natural tool for personal growth and transformation. We are not our feelings. By allowing our feelings to flow through us, we come to recognise what they are trying to tell us about our past, our present and our future. It is very important that re-birthers must have gone through their own rebirthing process before ever facilitating another. It is only through your own experience that you can support and guide another to re-experience, to pass through, to integrate and to grow from their unique experience. I have seen many transformations occur in people who have gone through the rebirthing process.

There was John, who could never bear to ask for support in any area of his life because of his fear of being manipulated and losing control, but through rebirthing he found that the cause of these feelings was his being stuck in the birth canal and 'rescued' by undergoing a very traumatic and painful delivery. There was Teresa, who had always felt unwanted, which led to a series of painful and unfulfilling relationships. The reasons for this pattern became clear when she re-experienced her feelings at the time of birth, when she had been left alone and separated from her mother for the whole night following her birth. In this way people can become aware that the old blueprint of their lives, which was formed and accepted as being true as an infant or child, was only true then but need not be true now. Rebirthing is personally challenging. It is an exciting and fascinating journey into the core of the self. It is both healing and life-enhancing.

Brenda can be contacted at Odyssey Healing Centre, 15 Wick-low Street, Dublin 2 (tel: 01 677 1021).

Case Study: Linda

Linda, a forty-one-year-old single mother of two children, thought about doing rebirthing for six months before she actually made an appointment to go and discuss the technique. It took her another four months to book her first session. Linda came from a large family. As a child she saw little of her father who worked as a taxi driver, and at fifteen she was forced to leave school to help her mother take care of the six younger children. At twenty, Linda took a job in a large clothing factory where she met her husband. The relationship was stormy even before they were married. Shortly after the wedding he became violent. The marriage lasted five years until Linda applied for a barring order after the birth of her second child. Over the fifteen years since the break-up of her marriage Linda had won a judicial separation, bought her own house, taken a job with a new and growing business, attended counselling and embarked on a live-in relationship with a new partner. She came to rebirthing suffering from exhaustion, and because relations at home between her children and her partner were not good. She felt that there must be more to life than working and taking care of the house, the children and her partner.

Linda's first session centred on helping her deal with her very real fear of change. This fear had paralysed her on many crucial occasions throughout her life and lay at the root of her caution about rebirthing. She knew instinctively that coming to rebirthing would involve changing herself in many fundamental ways, but she desperately needed to know that she was in control. One session was enough to show her that she was in total control of the process itself, and that any changes that took place within herself or in her life would come about only through her choice.

The focus of rebirthing for Linda was mainly her lack of recognition in her job. She had begun to take on managerial responsibilities in her new firm but had been given neither the title nor the appropriate increase in pay. She was putting in sixty hours a week and believed she had to do this because the people she worked with could not be relied upon to do their job. She talked at length, but it was not until she began to breathe with it in mind that she realised that her employer's attitude towards her was simply a reflection of the way she saw herself. This was a very empowering insight for Linda. It meant that if she changed her attitude, she could change her experience of life. Because this came to her while she was rebirthing it came to her on a physical and emotional, as well as an intellectual, level. In the three succeeding sessions Linda, through the breathing process, began to change her attitude towards herself. While breathing she began to recognise her own talents on a very deep level and once she began to value herself she commanded respect and recognition from her boss. Over the period in which she was rebirthing she asked for, and was given, a 25 per cent pay increase and a managerial title.

Another area that Linda wanted to tackle was her tendency to take on responsibility for everyone's work, as well as for her children's and partner's relationship. In her sixth session she came to the realisation that she had lost her sense of self early in life when she had been actively encouraged to take on the role of surrogate mother to her brothers and sisters. Breathing enabled her to feel and let go of the anger and resentment that followed this realisation. Subsequent sessions helped her build up a sense of who she was apart from any roles she might play in life. The experience was invigorating and enlivening. As she learned to step back from responsibility at work, the people she had been criticising began to do their own jobs, and her work-load shrank to thirty-eight hours a week. Similarly at home when she stopped trying to bring her partner and her children together, they sorted out their own relationship. As Linda's need to control, which was a by-product of her violent marriage, subsided, she began to let life flow and to accept the help and support that had been blocked by her belief that she had to do everything herself.

(Courtesy of Catherine Dowling)

Suggested Reading

Minett, G., *Breath and Spirit*, London: Aquarian/Thorsons, 1994.

Ray, S., *Celebration of Breath*, Berkeley, CA: Celestial Arts, 1983.

Ray, S., *Rebirthing in the New Age*, Berkeley, CA: Celestial Arts, 1983.

Sissons, C.P., *Rebirthing: Breath of Life*, Auckland: Total Press, 1984.

Sissons, C.P., *Rebirthing Made Easy*, Auckland: Total Press, 1985.

Reflexology

Foot reflexology works on the theory that there are areas on the feet which relate to areas in every part of the body. The practice of reflexology involves the manipulation of reflex points in the feet in a trained manner to bring about healing in any organs or systems in the body which may not be functioning to their optimum level.

The first known recording of a reflexology treatment is to be found on an Egyptian tomb drawing which dates from around 2330 BC. There is also evidence that reflexology was practised in ancient China, Africa and by the North American Indians. The practice in some cultures of walking barefoot was also a natural way of giving the body a reflexology treatment. A revival in the West began in New York in 1913 when Dr William Fitzgerald began experimenting and practising the art of reflexology or foot massage.

Principles and Uses of Reflexology

Reflexology divides the body into ten vertical and three horizontal zones. The feet are divided into corresponding zones. Each zone runs from a point in the head through the body, through each of the fingers and toes. The reflex zone for each organ and part of the body is located on the feet. For example, the zone for the heart is on the left foot, that for the appendix is on the right foot, the kidneys have a zone on each foot, as do the ovaries, brain, shoulders, etc. Reflexology sees the energy that flows between the feet and the rest of the body as life energy (or ki/chi). When the energy is at a low level, or when the body is out of balance, pain will be felt in a reflex zone on the feet, corresponding to the area that is affected in the body. When a zone is in good condition, no pain is felt in response to the massage of that zone. Reflexology can therefore be used to give a good indication of areas of the body that are diseased, damaged, or not working efficiently.

There are many different techniques used by a reflexologist. These include stroking, massaging, circling the ankle, shaking the ankle, stretching the Achilles' tendon, rubbing the foot, rubbing with the knuckles, pulling and rotating the toes, pushing the foot upwards or downwards, applying light or heavy pressure. For most reflexologists, however, the main tool is the thumb, which is used to manipulate the pressure points on each foot. The reflexologist can get a very accurate picture of the state of each of the body's organs while working on each area of the feet. Flabby, slack, tense, gritty or knotted areas of the foot may indicate a blockage of energy in the corresponding area of the body and may need a more invigorating movement to unblock energy. An experienced reflexologist can often tell a woman at what stage of the menstrual cycle she is, by feeling how tender the area is around the ankle; reflexology, however, is not advised if a woman is pregnant.

Benefits of Reflexology

The main purpose is to balance the body's energy flow and promote internal harmony. It can be a deeply relaxing treatment, helping to restore equilibrium to mind, body and soul. Like massage, it relieves congestion, aids circulation, relaxes muscles, calms over-activity in any part of the body and stimulates where there is under-activity. It can also be used in the treatment of constipation, pre-menstrual problems, inflammation, headaches, sinus trouble, insomnia and other complaints.

Practitioner: Miriam Brady

Miriam Brady works in private practice as a reflexologist. She combines this work with reiki healing, Indian head massage and her work as an actress on stage and television. Miriam holds the ITEC diploma in reflexology. She trained with the Holistic School of Reflexology and Massage, and has been practising as a reflexologist since 1992. Recently, Miriam was giving a reflexology treatment to a woman when she felt the area of her toes to be very tender. This is the area on the feet which corresponds to the sinuses. The patient could feel a lot of sensations in the region of her sinuses when her toes were being worked on, and admitted that she had been having a lot of trouble in this area for some time. Another problem that has shown excellent results when treated by reflexology is painful menstruation.

The incredible link between the feet and the body is again demonstrated by another of Miriam's patients: when Miriam was working on the area in the centre of the foot, corresponding to the stomach region, she felt a tiny lump, and asked the patient whether she was aware of any problems in this region. She was informed that the patient had a duodenal ulcer.

Miriam stresses, however, that reflexology is non-diagnostic. If she feels that there may be a blockage in some of the reflex points, she will sensitively explore any possible symptoms the patient may be experiencing, but will not give a medical diagnosis. She sees reflexology as being primarily a tool for detoxifying and cleansing the whole body, using different pressure points to access different regions. In this way the feet can be used as a mapping system for the rest of the body.

The difference between a reflexology treatment and a foot massage is that reflexology goes much deeper and concentrates on each of the pressure points in turn. There are fifty of these points on the right foot, for example. Talc is used in preference to oil during a reflexology treatment so that the thumb doesn't slip when working deeply on the pressure points. A reflexology treatment usually lasts fifty minutes. Before the initial session a case history of the person is taken. The number of sessions required to clear up particular problems depends very much on the severity of the problem. After an initial session, because of the power of the therapy, people can sometimes experience a healing crisis, but this is just the clearing out of the system taking place, and is typical of most therapies. Reflexology is very useful in the treatment of stress, as it is fundamentally a very relaxing therapy. Also it is excellent for treating headaches, as releasing toxins from the body is often all that is needed to restore balance to the body. 'People go floating out of here,' Miriam says. 'Reflexology is beneficial for both mind and body; it is rejuvenating, energising and uplifting.'

Miriam can be contacted for appointments at 7 York Avenue, Rathmines, Dublin 6 (tel: 01 496 7605).

Case Study: Mary

Mary initially went for a reflexology treatment because of her painful ulcer. She also felt very depressed and lonely at this time because she had just left Africa having taught in Kenya for thirty-five years. She had very few friends or relatives in Ireland, and she had also been recently bereaved by the death of a very close friend. During the first treatment session she found it hard to open up but talked a little about her feelings of loneliness. The reflexologist suggested tentatively that it might be a good idea if she went to see a counsellor as this would be a good adjunct to regular reflexology treatment. It was found during the first treatment that her adrenals, solar plexus and duodenum area felt very tender. Mary was advised to drink a lot of water and to try to cut out acidic foods to help clear out any toxins from her system in the week ahead.

During that week Mary contacted a counsellor, and began to be more careful with her diet. At the next visit to the reflexologist she felt a little better. The stomach, the adrenals, the pancreas and the lymph glands felt sensitive on this occasion, but Mary enjoyed the treatment and felt much more relaxed. By her fourth visit, Mary reported that her ulcer pain had eased considerably. She had been crying quite a lot during the previous week but she understood that this was a way of releasing a lot of her previously suppressed pain. She was also attending counselling; overall she felt much better in herself. Her adrenals, shoulder ridge and pituitary regions felt tender, indicating that some internal shift had taken place.

On the fifth visit, Mary talked a lot about her life — it was as though a release of grief and anger had been triggered by the treatment after so many years of bottled-up emotion. Mary's solar plexus and adrenal areas still felt tender but her original reason for coming to therapy — her ulcer — was now much less of a problem. Mary said that she enjoyed the reflexology treatment and could see quite clearly the benefits that she had received from it over a few weeks.

Suggested Reading

Kaye, A. and D.C. Matchan, *Reflexology Techniques of Foot Massage for Health and Fitness*, London: Thorsons, 1979.

Kunz, K. and B., *The Complete Guide to Reflexology*, London: Thorsons, 1984.

Kunz, K. and B., *Hand and Foot Reflexology*, London: Thorsons, 1986.

Norman, L., *The Reflexology Handbook*, London: Piatkus, 1996.

Oxenford, R., *Healing with Reflexology*, Dublin: Gill and Macmillan, 1996.

Stormer, C., *Reflexology: Headway Lifeguides*, London: Hodder & Stoughton, 1992.

Wagner, F., *Reflex Zone Massage*, London: Thorsons, 1987.

Reiki

Origins of Reiki

Reiki is a Japanese word meaning 'universal life energy', the energy of creation which is all around us. When activated and applied for purposes of healing, reiki addresses body, mind and soul. It accelerates the body's ability to heal physical ailments, and opens the mind and soul to the causes of dis-ease and pain. It thus proves the necessity for taking responsibility for our own life, the healing journey, and the joys of balance.

The Usui system of reiki was born out of the experience and the dedication of Dr Mikao Usui, a Japanese Christian Theologian, in the mid-1800s. Through travel, further study of Christianity, Japanese, Chinese and Tibetan Sutras (scriptures), Sanskrit texts and meditation, he discovered the healing system now known as reiki. He spent the rest of his life practising and teaching his method of natural healing, which involved attunement to the energy, and the laying on of hands.

What is Reiki?

Reiki is a natural healing art and science using universal life energy to promote balance, healing and consciousness. It is a precise technique to balance the energies throughout the physical, emotional, mental and spiritual levels. It supports and accelerates the body's own natural ability to heal itself, and it adjusts according to the needs of the recipient. It loosens up blocked energy and promotes a state of relaxation, vitalises body, mind and spirit, re-establishes spiritual equilibrium and mental well-being, and cleanses the body of toxins. It is an extremely pleasant and holistic method of healing. Reiki is not dependent on a belief system, and works on plants and animals. It can also be administered from a distance.

How Does Reiki Work?

Reiki always works where the recipient needs it most, therefore no general rule can be said to exist. The most common thing experienced during treatment is the sense of peace and relaxation, often combined with a feeling of security and of being enclosed in a fine sheath of energy. However, this won't be experienced every time. What can be stated with certainty is that reiki works holistically.

In a reiki healing session, the practitioner's hands are placed lightly on the patient's body, moving from one chakra to the next, to transmit healing. The recipient usually lies on a plinth. It is not necessary to remove any clothing. The reiki practitioner does not consciously direct the energy in any way. The energy goes to the area where it is most needed by the recipient. A treatment can last anything from thirty minutes to two hours.

What Happens During a Reiki Treatment?

Each individual experiences reiki in a unique way. The recipient may feel a kind of flowing sensation, often combined with a sensation of warmth, which can turn into heat, or become quite cold. The recipient will often feel the flowing of energy as acutely as the practitioner, as well as the sensations of hot and cold. On some occasions, the recipient may sense warmth in different parts of the body from where the practitioner does, or may experience as warmth what the practitioner experiences as cold.

Most reiki recipients relax during treatment and may even fall asleep, but this makes no difference to the effects of the treatment. On other occasions, old and unresolved experiences may become conscious again, and a release of emotions may occur. It has been known for experiences of a strongly visual character to occur. A series of treatments will bring about dissolution of inner barriers which have blocked a person's holistic growth, because reiki works on all levels.

Case Study: Marie

Having gone for counselling, I heard about reiki from a friend of my sister who was a reiki practitioner. I wanted to deal with issues from my childhood which kept on surfacing. I attended reiki initially every second week, and now I go about once a month. At first I found it very hard to relax. I did not like the feeling of someone being so close to me, or the idea of the practitioner laying her hands on me. As I attended a few times I began to trust and relax more. I found it very peaceful. Time seemed to pass too quickly, and I couldn't believe how good I began to feel.

The benefits I get from going to reiki are many. I'm able to deal so much better with my everyday life. I can cope better with the children, with my husband and friends. I don't get as sick physically as I used to. I feel a lot of healing has taken place. Now I'm trying to learn more about reiki, and maybe someday I will be able to help someone through reiki, in the way that I have been helped.

Suggested Reading

Baginski, B. and S. Sharamon, *Reiki — Universal Life Energy*, Mendocino, CA: Life Rhythm Publishing, 1988.

Brown, F., *Living Reiki, Takatas Teachings*, Mendocino, CA: Life Rhythm Publishing, 1992.

Haberly, H.J., *Hawago Takato's Story*, Olney, MD: Archedign, 1990.

Horan, P., *Empowerment through Reiki*, Twin Lakes, WI: Lotus Light, 1989.

Lubeck, W., *The Complete Reiki Handbook*, US: Shangri-la, 1995.

Lubeck, W., *Reiki for First Aid*, US: Shangri-la, 1995.

Stein, D., *Essential Reiki: A Complete Guide to an Ancient Art*, Freedom, CA: The Crossing Press, 1996.

Shiatsu

Shiatsu evolved in China, along with acupuncture and herbalism, over a period of three to five thousand years. It has been developed in its modern form during this century in Japan. Its unique characteristic is the application of healing touch to the body, based on highly developed intuition, together with theory, diagnostic methods, and treatment techniques. Touch is the medium that reaches into the physical, emotional, psychological and spiritual levels of being. The objective is always to work towards the deepest possible level of healing, beyond the physical and psychological symptoms. Shiatsu aims to open into our innate healing ability, and for treatment to be a catalyst for our healing empowerment.

The vehicle for this, and indeed for life itself, is what the Chinese call 'chi' and what the Japanese call 'ki'. This is best, though not absolutely accurately, translated as 'life-force'. It is more than what we usually call energy. It can be felt, and seen, and its constant movement can be tracked with shiatsu techniques. The skill of the shiatsu practitioner is the ability to feel the movement of ki in the meridians, or energy channels. Also to 'read' the quality of ki flow, to interpret that in terms of symptoms and underlying causes, and to know how to work so as to adjust the ki flow to promote better health and well-being.

'Shiatsu' literally means 'finger pressure'. Thumb pressure is the primary technique in shiatsu, but the pressure is also applied with the palms, elbows, feet, and knees, as appropriate. This pressure, which is firm but deeply relaxing, is applied to the meridians and pressure points on the surface of the body. Since the meridians connect to all the organs and body systems, the practitioner is able to make 'energetic evaluation' of the person's condition. Then by use of the appropriate techniques, the flow and quality of ki can be adjusted, so as to relieve discomfort and restore health and vitality.

Principles of Shiatsu

Shiatsu views the main organs of the body as being closely connected, and not as isolated parts. Each organ supports another. If one organ is not functioning properly, the other organs must work harder to try to maintain the body's overall level of functioning. The heart and small intestines, for example, control the functioning of the lung and large intestine, which in turn control the functioning of the liver and gall-bladder. Each pair of organs is related to the functioning of a particular sense.

The organs are also connected with the emotions. For example, the stomach area can relate to emotions of either calmness and contentment, or criticism and jealousy. Thus a person who is very critical and jealous may have problems with the stomach. The organs are linked to the five elements of fire, wood, earth, water and metal. For example, the kidney and bladder contain the properties of the element water, while the heart and small intestine contain the properties of fire.

Diagnosis in Shiatsu

Shiatsu is holistic, so if you go to the shiatsu practitioner with a stiff neck, the investigation is not of this area alone, but of all related areas where energy may have become blocked and need release. The cause of the problem will be traced and treated, leading to long-term relief from pain and discomfort.

The shiatsu practitioner uses a variety of diagnostic methods. Although the different methods are used in combination, the most important of these is touch diagnosis. Specific areas of the back and abdomen (hara) are related to the organs and the pairs of meridians. By gentle palpation of these areas the practitioner is able to determine the relative strength and weakness of ki in the related meridian/organ. This information is used together with your description of your state of health, and a review of your medical history, diet and lifestyle patterns. Other diagnostic techniques such as facial diagnosis and 'the five transformative theory' are also used to form a diagnosis. Each client is given a unique diagnosis, which may change in response to the treatment and to lifestyle changes made.

A Shiatsu Treatment

The practitioner gives a shiatsu treatment with the patient sitting or lying down on a mat on the floor. The client remains clothed throughout the treatment. The type of treatment given depends on whether the condition is acute or chronic, and whether the treatment is required for preventative measures or for reasons of illness or discomfort.

Techniques used to relieve pain and improve physical and emotional conditions are stretching, sotai (corrective exercises) and the application of pressure to energy points (tsuba). A session usually lasts for one hour. After the treatment the practitioner may recommend certain stretches or exercises that you can do between treatments. A change in diet or lifestyle may also be suggested to help improve the existing condition and supplement treatment. The shiatsu practitioner always helps you to feel comfortable at your current place in life. Gradually you are encouraged and guided to make positive changes which will greatly aid the body's self-healing ability, and increase your feeling of well-being.

Benefits of Shiatsu

Shiatsu is a starting point for health management, and a great way of preventing illness when used as part of day-to-day life. Many physical and emotional problems can be helped by shiatsu, including arthritis, asthma, bed-wetting, colitis, the common cold, constipation, diabetes, dizziness, epilepsy, eye problems, fainting and loss of consciousness, fatigue, headaches and migraine, heart problems, haemorrhoids, hiccups, high blood pressure, insomnia, labour pains, lactation, back and neck pain and stiffness, menopause and menstrual pain, neuralgia, nosebleeds, ringing in the ears, sciatica, sinus congestion, skin problems, sore throat, stomach cramps and spasms, stress and vomiting.

Who Goes for Shiatsu?

Back pain is one of the most frequent reasons for people initially going for a shiatsu treatment. Many backaches, however, do not originate in the spine. A practitioner usually does a lot of work on the back, as all the main organs have related treatment points along the spine. A pain across the hip area could be associated with large intestine energy and there could be a necessity to work on large intestine meridians in the arms as well. Diet is also a vital issue. For people who have problems with the large intestine, it is important that they avoid foods which irritate or stagnate in the colon.

A patient's lifestyle and attitudes are also important to investigate as sometimes practitioners can find that people who hold rigid thoughts or have rigid patterns of behaviour will have rigid, inflexible bodies. Working with a frozen shoulder may necessitate working on meridians in the legs. Pain in the left shoulder could be stomach-related, whereas pain in the right shoulder may be liver-related.

People with cystic fibrosis can also be helped by shiatsu. In these patients the upper body tends to be over-developed, and lungs and heart overworked. Often there is not enough energy for the person to take regular exercise. Simple stretches and shiatsu on the meridians in the legs can help to strengthen the lower body. Clients with cystic fibrosis, who have had shiatsu, have reported many benefits, such as increased energy levels, improved circulation and less stress in the upper body. Attention to diet and simple exercises help strengthen the body and improve the quality of life of these clients. They do, however, continue with their medication and remain under medical care.

Several people who had recently suffered the loss of partners presented for shiatsu with recurrent chest and lung problems. Emotions such as grief and depression are associated with the lung. The death of a partner requires a readjustment. Old habits are released and new boundaries are set. Work on the lung meridians helped greatly as did making the connections between the emotions and health.

What we are, think, feel and eat is held in the body. Shiatsu treats the person and not the symptom, by looking at all the vital factors such as emotions, diet, lifestyle and exercise which, if gradually changed, can lead to a greater sense of health and wholeness.

Suggested Reading

Downer, J., *Shiatsu*, London: Hodder and Stoughton, 1992.
Ferguson, P., *The Self-Shiatsu Handbook*, London: Newleaf, 1996.

Jarmey, C. and G. Mojay, *Shiatsu: The Complete Guide*, London: Thorsons, 1991.

Lundberg, P., *The Book of Shiatsu*, London: Gaia, 1992.

Ohashi, W., *Do-It-Yourself Shiatsu*, New York: E.P. Dutton, 1976.

Ridolfi, R., *Shiatsu: Alternative Health*, London: Optima, 1990

Shaw, E., *Sixty Second Shiatsu*, New York: Simon & Schuster, 1990.

Spiritual Healing

The Spiritual Tradition

Spiritual healing is the oldest type of healing known to humanity. In its broadest sense, it concerns the exploration, the awareness and the integration of spirit with our other physical, mental and emotional sides to create balance, harmony, wholeness and meaning in our lives. Spirit is that part of ourselves which is eternal and unique to each individual. Yet spiritually we are connected to all other life forms in a transpersonal way, each being a vital part of the whole. People who wish to explore their personal spirituality need not have any specific beliefs, as the spiritual experience can be viewed humanistically — as the link between the whole of nature, animals and human beings.

What is Spiritual Healing?

Spiritual healing is the channelling of healing energies through the healer to the patient. It re-energises and relaxes you to enable your own natural resources to deal with illness or injury in the best possible way. By directing energy, usually through the hands, the healer seeks to supplement your depleted energy, releasing the body's own healing abilities to deal with the problem in the most effective way for you. The healer asks for healing to be channelled from Spirit, God, the highest level of light. Unlike faith healing, it is not required that you have faith in the healer or in the healing process for healing to take place.

Benefits of Spiritual Healing

Spiritual healing can be beneficial for anyone who feels a lack of harmony of body, mind or spirit. It can be given for any illness, stress or injury. Healing always takes place in the manner in which it is needed. It can be helpful in a wide range of physical and psychological conditions, sometimes to a remarkable degree: case histories range from the relieving of everyday stresses and strains to the recovery of people who had previously been medically diagnosed as being terminally ill.

Spiritual healing has no side effects and is complementary to any other therapy. It is completely non-intrusive as there is no touch used by the healer, whose hands are raised about a foot from your body while you are sitting comfortably. In the UK spiritual healing can be obtained under the health service.

Absent Healing

Any person who asks for spiritual healing will receive it. If the healing is requested by one person for another, the healing chain is set in motion between the person who requested it, the person for whom it is requested, and Spirit. The person does not have to attend in this instance. Each person's name who requires healing is written in a special book, kept specifically for this purpose. Periodically the healer can read each new name entered in the book and ask for spiritual healing for that person. Each person is kept on the absent healing list for one month. Whatever healing is required then takes place. There have been many recorded cases of miraculous healing taking place using absent healing, even when recipients of spiritual healing were not aware that healing had been requested for them.

What Does Spiritual Healing Feel Like?

Many say that they experience some of the following sensations during spiritual healing: heat, cold, tingly feelings, the feeling of being really taken care of, a feeling of expansion and a new awareness of their spiritual being. Sometimes the recipient doesn't feel anything in particular, just a sense of deep relaxation and peace. A spiritual healing session usually lasts about thirty minutes. It is recommended that a person attend for spiritual healing at least three times, with approximately one week between each session.

The Irish Spiritual Centre

The Irish Spiritual Centre was founded by Brendan O'Callaghan in 1982 to promote spiritual awareness, and an understanding of the wider areas of human consciousness. The centre welcomes and respects the truths of spiritual traditions held by each and every individual. Besides Brendan there are three other spiritual healers in the centre: Sarah Branagan, Clara Martin and the author, all of whom are full healer members of the National Federation for Spiritual Healers (NFSH). Many workshops on spirituality are run at the centre.

Case Study — Gerry

It's about four years since I first attended the Irish Spiritual Centre for spiritual healing. I'd heard about spiritual healing from several friends who had experienced it and who seemed to be getting very good benefits from it. So I decided to give it a go. In hindsight I suppose I went because the spirit side of myself needed attention and emphasis. At this time I was starting out on the road of getting my life in order. I was searching for happiness and self-worth. I had a lot of problems coming to terms with my sexuality which were affecting my whole life. Initially I attended three times, once a week for three weeks. After that I'd just attend periodically whenever I felt I needed a boost, an uplift — about five or six times over the past four years.

During the healing I experienced many feelings and sensations. I felt a burning kind of sensation in different parts of my body, and I can remember very strong sensations especially over my heart and right wrist, and a kind of pain in my left shoulder. Also a pulling of energy down my legs, and a movement of energy all over. I could describe it as like a magnet going through an electric field. These feelings were all the more incredible because the healer never once touched me, but only placed his hands about a foot away from any part of my body which he seemed to be working on. There was also a feeling of deep relaxation, and a great feeling of being really cared about. It was quite an emotional experience. The whole healing process was completely focused on me. I felt a great comfort, a safety and a warmth. I felt in some way wide open. And afterwards the feeling of exhilaration, of being full of energy and 'high' was incredible. I felt like running down the street — a grown man — like a spring lamb!

I would attribute definite benefits in my life to spiritual healing. The healing gave me a greater awareness and interest in my spirituality, which led me to finding out more about it. I also went for counselling and I attribute this as a knock-on effect of spiritual healing. I got so much strength and security from the healing. I really felt I fitted in somewhere, I found my place in life. I realised I am a spiritual being, I am a worthwhile person, and the whole world has opened up for me. I have the right to be happy. Now I am in a happy relationship, my career has flourished and I'm much more confident and happy with myself.

Suggested Reading

Angelo, J., *Spiritual Healing Energy for Today*, Shaftesbury, Dorset: Element, 1991.

Bek, L. and P. Pullon, *The Seven Levels of Healing*, London: Rider, 1991.

Copland, D., *So you want to be a healer?*, Sunbury-on-Thames, Middlesex: National Federation of Spiritual Healers, 1981.

O'Callaghan, B., *Modern Medicine Man*, Dublin: ISM Publications, 1993.

Regan, G. and D. Shapiro, *The Healer's Handbook*, Longmead, Shaftesbury, Dorset: Element.

Traditional Chinese Medicine (Acupuncture and Chinese Herbal Medicine)

Traditional Chinese Medicine is one of the oldest and most sophisticated medical systems in the world. In China today over one thousand million people are exclusively treated by it. It has proven itself to be a safe and effective form of treatment for all types of illness. It is also an excellent way of preventing the premature onset of disease, and of remaining healthy.

History and Principles of Traditional Chinese Medicine (TCM)

The fundamental principles of TCM are embedded in Confucianism and Taoism. Taoism viewed the universe as a system of continually moving parts, all of which were aspects of the same unity or reality. The highest code was to act spontaneously in accordance with the Tao (the way of the universe) or one's own nature. The ancient Chinese sages and philosophers educated people in disease prevention: to obey the natural laws of the universe was their understanding of maintaining health.

The whole of the universe is made up of opposite forces: Yin and Yang. Yin is the negative, dark, cold and feminine energy, while yang is the positive, light, warm and masculine energy. Yin and yang is a continuous flow in which everything is expressed on the one hand, and recharged on the other. The balance between yin and yang is of utmost importance to life and health. In terms of illness, slow, lingering conditions or under-activity points to an excess of yin, while a strong sudden onset of illness or over-activity is an excess of yang. Likewise, all living things have qi (pronounced chi, and meaning 'breath' or 'air'). This is our life's energy. An excess or a deficiency can lead to illness. To be healthy and in balance we must have the correct balance of chi flowing through our system, and the correct balance of yin and yang.

A Holistic Approach to Treatment

Chinese medicine is completely holistic: it treats the whole person, and not just any one part of the body or mind where disease has manifested. If disease has occurred in the body or if there is emotional or psychological disharmony, a thorough diagnosis is carried out to ascertain the main cause or causes of the condition. The qi is central to all Chinese medicine as it is the life-force or energy source of the person. Meridian lines carry qi throughout the entire body and mind: there are millions of these energy points along the meridians, and several hundred of them are especially crucial to the health of the individual. If these main acupoints become blocked or damaged, disease results.

Diagnosis

TCM emphasises the use of natural and safe forms of therapy that do not carry any harmful side effects during or after treatment. Any treatment given by a Chinese medical practitioner is tailored to the uniqueness of the individual. The initial visit will usually last between an hour and ninety minutes. A full medical history is taken, including such details as previous diseases or operations, and the medical history of parents and siblings. The qualities of the presenting condition are ascertained by questioning the patient. When did it first occur? What was happening in your life at that time? Is the condition more painful on waking, or at a certain time in the day or evening? Is it a hot or a cold condition? Details of past physical or emotional traumas are taken, plus present dietary and sleep patterns.

Your tongue is inspected to ascertain your general state of health. The qualities examined are colour, coating, shape, length, whether or not there are cracks, protrusions, swellings, whether it deviates to the left or right, or has an upward or downward curl. For example, a red tongue indicates a yang condition, a pale tongue indicates yin; a white colour indicates cold, yellow indicates heat; cracks show heat, dryness, deficiency of yin and a lack of fluids; swollen with tooth marks on the side shows a deficiency of spleen qi. Your pulse is taken on both wrists in three positions, corresponding to the upper, the middle and the lower parts of the body. The overall quality of the pulse (whether quick or slow, throbbing or faint) shows whether there is a balance, an excess, or a deficiency of qi.

All problems in your body or mind are included in the diagnosis and treated concurrently. For example, you may suffer from headaches, PMT, a frozen shoulder, insomnia and periodic depression. To the Chinese medical practitioner these are all symptoms of an imbalance of qi, and are not seen as separate conditions. If you are a woman, details of your menstrual cycle are taken, including duration and heaviness. Touching areas of the body will indicate if an area is swollen, tender or painful. The abdomen is especially important to examine in this way as it is a good indicator of the state of qi in the body. The practitioner also listens to you, to your voice and your breathing. The sense of smell is used to ascertain whether certain types of condition are present. Also each part of the body is considered to be a hologram, or representation, of the whole. By examining one part, the health of the entire body and mind can be ascertained. For example, the examination of the ear, the foot or the hand by a skilled, experienced and intuitive practitioner can give a good indication of the state of health of the entire person.

There are many therapies which can be selected by a Chinese medical practitioner to use to treat a patient. These include acupuncture, moxibustion, massage, Qi Gong, T'ai Chi Chuan, cupping, nutritional therapy, therapeutic counselling, and Chinese herbal medicine. In the West, a person who studies traditional Chinese medicine will usually learn all of the therapies but will specialise in either acupuncture or Chinese herbal medicine. Each therapy is outlined below.

Acupuncture

Acupuncture consists of inserting very fine needles into the skin at certain specified points, called acupoints, selected in accordance with your diagnosis and basic state of health. The aim is to restore the proper flow of qi, the body's life-force, and the correct balance of yin and yang. The flow of qi can be controlled at various points along the meridian system which networks the body. Acupuncture stimulates the body's self-healing powers to restore its functioning to normal if any imbalance of energy has occurred, leading to the onset of illness.

There is great skill and knowledge required on the part of the practitioner to ascertain exactly which points need to be manipulated, based on the detailed diagnosis initially taken. The fine needles inserted into specific acupoints help to unblock the energy, leading to a greater flow of qi throughout the system. The needles manipulate the energy in a particular way, depending on which acupuncture point is used, and also on the way the needle is inserted, the depth of the insertion, and the position of the insertion, whether or not the needle allows a flow of energy with or against the energy channel. Before needles are inserted, the area is wiped with disinfectant. All needles used have been sterilised, usually by the manufacturers, and are disposable so that there is no risk of infection whatsoever. After the treatment, any points which have had needles inserted into them are wiped thoroughly with a disinfectant.

In acupuncture each person is seen as a unique creation which embodies the larger forces in the universe. The dynamic forces with which we are most familiar in the natural world, and in the cycle of life, are birth and growth, maturity, harvest and decline, rest and rejuvenation. Each of these is represented by an element or phase — wood, fire, earth, metal and water.

In this system the human being is also represented by the same elements of creation and nature. Certain areas of the body correspond to each of the five elements. Just as with yin and yang, it is the interrelationship and balance between the five elements, in the way they move together and integrate, that is the important question for the acupuncturist to investigate.

Illnesses and Diseases Treated by Acupuncture

Acupuncture is used to treat a range of illnesses and conditions, including acne, addictions, allergies, anaemia, angina, anxiety, arthritis, asthma, back pain, Bell's palsy, bowel problems, bronchitis, candida albicans, catarrh, childhood illnesses, common cold, conjunctivitis, constipation, cough, cystitis, dental pain, depression, diarrhoea, dizziness, drug addiction, duodenal ulcer, eczema, enuresis, frozen shoulder, gastritis, gum

problems, haemorrhoids, hay fever, headache, hiccups, hypertension, impotence, incontinence, indigestion, infertility, influenza, insomnia, lumbago, ME, menopausal problems, menstrual
problems, migraine, morning sickness, nausea, neck stiffness,
nervous problems, nosebleeds, obesity, painful periods,
palpitations, paralysis, peptic ulcers, polyuria, rheumatism,
rhinitis, sciatica, shock, sinusitis, skin problems, sore throat,
sports injuries, sprains, tennis elbow, tenosynovitis, thrush,
thyroid conditions, tinnitus, tonsillitis, trigeminal neuralgia,
urinary retention, urogenital problems, urticaria, and vertigo.

Moxibustion

Moxa, the dried leaves of the Chinese common mugwort, is
used in various forms to activate specific points or to warm
larger areas. Moxa can be rolled into sticks or cones and burnt
on the needle used during acupuncture, or directly on the skin.
A piece of ginger is often used between the moxa and the skin
to increase the healing quality, and to ensure that the skin is not
touched by the burning herb. You may be asked to take a moxa
stick to use at home between treatments, often on the lower
back or abdomen to strengthen the level of qi.

Cupping

Cupping is a traditional treatment which uses a bamboo or
glass cup with a lighted taper inside it to create a vacuum. The
taper is removed before the cup is placed on the skin. The skin
is drawn into the cup, in a suction effect. The cup is then moved
up and down, usually on the back area. Cupping can be used to
remove cold from an area, and is useful if you suffer from
asthma, arthritis, strained or tense muscles or the common cold.

Massage

Chinese massage is used to treat disease, to get the qi flowing
properly. The techniques used require a therapist to specialise in
this therapy alone. Some techniques work on muscles and other
tissue, some concentrate on the meridians to help the body's
energy flow, and some work directly on the acupuncture points.
In China this form of massage therapy is called Tui Na (pull and

grasp). A wide variety of illnesses can be treated effectively using Chinese massage, including digestive and bowel disorders, paralysis, infant diseases and deep muscle problems. Chinese massage can be quite painful, as the knuckles are frequently used to give a very deep massage.

Qi Gong

Qi Gong consists of repeating simple exercises which will aid the flow of qi around the system. Its success depends on mental attitude, correct posture, correct breathing and perseverance. In some hospitals in China, Qi Gong has been used successfully in the treatment of cancer. Patients can sometimes spend up to four hours a day practising the techniques. Regular practice of Qi Gong is believed to eliminate disease and prolong life.

T'ai Chi Chuan

T'ai Chi Chuan is a system of exercise and meditative therapy which, when practised regularly, can strengthen both mind and body, invigorate, prevent the onset of illness, and assist in the treatment of many diseases and illnesses.

It uses circular flowing movements which function in every direction. In China it is used by people all through their lives to keep them fit and healthy at all levels of their being. T'ai Chi Chuan is also used by some Chinese practitioners to keep their own qi balanced and flowing harmoniously, and is recommended to patients to learn as a form of preventative medicine.

Nutritional Therapy

The food we eat is important to a Chinese practitioner because it is part of TCM that food affects not only the body, but also the mind, the feelings and our personality. Also of importance is the selection, preparation and consumption of food. There are five distinct 'tastes' which Chinese practitioners speak of: sour, bitter, sweet, pungent and salty. Each of these tastes should be included at each meal, and as with all aspects of Chinese medicine, balance is important. Instructions as to food and drink suitable to help improve the health of the whole person will be included as part of the medical treatment.

172 Irish Guide to Complementary and Alternative Therapies

Therapeutic Counselling

The Chinese practitioner not only seeks to treat the presenting problem but wishes to educate the patient on ways to prevent a future onset of illness. The body or mind of the patient has become ill because of an imbalance in qi, or yin and yang, so it is important to discover what caused this imbalance in the first place. Possible causes of disease will be discussed, and changes in lifestyle to help prevent a recurrence will be explored.

Chinese Herbal Medicine

Many thousands of herbs can be used by a Chinese herbal practitioner. In China many herbalists are also acupuncturists, and so their initial diagnosis will lead them to choose either one method over another, or a treatment using both methods. The diagnosis that you receive from a Chinese herbalist addresses the same issues as that of the acupuncturist. This includes a full medical history, an outline of the presenting condition(s), an inspection of the tongue, the taking of the pulse, and the observation of your state of health through touching, listening, looking and smelling. While acupuncture works by manipulating the acupoints and thus releasing the flow of qi, Chinese herbs often work on building up your constitution. Different herbs will be prescribed depending on whether there is an excess or a deficiency of qi, whether there is an imbalance of yin or yang, and whether the condition is hot or cold.

The prescription is prepared by using at least five or as many as twenty different herbs, weighing them carefully and dividing them into equal portions for each daily dose. Usually you are instructed to boil the herbs for a set length of time, and then drink the remaining liquid. The herbal liquid is often strong and bitter, and needs some time to get used to. Modern-day research into herbs used by Chinese practitioners has led to the discovery that many contain chemicals similar to those used by orthodox medicine. It has also been found that many herbs contain several active ingredients which complement each other in such a way as to be safer and more effective than if individual ingredients were used. Herbs can be used to treat a range of problems including eczema, asthma, menstrual and menopausal problems, sinusitis, prostate gland problems, impotence, multiple sclerosis, arthritis, fungal infections and many other ailments. Herbs help to build up the immune system and to cleanse any toxicity in the blood. They can also be useful in the treatment of emotional problems, depression, insomnia, stress, anxiety, and in cases of addiction.

Acupuncture Practitioner: Irja Foley

Irja Foley is a Traditional Chinese medical practitioner and acupuncturist at Acupoint in Dublin. She studied Traditional Chinese Medicine and acupuncture with the Acupuncture Foundation of Ireland in Milltown. This course was three years in duration, and included a further post-graduate course in China before being awarded the Licentiate Diploma in Acupuncture. Irja completed her studies in 1994 and set up in private practice, but she admits that Traditional Chinese Medicine is such a complex and broad system of medicine that it is important for any serious practitioner to study and add to their store of knowledge on a continuous basis.

The question most often asked of Irja by new patients is: Does acupuncture hurt? There are two sensations in acupuncture: a tiny prick, like a mosquito bite, where the needle pierces the skin; and a second sensation of heaviness, tingling or numbness when the needle connects with the qi. As the treatment progresses, the patient may experience a stronger sensation, which shows that the energy is more abundant and flowing more easily. Any discomfort felt lasts for only a few seconds, because the needles are so fine that they are barely perceptible. The patient usually lies down for between thirty and forty-five minutes while the needles remain inserted. Most patients find this to be a very peaceful and relaxing time when they are left alone to allow their own self-healing abilities to come to the fore.

Irja has had many remarkable successes in her treatment of patients using acupuncture, moxibustion, cupping, herbal patents and other Chinese therapies. For example, three people came to Irja with Bell's palsy, a paralysis of one side of the face. This condition can take up to a year of Western medical treatment before improvement is seen. Within fourteen days, Irja's

174 Irish Guide to Complementary and Alternative Therapies

patients had made a full recovery. Irja can be contacted at Acupoint, the Traditional Chinese Medicine Clinic, 2–5 Johnson's Place, South King Street, Dublin 2 (tel: 01 677 4114).

Case Study: John

For nine months, I had been suffering with a sinus problem. I experienced severe nasal congestion, breathing difficulties, especially at night, and catarrh. This developed after a viral infection, which had been treated with antibiotics. After three months and a further dose of antibiotics, my doctor put me on a steroid inhaler. It seemed to help a little with my breathing, but my catarrh was worsening. My doctor suggested that I consult an ear, nose and throat specialist with a view to an operation and subsequent treatment with an inhaler. The prospects of success seemed uncertain and I decided to try something else. A cousin of mine had suffered for years from bad sinus headaches and had got relief through acupuncture, so I decided to try it for myself

At the initial consultation the acupuncturist welcomed me and asked me to fill out a short questionnaire. She asked me a long list of questions, not just about my state of health but about myself. Before a needle ever touched me, she had spent more time with me than my doctor ever had. This made a tremendous difference. The acupuncturist took care to show me the sterile, disposable needles before inserting any. The first session involved nine needles, primarily in the arms and legs. Each pin-prick was comfortably bearable and nothing to be apprehensive about. Once the needles were in, I was left alone for some time, listening to calming music, with the lights turned down. I felt very relaxed. After a few minutes I began to feel light and variable sensations at my extremities, and some slight localised numbness in my limbs. This was surprising. I hadn't expected to feel anything, especially during the first session. I lost touch of the time that I spent lying on the table, but then the acupuncturist returned to take out the needles and to ask me how I had found the experience. After the first session I felt a certain sense of wonder, and also a feeling of gentle euphoria. Emotionally I found it intensely positive. I felt no immediate change in my sinus problem, but the experience in itself was more than enough to make it worthwhile personally.

The second treatment was very different from the first. It was a difficult experience, physically and emotionally. The sensations were initially similar to the first time but soon changed to considerable discomfort. I felt aches and pains in my legs, sensations of pressure deep inside me, and even a spasmodic twitching of the muscles in my back. The session seemed extremely long. Afterwards I felt extremely low, as though I had been through a harrowing or shocking experience. The next day I was pretty much back to normal, but I felt apprehensive about returning for the third session. My condition seemed to have worsened. I had a constantly running nose and occasional headaches which I hadn't previously suffered from.

Before the third session I spent a long time discussing my experience of the previous week with the acupuncturist. She reassured me that although my response had been a strong one, it was following a normal pattern. This session was very relaxing and peaceful. I felt the energy for the first time flow through my body. Over the last few sessions I have felt this sensation becoming stronger. It's like a buzzing feeling coming deep from within. My fourth and fifth sessions were characterised by deepening relaxation. By the fifth session, things were improving. During my sixth session I experienced very deep rest and stillness and my sinuses were definitely much improved. Now I'm looking forward to the end of the road. It has been a wonderful experience, and I am extremely grateful to my acupuncturist who has been superb: skilled, giving, and tremendously open and helpful.

Suggested Reading

Firebrace, P. and S. Hill, *A Guide to Acupuncture (New Ways to Health)*, London: Hamlyn, 1988.

Hicks, A., *Principles of Chinese Medicine*, London: Thorsons, 1996.

Mole, P., *Acupuncture: Energy Balancing for Mind, Body and Spirit*, Shaftesbury, Dorset: Element, 1996.

Nightingale, M., *Acupuncture: Alternative Health*, London: Optima, 1991.

Peck, A., *An Introduction to T'ai Chi*, London: Optima, 1993.

Reid, D., *Traditional Chinese Medicine*, Boston, MA: Shambhala, 1996.

Warner, J.W., *A Manual of Chinese Herbal Medicine*, Boston, MA: Shambhala, 1996.

The Vega Test

The vega testing instrument was developed by Reinholdt Voll, a German doctor, in the early 1950s. The method relies on changes in the resistance to the flow of electricity over acupuncture points on the ends of your fingers or toes. These changes are brought about when particular substances, contained in glass phials or tubes, are inserted into the vega machine and are introduced into your 'circuit'. A tiny direct current voltage of .87 volts is applied via a small electrode. The electrode is positioned at an acupuncture point on your toe or finger, while at the same time you hold a silver-plated cylinder to complete the circuit. The electricity flows from the electrode through a complicated pathway in the body and out by the silver-plated cylinder. Usually your less dominant hand and foot are used.

Any substance can be introduced into your circuit and checked to see whether an intolerance to that substance in your system registers on the machine. Intolerance registers as a reading of less than 100 per cent. In this way you can become aware of any common foods or chemicals to which you may be 'allergic', and which may be contributing to physical or psychological problems. The entire process is completely safe and entirely painless. A full vega test usually lasts about two hours.

What Substances are Checked for Tolerance?

The vega test uses a set of phials which contain homoeopathic preparations of everything from specific foods and chemicals to organ tissues. The machine gives a mechanical display of how freely the bio-electricity in the patient is flowing. If you suffer from food allergies, sensitivity or intolerance, it will be shown clearly which substances or chemicals have an adverse affect on your system. It takes skill, sensitivity and experience on the part of the practitioner to be able to distinguish between true and false readings, and to get consistent results.

A more detailed vega test will test for tolerance to geopathic stress (for example, electrical, magnetic, and radioactive fields), petrol, gas fumes and lead, materials and fibres such as nylon, and many chemicals commonly found in our environment.

A detailed vega test will also test the energy or stress levels of each organ and nerve of the body, including the brain, heart, main arteries, liver, pancreas, stomach, colon and intestines, bowel, vagus nerve, sympathetic nervous system, and the spine. Again, if the level of energy in the organ being tested is satisfactory it will register 100 per cent on the machine, but if it is under stress, the reading will be somewhat less. Although the presence of stress does not necessarily mean that the organ is damaged, it does point to a potential problem, to which the patient is advised to pay attention. A test for possible infections or viruses that may be lingering in your system can also be administered. If you like, you can bring in a specific material, food or substance for testing, which you feel may be causing an allergy.

What Kind of Treatment is Advised?

At the end of the test any substances to which you have shown an intolerance are placed in the vega machine, and a combined reading is taken. Various homoeopathic remedies are then placed in the machine to ascertain which remedies will bring the reading up to 100 per cent. These remedies will alleviate the stress and help to eliminate toxins from your system, so that full functioning will be restored. When these remedies are found, they are prescribed to be taken daily for a month. Also foods or chemicals to which you have reacted are to be excluded, as much as possible, from your diet or environment during that period. In this way, damage to organs can be prevented from occurring in the future, and any present problems can be treated effectively. A follow-up test is usually done after a month. If the remedies have been taken and the dietary advice followed, there is usually a marked improvement in readings for any organs with which you had been having problems.

What Kind of Problems Will the Treatment Help Reduce?

There are many illnesses where food intolerance may be a factor. These include fatigue, headaches, intermittent poor memory, lack of concentration, gastro-intestinal diseases, skin diseases, respiratory diseases such as asthma, cardio-vascular diseases, musculo-skeletal diseases such as osteo- and rheumatoid arthritis, genito-urinary diseases, psychiatric diseases such as behaviour disorders and repressed learning ability.

Patients often crave food to which they are allergic — for example, chocolate, coffee or wheat. If you avoid the food for five days, any symptoms from which you have been suffering should disappear. For a few months afterwards you must be careful not to eat too much of this food. About eighteen months later, you may eat the food relatively freely as long as it is not on an excessive daily basis. The homoeopathic remedies help to clear out the system naturally when an irritating substance has been introduced over a period of time, or when toxins have built up and caused a lack of functioning to certain organs.

Vega Testing in Practice: Irja Foley

Irja Foley is an acupuncturist who also administers the vega test. Irja sees it as a way of helping people to gain insight into the foods and substances that are most suitable for keeping the body healthy and functioning to its maximum potential. As a way of preventing future problems it is also valuable, as organs and areas of the body that are increasingly coming under stress can be monitored and corrected with homoeopathic treatment and a greater awareness of substances to avoid in the future.

When a patient comes for a vega test, Irja asks about any current physical or psychological symptoms, such as headaches, skin problems, depression, food cravings or constipation. She notes if there are any foods or substances to which the person is aware of being allergic, whether any form of medication is being taken, or, if a female patient, whether the contraceptive pill is being taken. Irja uses the side of the second toe on the less dominant foot as the acupuncture point to place the electrode, as the skin here is very tender and sensitive so that a good reading can be obtained. The patient holds the silver-plated cylinder in the left hand. Irja wears a rubber glove so that her own energy won't interfere with the patient's readings.

The vega machine is simple to use and operate. It is the selection of remedies which takes a lot of experience, sensitivity and intuition on the part of the practitioner. It is also important, if any food items need to be avoided for a period of time, to advise the patient as to other foods which can be eaten, so that nutritional intake does not suffer. As well as using homoeopathic remedies to treat energy deficiencies in the patient's system, Irja also uses Chinese herbal remedies, which are also very effective and safe for boosting the immune system or clearing out toxins. She uses the full vega test, which takes about two hours, and is a completely pain-free experience. Irja can be contacted for appointments at Acupoint, 2–5 Johnson's Place, South King Street, Dublin 2 (tel: 01 677 4114).

Case Study: Maria

I had felt extreme fatigue, and had other symptoms of indigestion, acne, fluid retention and very painful periods before I decided to go for a vega test. The practitioner asked me to remove the sock on my left foot, and he placed a small electrode on the side of one of my toes. The electrode was connected to the vega machine, and I also held a silver-coloured cylinder in my hand which connected me to the circuit. The whole procedure was completely painless. It lasted about one hour. Samples of substances were placed in the vega machine. If there was any intolerance to the substance in my body, this registered on the machine. I was found to have a reaction to dairy products, soya, aspartame (an artificial sweetener), tartrazine (artificial colourant in yellow and red foods, and in chocolate), and to yeast. My adrenals registered as being low in energy. This was a sign of living under constant stress, that my 'fight or flight' indicator was on for long periods of the time. Probably this was caused by domestic problems, and by stress at work. My liver was also under par, and I had low blood pressure. The practitioner gave me homoeopathic tablets and four sets of drops to take each day, for a one-month period. Also I was asked to be careful with the foods and artificial substances which I had shown an intolerance to.

One month later I returned for a second visit. I had taken the tablets and drops. I felt a great improvement in my energy level. My period had been much less painful and much shorter than usual. The other symptoms had greatly subsided. This time the vega machine did not react to the foods and substances that I had previously been allergic to, except for chocolate and yeast. There were a few other foods and substances which my system showed a slight intolerance to: cigarette smoke, seafood, eggs, and chicken. My immune system showed up as being quite low, although my other organs seemed to have greatly improved. I was given some more drops and tablets to take. I am still taking them, and most of my former symptoms have not returned.

Suggested Reading

Kenyon, J.N., *21st Century Medicine: A Layman's Guide to the Medicine of the Future*, London: Thorsons, 1986.

Other Therapies

Anthroposophy

Anthroposophy (meaning 'wisdom of man') is an extension of the anthroposophical system of medicine, based on the work and teaching of Rudolf Steiner. Steiner advocated a view of humankind, and healing, which recognised and helped to integrate the physical, mental, creative, emotional, and spiritual aspects of an individual. He also initiated and developed anthroposophical medicine. This system of treatment involves both patient and doctor working together to find a form of healing that is uniquely suited to the patient, as well as seeking ways of preventing any future occurrences of illness.

Today many therapies use the principles of Steiner in their work. These include nursing, rhythmical massage, hydrotherapy, music therapy, dance therapy (curative eurhythmy), speech therapy and art therapy. Also the principles of anthroposophy are used by some medical doctors, in schools, in agricultural communities (biodynamic farming and gardening), and in child-rearing practices. Worldwide a system of general education has also been developed. In England the Anthroposophical Medical Association can be contacted for further information at Rudolf Steiner House, 35 Park Road, London NW1 6XT. In Ireland there are several anthroposophical schools offering education in a therapeutic environment for children, adolescents and adults who are in need of special care.

Camphill Communities

There are eight Camphill communities in the Republic, and three in Northern Ireland. They were founded by Dr Karl König in 1940 and offer children, adolescents and adults who are in need of special care a supported environment, in which their educational, therapeutic and social needs can be met. A home is provided for people with a wide range of needs, varying from cerebral palsy, Down's Syndrome, autism, epilepsy, to social and behavioural difficulties. Schools are provided for children aged from six to nineteen, where a balance is sought between academic and working skills, crafts and leisure pursuits. The aim is to foster the harmonious development of the whole human being: body, mind and spirit. Therapies involving music, art, movement and speech are undertaken in close co-operation with the school doctor, and are supported by the use of anthroposophical and homoeopathic medicines. Further education and training is available for adults. In time, some people choose to leave, to seek new experiences or to return to their families. Some adults with special needs continue to live and work in the community, together with their co-workers, families and children. The communities are listed in the Directory.

Schools

Founded in 1986, Coolenbridge School in Scariff, Co. Clare, was the first Steiner school in the Republic of Ireland. It works together with the Steiner Schools Fellowship in the UK and other international bodies. It is co-educational, and has a kindergarten and four classes up to age thirteen. Subjects are developed and taught in an interdisciplinary way. The curriculum includes a balance of practical life skills with work experience. A wide range of artistic activities is also taught.

Founded in 1988, the Dublin Rudolf Steiner School is co-educational and caters for children from four to twelve years of age. In kindergarten, the emphasis is on creating an environment akin to a harmonious and loving home. The relationship between child and teacher is central to all teaching. Domestic and artistic activities are fostered, as well as the qualities of lively imagination and will-activity, and learning techniques of rhythm and repetition. Reading, writing, arithmetic, foreign languages, Irish, music, history, geography, and handwork are introduced at a later stage. Festivals are held throughout the school year, where children, teachers, parents, and their family and friends can celebrate together.

Body Harmony

Body harmony is a hands-on form of body-work, which acknowledges our physical, mental, emotional and spiritual dimensions. It was developed by Don McFarland, based on the theory that our bodies record every experience that we have. A body harmony practitioner specialises in listening touch — following any instructions given by the body physically, emotionally or intuitively. This can lead to the unblocking of tensions, and freedom from redundant patterns of thinking, feeling, moving and living. Change and letting go are gently encouraged and supported by the practitioner. Body harmony teaches us to love and respect the intelligence and magnificence of the body, and to experience the joy and beauty of our own uniqueness.

Cranio-sacral Therapy

This is a specialised form of osteopathy which follows the teachings of Dr William Garner Sutherland. It is based on the premise that the bones in the skull are not fixed, but can move slightly. Although the degree of movement may be small, it can still be measured by an oscilloscope and can be detected by a trained therapist. The brain is suspended by sheets of fascial tissue, called meninges, held in tension by attachments. The meninges extend all the way down the spine to the sacrum at the base. Along the spine there is the cerebro-spinal fluid which bathes both the brain and the spinal column. Trained craniosacral therapists maintain that this fluid creates a rhythmic pulse, called the cranial rhythmic impulse. Any disturbance to the normal cranial bone movement leads to a corresponding disturbance of the normal cranial rhythm and thus disturbs the normal fluid flow. Cranio-sacral therapists use these disturbed patterns of movement to diagnose and treat disorders in a gentle and non-invasive way. They also seek to balance the rhythmical forces at work in the body, by helping to release any tension trapped in the tissues. It is a gentle but powerful form of therapy, and can be beneficial in the treatment of many disorders including arthritis, asthma, back pain, migraine, sinusitis, spinal curvature, stress-related illnesses, and whiplash injuries.

Drama Therapy

Drama therapy has its theoretical base in psychology, anthropology, theatre and psychoanalysis. An opportunity is provided in a drama therapy session to process the difficulties encountered in life, through the safety of dramatic distance, and re-enactment of real-life events. Role-play, improvisation, dramatic representation and other techniques are utilised for therapeutic exploration and growth.

The need for a dramatic talent is not essential to participation, as the vehicle of change and exploration is often through the re-emergence of the world of play and the re-capturing of those times of childhood freedom. The therapeutic process can evolve through enjoyment, as well as through the painful confrontation of life and its problems. A list of drama therapists who are members of the Irish Association of Drama, Art and Music Therapists is contained in the Directory. (See also Art Therapy and Music Therapy.) They can be contacted by writing to the association address: PO Box 4176, Dublin 1. Another form of psychotherapy which uses drama to facilitate healing is psychodrama (see individual section).

Faith Healing

Faith healing has had a long tradition in Ireland, practised both inside and outside religion. Individuals are believed to have been given the gift of healing by God, and to have the ability to heal others from a young age. Some faith healers are seventh sons of seventh sons and are sought by members of their community for their healing abilities. The faith of the healers is of most importance — the faith that God will use them as a channel for healing. In many cases the faith of the recipient of healing is also crucial, as it is usually believed that the more faith you have, the greater the likelihood that you will be cured.

Energy Healing

Energy healing is another form of faith healing. A postal request service is offered at Tony Quinn Centres. This is part of Tony Quinn's EDUCO (to lead out from within) formula, which states: 'If you want something, believe you have it without any inner doubt and it will come to you.' This system claims to obtain results in every aspect of a person's life. Those with a request for healing or to achieve some special goal are asked to write down their request and to send it, with a photograph, to the Tony Quinn Centre. This request is worked on for a month, to help bring about the desired results. A specific goal will be worked on and the belief assumed that it has already happened.

The 'Successful Living' sessions in the Tony Quinn Centres use relaxation and positive thinking to help to draw out the potential of the individual and to boost their own self-healing. The initial session usually takes place in a one-to-one session with a trained healer. Here you are helped to learn how to relax, and to request the goals or healing which you want to achieve. You can then attend a weekly group session where relaxation and positive thinking help you to make the desired changes. (See Directory for details of the postal request service and the Successful Living sessions.)

Indian Head Massage

Indian head massage has been practised for a thousand years informally in the homes of Indian women. It is believed in India that head massage keeps hair healthy and delays the onset of greying. Various oils such as coconut, sesame, almond and olive oil contribute towards lustrous growth. Scalp massage revitalises circulation at the hair roots and oil nourishes the growing hair. One of the main features of Indian head massage is the easing of tension and the sense of relaxation that it brings. Headaches and heaviness are relieved, muscles are unknotted and other parts of the body also respond to this relaxed state.

A treatment usually takes about twenty to thirty minutes. Sometimes the upper part of the body, the neck and shoulders are also worked on. The receiver of the massage need only sit in a chair, so it can be done anywhere. The upper part of the body can be worked on through the clothes, but it is most effective when the practitioner works directly on the skin. Usually the massage is done with dry hands, but if an oil is used it should be left for eight hours before shampooing. Some of the benefits of Indian head massage are improved scalp circulation, which promotes texture, strength and growth in hair; relaxing the scalp and muscles; soothing and rebalancing the energy flow in the face; easing muscle tension and stimulating circulation in the neck and shoulders; restoring joint movement and mobility; and stimulating lymphatic drainage.

Iridology

Iridology is the interpretation of the patterns, textures, colours and markings of the iris to analyse a person's health. The word *iris* is Greek for 'rainbow'. The iris is our own personal rainbow, which reveals much valuable information about our physical, physiological and psychological make-up. An iridologist will have learnt to focus on the whole person and will build an individual picture of each patient based on what is seen in the eyes. Iridologists use an iris chart to map the markings of the eye. This shows the areas of the iris which correspond to the different parts of the body. The map is obtained by photographing the magnified eye. When the iridology analysis is completed, the results are discussed with you, and a treatment programme is prescribed. This may consist of a change of diet, a course of therapy such as acupuncture or aromatherapy, homoeopathic or herbal remedies, an exercise programme, a visit to your GP, or a combination of these. A follow-up session, about eight or ten months after the initial session, is advised to see how you are responding to the treatment. Many benefits in health and well-being are reported by patients who have had an iridology test and followed prescribed treatment. A session takes about forty-five minutes and is completely painless.

Meditation

Meditation, meaning 'to centre the self', is a way of expanding our awareness. It is a systematic narrowing of attention, which leads to increased concentration and relaxation. During meditation you just sit, with your eyes closed, and turn your attention inwards. Some people like to spend time staring at a candle to assist meditation. Others use a mantra, which is a word or phrase that is repeated to keep the conscious mind occupied. This helps the subconscious mind or higher self to come to the fore. Guided imagery, or paying attention to your breathing, can also be used as focusing techniques.

Regular meditation brings many healing benefits to both

body and mind. It aids concentration, alleviates stress, decreases blood pressure and respiration, activates your creative and intuitive side, and brings a feeling of calm and peace to your day-to-day life. Being more relaxed and less anxiety-prone often leads to a marked improvement in your health. The best results come about when meditation is practised consistently, for fifteen to thirty minutes, two or three times a day. There are several groups where you can learn to become familiar with the feelings and techniques of meditation in a safe and supportive environment (see Directory).

Metamorphosis

Metamorphosis is a means of re-educating the unconscious mind and of eliminating deep-seated influences of genetic, karmic and other sources. Based on the ancient system of reflexes, practitioners use those of the feet, the hands, and the head, as well as the more abstract hand symbol, to gain access to the patterns formed by your pre-natal conditioning. The illnesses of the mind and the body stem from the primary attitudes of mind created at conception and developed during gestation. Metamorphosis enables you to contact these primary conditioning factors and to effect changes which finally eliminate many long-standing problems.

There is no limit to age or to severity of the trouble. It is the patient who effects the change, and it is this inner change that alters the attitude of mind, and heals illness of mind and body. Metamorphosis can be taught to anyone who has the desire to effect a real and permanent change in their behaviour patterns.

Muscle Effect Therapy

Muscle effect therapy is a gentle system of using light and precise touch, to enable you to change your body and break out of old and painful patterns of behaviour. It has evolved as a synthesis of the best elements from several therapies, including rolfing, deep-tissue therapy, and co-counselling. An entirely non-verbal form of therapy, it melts frozen muscles so that you can regain flexibility and move more easily. It opens a path into memories held in tight muscles, which may have been completely blocked out of the conscious mind, and enables you to regain these memories gradually, leave behind pain, anger or grief associated with them and move on into a more balanced state of being. The therapy is client-directed, which means that you are in charge at all times, and decide how far to go, when to stop, how much feels safe.

Muscle effect therapy can be used by therapists and health-care professionals, as well as by individuals for personal growth. It works as well for growth as it does for repair. Some of the benefits include: an increase in lung capacity for asthmatics and for people active in competitive sports; an increase in flexibility and ease of movement; the ease of long-term pain held in the muscles after injury, surgery or other physical trauma, and the promotion of healing; the ease of stress-related headaches, period pains and depression. It improves coping strategies with problems at work, and in the client's personal life. After receiving muscle effect therapy, people feel more comfortable in their bodies and have a better self-image.

Music Therapy

The ability to appreciate and respond to music is an inborn quality in human beings. Music therapy involves the creative use of music, and its elements of pitch, rhythm, and timbre, to facilitate change in an emotional, intellectual or physical capacity. In a music therapy session the client and therapist may engage in voice-work, playing instruments, improvising vocally or instrumentally, moving to music, composing and listening. You are introduced to a variety of percussion, keyboard and stringed instruments. No prior experience of performance is required and your innate response to rhythm, pitch, melody and dynamic is employed as a basis for communication. Music therapy can be experienced by any individual, regardless of age, disability or musical background.

The types of clinical problems addressed by the music therapist include emotional disturbance, language delay and disorder, sensory impairment, and poor physical co-ordination. Depending on the clinical setting, the therapist will liaise closely with parents, medical or educational staff and other members of the therapeutic or multidisciplinary team. See Directory for a list of music therapists who are members of the Irish Association of Drama, Art and Music Therapists. They can be contacted by writing to the association address: PO Box 4176, Dublin 1 (see also Art Therapy and Drama Therapy).

Naturopathy

Naturopathy works on the basis that healing depends upon the action of natural healing forces present in the human body. It does not seek to suppress symptoms, but to discover and remove the root cause of disease, whether it be chemical (caused by faulty eating, excessive drinking, problems with breathing or elimination), mechanical (poor posture, stiff joints, spinal misalignment, muscular tension) or psychological/emotional. It is holistic, and encourages prevention just as much as cure.

The naturopath, although not medically trained, undergoes a long and technical training before becoming qualified. During an initial consultation, a lot of the naturopath's time is spent taking a detailed medical history. Blood-tests, X-rays and other minor medical procedures may be conducted, to ascertain your general state of health. Naturopathy views illness and disease as the manifestation of the healing forces' effort to bring the system back into balance. Your lifestyle, diet, posture, emotional outlook, and exercise routine are all assessed. Naturopathy uses natural and safe techniques of diet and fasting, exercise and massage, to help the body return to a state in which it begins to rid itself of illness, and becomes healthier and fitter. Many conditions can be successfully treated, including sore throats, colitis, gastritis, bronchitis, haemorrhoids, digestive and liver problems, and serious diseases such as tuberculosis.

Rolfing

Rolfing is a deep massage and manipulation therapy in which the hands work on the fascia (the elastic tissue between the muscles and under the skin) and the muscles, to stretch and remodel the body, so that the posture and overall structure are greatly improved. The system was developed by Ida P. Rolf. At the beginning of treatment you are observed and photographed in your underwear, to ascertain the structure and the degree of vertical alignment of the body. During treatment you lie on a cushioned surface while the therapist uses hands, knuckles and an occasional elbow to assist the movement and re-positioning of tissue. There may be some discomfort, but once the tissue is released, this disappears. Emotional release can accompany this process. Usually it takes about ten sessions to correct structural problems, with each session lasting about an hour. Benefits reported include a feeling of lightness, more freedom in movement, increase in energy, a greater feeling of confidence and a more positive self-image.

SHEN® (Specific Human Emotion Nexus)

SHEN® works on the bio-field of the patient, to help release and clear away blocked emotions from mind and body. Many painful emotions are stored in the body. We may feel discomfort in our stomach, head, shoulder and neck areas; our hearts may ache and we may find it difficult to breathe. All kinds of physical problems such as migraine, eating disorders, PMT and upset bowels often have psychosomatic causes. This therapy is a unique hands-on bio-field intervention that seeks to release painful emotions directly from the body so that emotional health can be regained.

During SHEN® the practitioner's hands are placed, without applying any pressure, on your clothed body and a naturally occurring energy is directed through the emotional centres in carefully planned patterns. This subtle process gently releases painful, trapped emotions and uncovers empowering emotions such as confidence, joy and a sense of well-being. Often, previously hidden memories are recalled during a treatment. Feelings such as anger, sadness or rejection may build up in certain areas of the body during a treatment. When these feelings peak they are gently dissipated, without the need for screaming or getting caught up in any physical action. SHEN® was developed by Richard R. Pavek in 1977, after much research into the effects of the bio-field on bodily-held emotion.

Shen Tao Acupressure

Shen Tao acupressurists receive essentially the same training as classical Chinese acupuncturists, with the addition of Western anatomy and physiology. However, instead of needles, the tip of the middle finger of each hand is used to palpate the acupoints. Pressure, as such, is seldom used. Recipients are reassured that they need remove only shoes, watch, belt and heavy jewellery.

As a form of vibrational medicine, Shen Tao adjusts the subtle electro-magnetic flow in the energy pathway, or meridian system, and is useful to treat a broad range of disorders. It addresses all four aspects of being: physical, emotional, mental, and spiritual, simultaneously. The chosen emphasis on any one of these levels is determined by the combinations and sequences of points used in the treatment session.

Practitioners of Shen Tao, like all practitioners of Chinese medicine, use a holistic approach, and will guide people toward changes in lifestyle where necessary. They may recommend appropriate diet, exercises, such as Qi Gong, T'ai Chi and meditation, as well as using moxa and sometimes herbs. Health maintenance is an aim among Shen Taoists too. Practitioners use patterns of acupoints that assist seasonal transitions, as well as supporting the individual's immune system, at a time when we are all constantly threatened by our compromised environment.

Spinology

For thousands of years many cultures and peoples have recognised the importance of the spine and nervous system for an individual's health and well-being. Spinology is a method of maintaining and restoring health by means of specific adjustment of the bones of the spinal column (spinal vertebrae). It has as its focus, correct alignment and function of the spinal column, thereby reducing nerve interference, and allowing the body to function naturally more efficiently and harmoniously.

Our spinal column consists of twenty-four movable vertebrae, the sacrum and coccyx. It is designed for support, flexibility, strength and protection of the nervous system. When the vertebrae are correctly aligned, and the joints of the spine retain their proper mobility, they serve their purpose well. But we may be subjected to various forces that sometimes result in misalignment, which can adversely affect the nerve tissue the spine is designed to protect, and is called spinal obtrusion.

Falls, car crashes, physical strain or stress, emotional stress, improper posture, poor eating habits, incorrect lifting, over-work, lack of suppleness, trauma of childbirth and sports injuries can all cause spinal obtrusion. Spinology identifies, analyses and, when possible, adjusts these obtrusions, thus removing the nerve interference. To assess the condition of the spine, a spinologist uses palpation. With the hands, the practitioner will make a corrective adjustment using a highly-skilled, precise, safe and painless technique.

People consult a spinologist with a specific problem, such as back pain, neck pain, headaches, sciatica, numbness or tingling in the arms or legs, arthritis, loss of strength, tension, or other problems. Spinologists seek to restore better function and alignment to the spinal column, thus releasing nerve pressure which can cause many of the above problems. Spinologists do not diagnose and treat symptoms, but rather attempt to correct the cause of the nerve interference, thus allowing the body to exercise its own healing potential. People who have attended a spinologist for a specific problem have reported other benefits arising from the treatment, as well as the alleviation of their original symptoms. Some of these benefits reported are improved digestion, better circulation, improved mental clarity, increased energy, easier breathing, and a general feeling of well-being. Spinologists also encourage people to have their spines checked regularly, to prevent the onset of pain and illness.

Voice Therapy

Voice therapy allows the individual to uncover the self through healing sounds. There are remarkable similarities between sounds in many cultures which have been used for healing and sacred purposes through the ages.

Voice therapy can help to retune the body, to clear and balance the chakras or energy systems. It can help us to reclaim our natural voice, which reveals a lot about our physical, emotional, mental and spiritual well-being. Often in the past we may have been silenced by those who did not wish us to speak the truth of our experiences. We may have smothered and choked back our voices, through fear, grief, anger, hurt or confusion. By giving ourselves permission to speak, to chant, to screech, and to sing, we can release suppressed emotions and reclaim our creativity, spontaneity and feelings of joy. When we begin to free the voice, we give ourselves permission to let go of inhibitions, and to cry and laugh in full-bodied voice. Using the voice is a great way of connecting with others, and raising the vibration of the whole group. Voice work can be combined with dance and movement, drama, breathing and relaxation, meditation and body-work.

Yoga

Yoga, taken from the Sanskrit, means 'union with the source', or 'oneness'. It is based on ancient Indian traditional beliefs about human existence, in which there are five levels of existence *(sheats)*: the physical frame; the vital body which is made up of *prana* (the life energy that flows through invisible channels known as *nadis*); the mind (emotions and thoughts); the highest intellect (perfect thought and knowledge); and the abode of bliss and inner peace. Disease arises when an imbalance occurs in the three lower sheats, in the realm of the ego consciousness, and can show itself as physical, mental or psychosomatic pain and illness. The fourth and fifth sheats are permeated by a wider universal consciousness and cannot be disturbed, although disharmony in the lower physical/mental levels will block the flow of peace and happiness throughout the system.

Yoga aims to treat illness by improving health on all levels simultaneously and by restoring inner harmony. It uses different kinds of specially designed physical and mental exercises to work on all of these levels. *Asanas* relax and tone the muscles and massage the internal organs. *Pranayama* slows breathing and regulates the flow of prana (life energy). Relaxation and meditation calm the mind and emotions, and heal the spirit. The different types of exercises augment each other and are more effective when done together. For example, asanas stretch the muscles, muscle tension is released and therefore it is easier for

194 Irish Guide to Complementary and Alternative Therapies

the body to relax and become more balanced. The daily practice of a complete yoga session is believed to restore natural balance and harmony, helping to clear out toxins and heal damaged tissue much more quickly. It also brings positive good health to all parts of your life — physical, mental and spiritual. Some of the benefits are increased flexibility, improved posture and muscle tone, increased vitality, a sense of well-being, improved blood circulation, lower blood pressure, improved respiration, and increased awareness of the beauty of life in all its forms.

Zero Balancing

Zero Balancing is a gentle yet powerful hands-on method of balancing body structure. Using finger pressure and held stretches, it enables the release of tension accumulated in the deep structures of the body. It provides a point of stillness around which the body can relax, giving you the opportunity to let go of pain. One of the main benefits of zero balancing is the reduction of stress. The energy is unblocked, allowing it to flow smoothly through the structures of the body, helping to release stressful patterns and knots of tension. Often this leads to a healing of the physical body and to freedom from pain.

Zero balancing focuses on a particular group of joints which are involved with the smooth transmission of forces through the weight-bearing skeletal structure. It enhances the way they relate to each other in the whole body allowing natural re-alignment and improved flexibility and posture.

Glossary

Other Treatments and Services Offered by Therapists

Active Balancing: Uses gentle manipulation to realign and strengthen the spine, and to balance the energy centres.

Astrological Readings: Ancient system which charts the date, time and location of your birth, and maps the position of the planets and solar system at that exact moment. The chart is then interpreted with regard to personality tendencies, life purpose and future.

Chelation: Form of hands-on healing which aims to instil relaxation, and to balance the energy centres, by channelling earth energies.

Colonic Irrigation (also called *Colon Hydrotherapy*): An internal bath which cleanses the large intestine of toxins, excess mucus, bacterial overgrowths and parasites, promoting effective elimination and general health.

Dream Interpretation: Interpreting symbols in dreams to help you gain insight into your subconscious fears, motivations, and emotions. There are many schools of dream interpretation, including Freudian and Jungian.

Enneagram: Based on an ancient Sufi teaching which describes nine different personality types and their interrelationships. Recognising your own 'type' is said to promote a greater awareness of your motivations, and those of family, friends and partners.

Feng shui: An ancient Chinese art of placement, for home and work environment.

Flotation Therapy: A relaxation technique based on the removal of environmental stimuli. Research has shown that profoundly deep relaxation and improved brain functioning are easily achieved through floating in a flotation tank.

Lymphatic Irrigation: A method of internal cleansing which removes blockages from the lymphatic system, hence fortifying the tissue system and preventing swelling caused by accumulated fluid. Usually used in conjunction with massage.

Numerology: System of using numbers and ascribing numbers to letters, to help unravel the complexities of human personality and life. Each number is linked to particular characteristics.

Palmistry: System which studies the lines on the palm to ascertain your life map and future.

Past-Life Regression: Deep relaxation techniques are used to facilitate the release of memories of past incarnations.

Polarity Therapy: Based on the five elements of ether, air, fire, water and earth. It combines counselling, nutrition and exercise, to assist in achieving optimal health on all levels.

Somato Emotional Release: Encouraging emotional release through working with cranio-sacral rhythm and the use of imagery.

Spiritual Readings: Using intuition and the channelling of spiritual energies to predict future events, and to guide you into finding your true purpose in life.

Tarot Card Readings: Using tarot cards to predict future events, and to give you insight into your life.

Thalassotherapy: Sea-based healing treatments, using mainly seaweed products. Treatments for aches and pains, and skin and beauty enhancement.

Visceral Manipulation Techniques: Working with rhythms generated by the movement of organs, to encourage mobility.

Index of Therapies, Treatments and Techniques

Index of Problems, Ailments and Symptoms

Healing Centres

Co. Antrim

Formula Health, 1–4 Hipark Centre, High Street, Belfast BT1 2JZ (☎08 01232 231 002). Centre offers homoeopathy, aromatherapy, chiropractic, osteopathy, acupuncture, herbalism, reflexology, nutrition therapy, vega testing.

Framar Health, The Jan de Vries Clinic, 595 Lisburn Road, Belfast (☎08 01232 681 018/5). Offers acupuncture, nutrition therapy, homoeopathy, herbalism, allergy testing, aromatherapy, reflexology.

Lifespring Centre, 111 Cliftonville Road, Belfast BT14 6JQ (☎08 01232 753 568). (Classes held in Belfast, Cork, Dublin, Galway, Limerick, and Sligo.) Accredited practitioner diploma courses in psycho-social aromatherapy, remedial massage, reflexology; post-graduate diploma courses include aromatherapy, counselling. Mary Grant Associates Practice provides high-quality therapies in psycho-social aromatherapy, reflexology, counselling, osteopathy, short courses for stress management.

Quintessence, 327 Antrim Road, Belfast (☎08 01232 351 590). Offers homoeopathy, aromatherapy, reflexology and kinesiology.

Co. Clare

Lisdoonvarna Spa Wells and Health Centre, Lisdoonvarna (☎065 74023). Therapies available include sulphur baths, saunas, massage, aromatherapy and reflexology. Open from June to October.

Co. Cork

The Alpha Centre, 29 Parnell Place, Cork (☎021 273467). Therapies include massage, reiki, bio-energy, shiatsu, healing touch massage and divine spirit healing.

The Beara Circle, Clinic for Natural Medicine, Castletownbere (☎027 70744/70745). Therapies include reflexology, allergy testing and therapy, colon hydrotherapy, counselling and psychotherapy, herbalism, homoeopathy, massage, nutrition, vega test, iridology, yoga, metamorphosis, proven candida and mycosis treatments, mercury detoxification, water therapy, cell therapy, Bach flower remedies. Lecture and workshop facilities available. Wholefood dining room. Sauna and meditation facilities.

Evergreen Clinic of Natural Medicine, 79 Evergreen Road, Cork (☎021 966 209). Some of the therapies offered at the clinic are acupuncture, herbal medicine, aromatherapy and massage, aromatology, and reflexology.

Freedom Holistic Centre, Church Lane, Midleton (☎021 642 466). Therapies include kinesiology, nutrition and allergy testing.

Inner Healing Centre, 46 Sheares Street, Cork (☎021 278 243). Aromatherapy consultations, treatments and home-use classes. Essential oils and aroma-therapy materials, also reiki, metamorphosis and food-allergy testing.

Natural Healing Centre, Thompson House, McCurtain Street, Cork (☎021 501 600). Offers aromatherapy, massage, osteopathy, acupuncture, T'ai Chi. Also workshops in reflexology, massage and aromatherapy.

Natural Medicine Clinic, Main Street, Carrigaline (☎021 372 787). Offers homoeopathy and reflexology.

Natural Therapy Centre, Main Street, Macroom (☎026 41916). Therapies include aromatherapy, massage and reflexology.

The Self-Healing Centre, Chapel Street, Dunmanway (☎023 47042). Shiatsu therapy, dietary advice and macrobiotic consultations are available at the centre.

Thalassotherapy Centre, Rochestown Park Hotel (☎021 894 949).

Co. Dublin

Astrea Psychic Services, 33 Lower Pembroke Street, Dublin 2 (☎01 662 5669). Astrea offers palmistry, tarot card readings, past life regression, insight readings and other services including courses in freeing the writer within, talking with angels, meditation, guided visualisation and spiritual healing.

The Beaumont Institute of Complementary Therapies, Beaumont Convent, Beaumont Road, Dublin 9 (☎01 836 8363). Full-time courses in reflexology, touch for health (an introduction to applied kinesiology) and educational kinesiology.

Celtic Healing and Natural Health Clinic, 117–119 Ranelagh, Dublin 6 (☎01 491 0689). The centre offers courses and therapies, including acupuncture, aromatherapy, osteopathy, reiki, reflexology, bio-energy, remedial massage, counselling, complex homoeopathy and hypnotherapy.

Clinic of Wholistic Medicine, 50 Merrion Square, Dublin 2 (☎01 676 4640). Therapies offered are homoeopathy, acupuncture and nutrition.

Clondalkin Holistic Healing Centre, Desmond House, Boot Road, Clondalkin, Dublin 22 (☎01 464 0628). Courses include dream analysis, meditation (stages 1 and 2), development course, certificate and diploma courses in massage, aromatherapy workshop, and holistic healing diploma course (3 stages). Therapies available include shiatsu, holistic healing, reflexology, aroma-therapy, homoeopathy, massage, nutrition, active balancing, and counselling.

College of Metaphysicians, Park Centre, 120 Sundrive Road, Dublin 12 (☎087 445 516). Courses offered by Jay Silver are: 'Teachings of the Inner Christ', 'Women who Run with the Wolves', and 'The Celestine Prophesy'. Therapies available include cutting the ties, working with the inner child and psychotherapy.

Complementary Healing Centre, Hilltop, Station Road, Raheny, Dublin 5 (☎01 851 0077). Therapies include active balance, kinesiology, massage, hypno-therapy, spiritual readings. Also courses and workshops including dance.

Complementary Healing Centre, 91 Terenure Road North, Terenure, Dublin 6 (☎01 492 9077). Courses offered include 'Reach for the Stars', 'Find the Soul's Purpose', 'Exploring Masculinity', Indian head massage, 'Inner Child', meditation, and reflexology. Also a certificate course in healing massage.

Complementary Healing Therapies, 136 New Cabra Road, Dublin 7 (☎01 868 1110). Courses run at the centre include ITEC Diploma in Holistic Massage, diploma in reflexology, stress management, anatomy and physiology; certificate courses in Indian head massage, reiki and seichem.

Donnybrook Medical Centre, 6 Main Street, Donnybrook, Dublin 4 (☎01 269 6588). ITEC diploma courses. Therapies include aromatherapy, reflexology, holistic massage, sports massage.

Hands of Light Institute of Healing, 160 Pembroke Road, Dublin 4 (☎01 668 1809). The following are available: public healing clinics, individual healing sessions, certificate introductory healing and personal development course, diploma advanced healing course (2 stages), reiki healing courses (parts 1, 2 and 3), assertiveness and stress management workshops.

Harvest Moon Centre, 24 Lower Baggot Street, Dublin 2 (☎01 662 7556). Courses in massage, metamorphosis, dream interpretation, healing, and Indian head massage. Flotation Tanks and a range of therapies available.

The Healing Place, 61 St Assam's Park, Raheny (☎01 848 4270; 087 461 853). Therapies available are cranio-sacral therapy, shiatsu, and hands-on healing.

Holistic Healing Centre, 38 Dame Street, Dublin 2 (☎01 671 0813). Courses and therapies are offered including massage (diploma course), yoga, reflexology and aromatherapy. Daily clinics.

The Holistic Health Centre, 197 Lower Kimmage Road, Dublin 6W (☎01 492 9279/). Therapies available include reflexology, osteopathy, acupuncture, allergy testing, aromatherapy, ki massage, holistic beauty therapy, and psychotherapy. Also yoga classes and relaxation and positive thinking.

The House of Astrology at Temple Bar, 9 Parliament Street, Dublin 2 (☎01 679 3404). The following therapies are available: reiki, Indian head massage, healing massage, shiatsu, cranio-sacral therapy, metamorphosis, childhood trauma counselling, astrological and tarot readings.

Irish Association of Holistic Medicine, 9–11 Grafton Street, Dublin 2 (☎01 671 2788). Therapies and diploma courses are offered in ki massage and aromatherapy (also certificates from City and Guilds in London), holistic preventative medicine, yoga, holistic dietetics, psychotherapy, anatomy and physiology, and business course; also postal requests, Successful Living sessions, and health stores.

The Irish Spiritual Centre, 30–31 Wicklow Street, Dublin 2 (☎01 671 5106). Courses offered include NFSH (National Federation of Spiritual Healers) training in spiritual healing; probationary spiritual healers' group; meditation open group (weekly); developmental meditation group; spiritual and psychic development; dream interpretation course; discover the power of colour; ethnic meditations; life cycles; insights into astrology; winter solstice celebration; summer solstice; spiritual emergence. Therapies available include spiritual healing, spiritual readings, counselling and reality therapy, hypnotherapy, physiotherapy, osteopathy, astrological readings and cutting of the ties.

LifeChanges, Unit 1, Blackrock Centre, Blackrock, Co. Dublin (☎01 278 0093). Therapies include: hypnosis, time-line therapy and Neuro Linguistics.

Mary Anderson Healing Centre, Hamilton House, 13 Trafalgar Terrace, Monkstown (☎01 280 3635). Professional training courses to international diploma standard are offered in aromatherapy, anatomy and physiology, colonic irrigation therapy and reflexology. Therapies available are reflexology, massage and aromatherapy, kinesiology, colonic irrigation, lymphatic irrigation and nutritional therapy. Also yoga classes and introductory courses in aromatherapy and reflexology are regularly offered at the centre.

MELT Temple Bar Natural Healing Centre, 2 Temple Lane (Sth), Dublin 2 (☎01 679 8786). This centre provides therapies including aromatherapy, cranio-sacral therapy, reiki, reflexology, iridology, healing massage and courses in yoga, art therapy, reiki, body talk, T'ai Chi Chuan and polarity therapy.

Moytura Healing Centre, 2 Lower Glenageary Road, Dún Laoghaire (☎01 285 4005). Diploma courses are offered in massage and in energy healing.

A healing clinic in chelation and meditation is also available at the centre.

The Natural Health Clinic, The Mews, 154 Leinster Road, Rathmines, Dublin 6 (☎01 496 1316). Therapies offered at the clinic include aromatherapy, holistic massage, reflexology, crystal therapy, herbal medicine, counselling and hypnotherapy, nutrition, shiatsu, traditional Chinese medicine and acupuncture.

Natural Living Centre, Walmer House, Station Road, Raheny, Dublin 5 (☎01 832 7859/832 7861). International diplomas (mainly ITEC) are offered in holistic massage, aromatherapy, reflexology, anatomy and physiology, nutrition and diet, colour therapy and healing. Classes are held in yoga, T'ai Chi Chuan, basic massage, sports massage, assertiveness, stress management, tarot card readings, holistic living and herbal medicine. Therapies on offer include acupuncture, chiropractic, herbal medicine, aromatherapy, holistic massage and homoeopathy.

Odyssey Healing Centre, 15 Wicklow Street, Dublin 2 (☎01 677 1021). Therapies offered include rebirthing, bio-energy, and body harmony. Courses include bio-energy therapy.

The Sweet Earth, 69 Upper George's Street, Dún Laoghaire (☎01 280 9873). Offers kinesiology, aromatherapy, massage, reflexology and osteopathy.

Teach Bán (Patrick Duggan and Ann Currie), 6 Parnell Road, Harold's Cross, Dublin 6 (☎01 454 3943). Courses offered include shiatsu healing therapy (2 years), alternative medicine (8 weeks), feng shui, and wholefood cookery (8 weeks). Therapies include shiatsu treatments, and macrobiotic consultations.

The healing house, 24 O'Connell Avenue, Berkeley Rd, Dublin 7 (☎01 830 6413). Courses and workshops include journey to the light; money magnetising; healing the heart; self-healing group; reiki; ceremony of light (winter solstice); numerology; African drums; awareness and relaxation; becoming psychic safely; gatherings; personal development; reflexology; tarot card classes; 'You Can Heal Your Life'; 'The Joy of Sound'; the Well Woman centre. Therapies include spiritual life readings, active balance clinic, cranio-sacral therapy, counselling, Indian head massage, memory integration, past-life regression, spiritual healing, stress management, past life healing and regression therapy.

Co. Galway

Acupuncture, Osteopathy and Allergy-Testing Clinic, 1 McDara Road, Shantalla (☎091 522 631).

Clinic of Complementary and Natural Medicine, Kiltartan House, Forster Street, Galway (☎091 568 804). Therapies include homoeopathy, Traditional Chinese Medicine, chiropractic, hypnotherapy, nutrition, and allergy testing.

Clinic of Wholistic Medicine, 34 Upper Abbeygate Street, Galway (☎091 567 416). Therapies offered are acupuncture, homoeopathy and nutrition.

Co. Kildare

Alternative Treatment Centre, Crookstown, Athy (☎0507 23231). Offers treatments in aromatherapy, reflexology and massage.

The Complementary Medical Centre, Fairgreen, Naas (☎045 874 477). Therapies include homoeopathy, aromatherapy, massage and reflexology.

Co. Kilkenny

Kilkenny Acupuncture and Reflexology Clinic, 20 Upper John Street, Kilkenny (☎056 62196).

Co. Laois
Body Works, Railway Street, Portlaoise (☎0502 60610). Treatments include Swedish massage, aromatherapy and reflexology.

Co. Limerick
Limerick Natural Healing Centre, 64 Catherine Street (☎061 400 431). Therapies include aura soma, colour therapy, healing energy and reflexology. Natural Harmony, 26 William Street (☎061 419 455). Treatments in aromatherapy, massage and reflexology.

Co. Louth
Iomlánú, Roden Place, Dundalk (☎042 32804/27253). Courses in spirituality, hypnotherapy, NLP, vegetarian cookery, assertiveness, parenting, psychology, mythology, theology, hands-on rhythm (drumming), astrology, colour therapy, letting go of fear, reiki, seasonal celebrations, de Mello awareness, sex education, bereavement, T'ai Chi Chuan, enneagram, the way of the Shaman, movement and dance, ecology and earth wisdom. Therapy clinics and groups include reiki, yoga, health options, self-esteem, meditation, massage and healing.
Progressive Hypnotherapy Clinic, Dundalk (☎042 31406). Therapies offered include hypnotherapy and psychotherapy. Brochure available.

Co. Mayo
Tir na nÓg, Holistic Beauty Centre, The Square, Claremorris (☎094 62678). Therapies include aromatherapy, massage and reflexology.

Co. Westmeath
Clinic of Wholistic Medicine, Church Street, Athlone (☎0902 78750). Therapies available are acupuncture, homoeopathy and nutrition.

Co. Wexford
Centre for Natural Therapies, 16 George's Street, Wexford (☎053 21363). Therapies offered include acupuncture, nutritional therapy, homoeopathy, massage, reiki, reflexology, iridology, spinal healing, guided visualisation.

Co. Wicklow
Amethyst, Curtlestown, Enniskerry (☎01 286 2428). Courses are offered in: introduction to healing; healing body, mind and spirit; primal integration and regression therapy training; the healing journey; healing for the new age; diploma in pre- and peri-natal psychotherapy; regression therapy; chelation treatments. Also a diploma in prenatal and peri-natal psychotherapy (2 years).
Chrysalis, Donard (☎045 404 713). Chrysalis, formerly a Church of Ireland rectory dating back to 1711, is set in three acres of tree-filled grounds within a short walk of an ancient stone circle. Vegetarian food and accommodation are included in the cost of weekend and five-day residential courses. Courses include: body-work; 'Touch for Healing'; 'Find your Gift'; Alexander Technique; stress management and massage; 'Risk Go Deep' and 'Own Your Truth'; facing co-dependency; gestalt therapy; freeing the voice; Anthony de Mello; 'Your Body Speaks Your Mind'; the dynamics of inner peace; healing and transformation; reiki; 'Making Peace with the Past'; 'Find Your Inner Rhythm through Drumming'; and 'Dancing the Rainbow'. Day workshops include: bellydancing, nutrition, vegetarian cooking, meditation, colour, and many other areas. Counselling is also available at the centre.

Residential Healing Centres

Co. Cork

The Beara Circle, Clinic for Natural Medicine, Castletownbere (☎027 70744/70745). For details of treatments offered, see entry under Healing Centres (p. 201).

An Sanctóir, Bawnaknockane, Ballydehob (☎028 38287/37155). Workshops run at the centre include circle and peace dances, chants, painting, and others.

Co. Donegal

Centre for Natural Health Therapies and Healing, Ardun House, Glenties (☎075 51147). At the foot of the Bluestack Mountains, the centre offers healthy food, with an option for vegetarians, and yoga, shiatsu, reflexology, massage and reiki.

Co. Kerry

Lios Dána, The Natural Living Centre, Inch, Annascaul (☎066 58189). Lios Dána offers a diverse range of courses suitable for those on a path of personal or spiritual development. The centre is located on the southern shoreline of the Dingle peninsula, and offers panoramic views of Ireland's highest mountain range, plus the beauty and tranquillity of country lanes, and four miles of Atlantic shoreline. Courses and therapies offered, including accommodation, are shiatsu, yoga, the Alexander Technique, and creative writing.

Co. Galway

Loughaunrone, Oranmore, Rinville West (☎091 790 606). Loughaunrone Health Farm offers a place where people can rejuvenate their bodies and relax their minds. The main residence is set in a beautiful Georgian house, in the midst of a fifty-acre deer farm on the shores of Galway Bay. A residential stay of three or five days includes healthy balanced meals, an exercise programme which includes a workout in a gymnasium or yoga, walks in woodlands or along the sea coast, swimming (optional), therapeutic massage and sauna. Other therapies and activities of which guests can avail are reflexology, stress management classes, aerobics and stretch classes, tennis, horse riding, golf, aromatherapy and beauty treatments.

Co. Mayo

Cloona Health Centre, Westport (☎098 25251). The Cloona Centre is an old woollen mill which was renovated in the early 1970s, situated in a hilly, rural area away from main roads. Courses offered at the centre run from Sunday to Friday, with some weekend courses. They include a carefully regulated diet to encourage inner cleansing, and a daily programme of yoga, walking, sauna and massage.

Co. Sligo

Rainbow's End Healing Centre, Castlebaldwin (☎071 65728). Rainbow's End is set in the Bricklieve Mountains, home of the Carrowkeel Passage Tombs, one of the oldest sites in Ireland. It offers a whole range of natural therapies, including reiki and seichem, and also workshops. Details are available from the centre.

Co. Tipperary

An Tearmann Beag (The Small Sanctuary), Mooresfort, Kilross, Tipperary (☎062 55102). This centre is located on an organic farm in the heart of the Golden Vale, near the Glen of Aherlow. It offers weekend and midweek breaks in a fully equipped self-catering cottage or apartment. A free therapy is included in the price for each guest. Weekend courses offered include a journey towards wholeness. Therapies available are aromatherapy, allergy testing, rebirthing, reflexology, kinesiology, energy body-work, and vega testing (including homoeopathic remedies).

Co. Wexford

The Kilimanjaro Cakehouse and Soul Centre, Ballyhearty, Kilmore Quay (☎053 29780). Workshops in various therapies are offered at the centre. Details available on request.

Co. Wicklow

Avoca Holistic Centre, Knockanode House, Rathdrum (☎0402 35364, 01 473 1924 or 01 831 7888 Unit 124800). The Avoca Centre, located in the vale of Avoca, overlooks the tranquil natural splendour of the meeting of the waters and is surrounded by fifteen acres of woodland. The house is being developed as a centre for holistic healing, personal growth and spiritual development for the practice, teaching and appreciation of alternative and complementary medicines. Workshops and training courses are regularly run at the centre, in areas such as spiritual healing, women's self-help, relationships, personal development and self-awareness.

Avon Park, Glendalough Road, Rathdrum (☎0404 46610). Avon Park is a restored Georgian building which looks out over a small lake where wild duck are resident most of the year. It provides weekend and week-long programmes for those who wish to experience the benefits of a cleansing detox-diet as well as alleviating stress and restoring balance. All food is organically grown. Some of the treatments available are massage, yoga exercises, meditation, reiki healing, reflexology, and Indian head massage.

Chrysalis, Donard (☎045 404 713). For details of treatments offered, see entry under Healing Centres (p. 205).

Professional Associations

Where possible, you are advised to check with the relevant society whether your practitioner is registered and insured.

Acupuncture Foundation of Ireland
Dominick Court, 41 Lr Dominick Street
Dublin 1 *or*
60 Lr Baggot St, Dublin 2. ☎01 662 3525

The Association for Dance
   Movement Therapy
c/o Arts Therapies Department
Springfield Hospital, Glenburnie Rd
Tooting, London SW17 7DJ, UK

Association of Colour Therapists
c/o ICM, 21 Portland Place
London W1 3AS, UK

The Association of Irish Rebirthers
   (AIR)
33 Inchicore Road, Dublin 8
Catherine Dowling (Secretary)
☎01 453 3166

The Association of Rebirther
   Trainers International (ARTI)
Rere No. 4 Crofton Terrace
Dún Laoghaire, Co. Dublin
Patsy Brennan. ☎01 284 1660

The Association of Reflexologists (AOR)
Membership Admin., 5 Robart House
Lodge Lane, London N12 8JN, UK
☎0044 181 445 0154

The Association of Systematic
   Kinesiology
c/o Siobhan Barnes, 48 Percy Place
Ballsbridge, Dublin 4. ☎01 660 2806

An Bord Altranais (The Irish
   Nursing Board)
31/32 Fitzwilliam Square, Dublin 2

British Association for Psychotherapy
121 Hendon Lane, London NW3 3PR
UK

British Association for Counselling
37a Sheep Street, Rugby
Warwickshire CU21 3BX, UK
☎0044 1788 550 899

The British Chiropractic Association
29 Whitley Street, Reading, UK
☎0044 118 9757 557

The British Psychodrama Association
8 Rahere Road, Crowley, Oxford
OX4 3QG, UK. ☎0044 1865 715 055

Chiropractic Association of Ireland
☎01 833 4026

Confederation of International
   Beauty Therapy and
   Cosmetology (CIBTAC)
The Parabolo House, Parabolo Road
Cheltenham GL50 3AH, UK
☎0044 1242 570384

Council for Hypnotic Psychotherapy
   and Counselling (CHPC)
52a Main Street, Swords, Co. Dublin
☎01 840 4161

Dev Aura Foundation
Little London, Tetford
Lincs LN9 6QL, UK
☎0044 1507 533 581

The Dr Edward Bach Foundation
Mount Vernon, Sotwell, Wallingford
Oxon. OX10 0PZ, UK

The Family Therapy Association of
   Ireland
c/o Ann Daly, 17 Dame Court
Dublin 2. ☎01 679 4055

The Gestalt Psychotherapy Institute
PO Box 620, Bristol BS99 7DL, UK

Institute for Reality Therapy in Ireland
c/o Eileen Hearne
24 Glendown Court, Templeogue
Dublin 6w. ☎01 456 2216
or Brian Lennon, 6 Red Island
Skerries, Co. Dublin ☎01 849 1906

Institute of Psychosynthesis and
   Transpersonal Theory
19 Clyde Road, Dublin 4
☎01 688 4687

The Institute of Spinologists in
   Ireland
c/o Brigid McLoughlin,
4 Summerhill North, Cork
☎021 509 075

The International Association for Colour Therapy
73 Elm Bank Gardens
London SW13 0NX, UK
International Association of Clinical Iridologists
853 Finchley Road
London NW11 8LX, UK
The International Federation of Reflexologists (IFR)
76–78 Edridge Road, Croydon
Surrey CR0 1EF, UK. ☎0044 181 667 9458
International Taoist Society
☎01 855 7699
International Therapy Examination Council (ITEC)
James House, Oakelbrook Mill, Newent
GL18 1HD, UK. ☎0044 1531 821875
Irish and International Aromatherapy Association (IIAA)
Roscore, Blueball, Tullamore
Co. Offaly. Markie Walsh (Secretary)
Irish Association for Improvements in Maternity Services (AIMS)
Raheen House, Meath Road, Bray
Co. Wicklow. ☎01 286 4585
Irish Association of Counselling and Therapy, The (IACT)
8 Cumberland Street, Dún Laoghaire
Co. Dublin. ☎01 230 0061
Irish Association of Drama, Art and Music Therapists
PO Box 4176, Dublin 1
Irish Association of Health Stores
Unit 2d, Kylemore Industrial Estate
Kileen Road, Dublin 10. ☎01 623 6828
Irish Association of Holistic Medicine
9–11 Grafton Street, Dublin 2
☎01 671 2788
Irish Association of Humanistic and Integrative Psychotherapy
82 Upper George's St, Dún Laoghaire
Co. Dublin ☎01 284 1665
Irish Association of Hypno-analysts (IAH) (*Associated to the International Association of Hypno-analysts*)
Therapy House, 6 Tuckey Street, Cork
☎021 275 785

The Irish Childbirth Trust
17 Dame Court, Dublin 2
☎01 679 4055
Irish Council for Acupuncture
Dublin 7. ☎01 838 8196
Irish Council for Psychotherapy
17 Dame Court, Dublin 2. ☎01 679 4055
Irish Health Culture Association (IHCA)
66 Eccles Street, Dublin 7
☎01 820 4029
Irish Institute of Counselling and Hypnotherapy
118 Stillorgan Road, Dublin 4
☎01 260 0118
Irish Institute of Psychoanalytic Psychotherapy
124 Ranelagh, Dublin 6. ☎01 497 8896
The Irish Massage Therapists Association
Ard Lynn, Mount Rice, Monasterevin
Co. Kildare. ☎045 525 579
Irish Medical Homoeopathic Association
c/o 16 Oaklands, Ballsbridge
Dublin 4. ☎01 668 9242
The Irish Nutrition and Dieticians Institute (INDI)
17 Rathfarnham Road, Dublin 6w
☎01 490 3237
The Irish Osteopathic Association (IOA)
c/o 17 Windsor Terrace, Portobello
Dublin 8, ☎01 473 0828
Irish Psycho-analytical Association
2 Belgrave Terrace, Monkstown
Co. Dublin. ☎01 280 1869/496 7288
The Irish Reflexologists Institute (IRI)
3 Blackglen Court, Lambs Cross
Sandyford, Dublin 18. ☎01 295 2238
4 Ruskin Park, Lisburn, Co. Antrim
☎08 01846 677 806
Irish Society of Homoeopaths
66 Mount Anville Wood, Goatstown
Dublin 14. ☎01 278 3161;
Fax: 01 288 6344
Irish Yoga Association
108 Lr Kimmage Rd, Harold's Cross
Dublin 6W. ☎01 492 9213

La Leche League of Ireland
☎01 282 9638/835 4469
National Federation of Spiritual Healers (NFSH)
Old Manor Farm Studio
Church Street, Sunbury-on-Thames
Middlesex TW16 6RG, UK
☎0044 1932 783 164
The National Institute of Medical Herbalists
56 Longbrook Street, Exeter EX4 6AH
UK. ☎0044 1392 426 022
Nature's Way, New Life Foundation of Ireland
Hebron Road, Kilkenny. ☎056 65402
Osteopathic Information Service
PO Box 2074, Reading, Berks RGI 4YR
UK. ☎0044 1734 512 501
Register of acupuncture and Traditional Chinese Medicine practitioners of Ireland (RTCMI)
☎01 679 4216
The Reiki Association
Secretary: Kate Jones
2 Manor Cottages, Stockley Hill
Peterchurch, Hereford HR2 0FF, UK
☎0044 1432 550 824
Republic of Ireland:
c/o Regina O'Mahoney
8 Kilmoney Heights, Carrigaline
Co. Cork. ☎021 372 519

Shen Tao Practitioners Association (SPA)
c/o Judith Hoad, Room for Healing
Inver, Co. Donegal. ☎073 36406
The Shiatsu Society of Ireland
c/o Patricia O'Hanlon
12 The Cove, Malahide, Co. Dublin
☎01 845 3647
The Society of Applied Cosmetology
47 South William Street, Dublin 2
☎01 679 8018
Society of Teachers for the Alexander Technique
20 London House, 266 Fulham Road,
London SW10 9EL, UK
☎0044 171 351 0828
T'ai Chi Chuan Association
c/o St Andrew's Resource Centre
114–116 Pearse Street, Dublin 2
☎01 677 1930
Veterinary Homeopaths Association of Ireland
Inisglas, Crossabeg, Co. Wexford
☎053 28226

Training and Workshops

Alexander Technique

Chrysalis
Donard, Co. Wicklow
☎045 404 713
Residential courses.

Society of Teachers for
the Alexander Tech-
nique (STAT)
20 London House
266 Fulham Road
London SW10 9EL, UK
☎0044 171 351 0828
*Three-year full-time
professional training
courses. Minimum of
1,600 hours of tuition.*

Aromatherapy

Co. Antrim
Lifespring Centre
111 Cliftonville Road
Belfast BT14 6JQ
☎08 01232 753 658
*Aromatherapy practitioner
diploma course. Classes held
in Belfast, Cork, Dublin,
Galway, Limerick, and Sligo.
Post-graduate diploma
courses also available.*

Roberta Mechan
College of Beauty
17 Castle Arcade
Belfast BT1 5DG
☎08 01232 664 960
ITEC diploma.

Co. Cork
Nicola Darrell
Evergreen Clinic of
Natural Medicine
79 Evergreen Road
Cork. ☎021 966 209
Courses affiliated to the

London School of
Aromatherapy (LSA).

Johanna Gubbay
The Old Forge, Ahiohill
Ennisheane
☎023 39250
ITEC diploma.

Co. Dublin
Academy International
48 Upr Drumcondra Rd
Dublin 9. ☎01 836 8201
Rosemary Campbell
ITEC diploma.

Celtic Healing and
Natural Health Clinic
117–119 Ranelagh
Dublin 6. ☎01 491 0689
Aromatherapy, massage.

Bronwyn Conroy
40 Grafton Street
Dublin 2. ☎01 677 9184
ITEC diploma.

Coogan-Bergin Clinic
and College
Glendenning House
6–8 Wicklow Street
Dublin 2. ☎01 679 4254
ITEC diploma.

Donnybrook Medical
Centre
6 Main St, Donnybrook
Dublin 4. ☎01 269 6588
ITEC diploma.

Galligan Beauty Group
12 Hume Street
Dublin 2. ☎01 661 1122
ITEC diploma.

Holistic Healing Centre
38 Dame Street
Dublin 2. ☎01 671 0813
Diploma periodically.

Holistic School of
Reflexology and
Massage
2 Laurel Park
Clondalkin, Dublin 22
☎01 459 2460
Olive Gentleman
Diploma (five months)

Irish Association of
Holistic Medicine
9–11 Grafton Street
Dublin 2. ☎01 671 2788
*Diploma in aromatherapy
(IHCA) and diploma in
aromatherapy massage
(City and Guilds).*

Mary Anderson
Healing Centre
Hamilton House
13 Trafalgar Terrace
Monkstown
☎01 280 3635
*Awards international
diploma in aromatherapy.*

Massage Ireland
Lonsdale House
Avoca Rd, Blackrock *or*
16 Oaklands
Ballsbridge, Dublin 4
☎668 9242
Cathie Hogan
ITEC diploma.

Natural Living Centre
Walmer Hse, Station Rd
Raheny, Dublin 5
☎01 832 7859/832 7861
ITEC diploma.

Senior College Dún
Laoghaire
Eblana Avenue
Dún Laoghaire
☎01 280 0385
*CIBTAC (Confederation
of International Beauty*

*Therapy and Cosmetology)
Certificate in Aroma-
therapy — 1 year.*

Shirley Price Inter-
national College of
Aromatherapy
PO Box 16, Wicklow
☎0404 47319
Diploma/advanced dip.

The healing house
24 O'Connell Avenue
Berkeley Rd, Dublin 7
☎01 830 6413

Co. Galway
Galligan College of
Beauty
Lismoyle House
St Augustine Street
Galway. ☎091 565 628
IFA diploma.

Co. Limerick
Foxall College of
Beauty Therapy
136 O'Connell Street
Limerick. ☎061 410 996
ITEC diploma.

Galligan College of
Beauty
123 O'Connell Street
Limerick. ☎061 410 628
ITEC diploma.

Co. Louth
Marygold
Aromatherapy Clinic
90 Bridge Street
Dundalk. ☎042 32154
ITEC diploma.

Co. Monaghan
Olivia Keenan Beauty
Salon
22/24 Glaslough Street
Monaghan. ☎ 047 83320
ITEC diploma.

Further details from:

The Confederation of
International Beauty
Therapy and
Cosmetology
Parabolo House
Parabolo Road
Cheltenham, GL50 3AH
UK. ☎0044 1242 570 384

ITEC: International
Therapy Examination
Council
James House
Oakelbrook Mill
Newent GL18 1HD, UK
☎0044 1531 821 875

Art Therapy

There is no professional
training in art therapy
in Ireland. Crawford
College of Art and
Design plans to run
courses (two-year full-
time, and three-year
part-time) in September
1997. Trinity College
and DIT have plans for
a course (three-year
part-time) in 1998.
Neither has been
finalised at time of
going to press. For
information, contact:

Noreen Hayes
DIT, Rathmines
Dublin 6. ☎01 402 3455

Louise Foott
Crawford College of
Art and Design
Sherman Crawford St
Cork. ☎021 966 777
*Crawford College offers
an art therapy summer
school (five-day work-
shop) and a foundation*

*course in art therapy
(eight weekends).*

Professional post-grad.
courses are offered by
the following in the UK:

Art Psychotherapy Unit
Goldsmith College
23 St James
London SE14
☎0044 181 692 1424

Centre for Art and
Psychotherapy Studies
Floor 0
Dept. of Psychiatry
Royal Hallamshire
Hospital
Glossop Road
Sheffield S10 2JF
☎0044 114 271 1900;
ext: 2422

Post-grad Art Therapy
Programme
University of
Hertfordshire
Hatfield AL10 9TL
☎0044 1707 285 300

MELT, Temple Bar
Natural Healing
Centre
2 Temple Lane South
Dublin 2. ☎01 679 8786
Courses and workshops

Aura Soma

Dev Aura
Little London, Tetford
Lincolnshire LN9 6QL
UK. ☎0044 1507 533 581
*Training worldwide.
Three modules in diploma
awarded by International
Academy of Colour
Therapeutics (Dev Aura)
— foundation, inter-
mediate and advanced*

(six days each). An essay of 2,000 words is a prerequisite for attending advanced course. Courses run periodically in Ireland. Training to become a teacher is open to those who have successfully completed the diploma course, and it takes four modules to complete — includes introductory evenings and weekends, foundation level, intermediate level and advanced level (each of six days' duration).

Bach Flower Remedies

The Dr Edward Bach
Foundation
Mount Vernon, Sotwell
Wallingford
Oxon. OX10 0PZ, UK
Practitioner course is intended for practising therapists (aromatherapists, reflexologists, counsellors and nurses) who wish to incorporate the remedies into their work. Part 1 is an intensive three-day course, with examination on the last day. Successful graduates of Part 1 can study Part 2. This consists of three months' fieldwork practice, during which time the theoretical knowledge learned in Part 1 will be put to practical use. Two in-depth case studies must be presented at the end of the three-month period, together

with an extended essay. Successful completion of Part 2 entitles inclusion on the register of counsellors of Bach Flower Remedies. Counsellors are subject to a code of ethics.

The Natural Medicine
Company
Burgage, Blessington
Co. Wicklow
☎045 865 575
In Ireland introductory and professional courses are run by The Natural Medicine Company in association with the Dr Edward Bach Foundation.

Bio-energy

Michael D'Alton
Odyssey Healing Centre
15 Wicklow Street
Dublin 2. ☎01 677 1021/
087 231 7984
One-year course.

Plexus European
Institute of Bio-Energy
Enterprise House
Aidan Street, Kiltimagh
Co. Mayo *or*
Lismoyle House
Merchant's Road
Galway. ☎091 568 855
Plexus diploma courses (one year) held in Dublin and Ennis.

Biofeedback

Kevin Gray
2 Old Row
Burton Upon Stather
Scunthorpe, DN15 9DL
UK. ☎0044 1724 720 909
The monitor, plus the necessary training, can be

obtained from Kevin Gray. Used by complementary therapists, especially hypnotherapists, to gauge the level of relaxation of their clients.

Body Harmony

Rosemary Khelifa
☎01 833 0656
It takes 100 hours of training to become a practitioner (basic level), 1,000 hours to become an international practitioner, and a further 1,000 hours to become a teacher.

Chiropractic

As there is no school of chiropractic here, Irish people must attend full-time study overseas. There are chiropractic colleges in the US, Canada, Australia, New Zealand, South Africa, the UK, France and Japan. Five or six-year full-time degree or postgraduate degree course, covering all the basic sciences — anatomy, physiology, pathology, biochemistry, and microbiology — as well as more specific chiropractic-oriented subjects in neurology, spinal anatomy and biomechanics and orthopaedics. Students also trained to take and analyse X-rays. Hands-on training includes internship under college guidance, and externship period working in the field. Please contact:

Chiropractic Association of Ireland
c/o Dr Christopher Barnett
85 Glasnevin Avenue
Dublin 11. ☎01 842 9211
or
Anglo European College of Chiropractic
13–15 Parkswood Road
Bournemouth, Dorset
BH5 2DF
☎0044 1202 436 200

Colour Therapy

The Hygeia College of Colour Therapy Ltd.
Brook House, Avening
GL8 8NS, UK
and
Nuala Kiernan
22 Treesdale
Stillorgan Road
Co. Dublin
☎01 283 5648
and
John Quinlivan
The National Health Clinic
64 Catherine Street
Limerick. ☎061 400 431
International certificate, higher certificate and diploma in colour therapy. Certificate is awarded on attendance at six weekends (which explore colour and form, sound, therapy, counselling, and colour's practical application to health), a ten-day

residential course (further study in crystals, aromatherapy, dance and art work) and a written examination. Higher diploma is awarded to certificate holders who have also completed a one-year probationary period as colour therapists, where case histories must be submitted for analysis, and where students have obtained an ITEC qualification in anatomy and physiology. Graduates of this course can practise as colour therapists. Candidates for diploma must have had two years' practical experience, as well as the certificate. They must also submit a thesis on an in-depth study of their own research. Courses in both Dublin and Limerick.

The Natural Living Centre
Walmer Hse, Station Rd
Raheny, Dublin 5
☎01 832 7859/832 7861
Diploma in colour therapy. Qualification in anatomy and physiology, and completion of Dr Christine Page's course in esoteric anatomy necessary before students can qualify for diploma. Course held over six weekends includes history and psychology of colour, art as therapy, colour and form, sound, reflexology, aromatherapy, massage, spiritual healing, dress, décor, practical treatments and counselling.

A 5,000-word thesis and a written examination compulsory.

UK
Association of Colour Therapists
c/o ICM
21 Portland Place
London W1 3AS
Information on training courses.

Colour Bonds Associates (Lilian Verner Bonds)
137 Hendon Lane
Finchley
London, N3 3PR
Information on training courses.

The International Association for Colour Therapy
73 Elm Bank Gardens
London SW13 ONX, UK
Information on courses.

Know Yourself Through Colour
c/o Marie Louise Lacy
3a Bath Road, Worthing
Sussex BN11 3NU, UK
Periodically runs courses in Ireland.

Living Colour
33 Lancaster Grove
London NW3 4EX, UK
Information on training courses.

Universal Colour Healing
67 Farm Crescent
Wrexham Court
Slough SL2 5TQ, UK
Information on courses.

Counselling and Psychotherapy

Co. Antrim
Lifespring Centre
111 Cliftonville Road
Belfast BT14 6JQ
☎08 01232 753 658
Courses offered in counselling and transpersonal psychology. Postgraduate diploma course in counselling.

Co. Cork
The Counselling Centre
7 Matthew Street, Cork
☎021 903 000
Diploma in counselling.

Dept. of Applied Psychology
University College Cork
☎021 296 871
Post-graduate higher diplomas in counselling, and in gestalt therapy.

Co. Dublin
ACCEPT Counselling Association of Ireland
Newpark Counselling Training Centre
Newtownpark Avenue
Blackrock, Co. Dublin
☎01 280 0280
Diploma in community and voluntary counselling (two years); diploma (two years) and certificate (one year) in counselling, psychology and therapy (by distance learning).

Bereavement Counselling Service
St Anne's Church
Dawson Street
Dublin 2, ☎01 676 7727
Courses in counselling skills.

C.J. Jung Centre
29 Manor St, Dublin 7
☎01 868 4363
Diploma (three years) and certificate in Jungian Studies (one year).

Celtic Healing and Natural Health Centre
117–119 Ranelagh
Dublin 6. ☎01 491 0689
Theory and practice of counselling skills; introduction to hypnotherapy.

Clanwilliam Institute
Clanwilliam Terrace
Grand Canal Street
Dublin 2. ☎01 676 1363
Foundation course.

Creative Counselling Centre
82 Upper George's St
Dún Laoghaire
☎01 280 2523
Diploma in humanistic integrative psychotherapy (four years); diploma in humanistic integrative counselling (three years); introductory course in counselling and psychotherapy (one year); certificate in counselling skills (one year).

Dublin Counselling and Therapy Centre
41 Upper Gardiner St
Dublin 1. ☎01 878 8236
Diploma in therapeutic counselling (three years).

The Irish Forum for Child and Adolescent Psychotherapy
Child and Family Centre
59 Orwell Road
Rathgar, Dublin 6
Diploma in child and adolescent psychotherapy (three years).

Irish Institute of Counselling and Hypnotherapy
118 Stillorgan Road
Dublin 4. ☎01 260 0118
Two-year diploma course in counselling, NLP and Hypnotherapy; City & Guilds and BTEC certification; NLP practitioner certificate.

Irish Institute of Integrated Psychotherapy
26 Longford Terrace
Monkstown. ☎01 280 9313
Diploma of Irish Institute for Integrated Psychotherapy (three years).

Irish Institute of Psychoanalytic Psychotherapy
124 Ranelagh, Dublin 6
☎01 497 8896
Diploma in psychoanalytic psychotherapy (three years).

Liberties College
Bull Alley Street
Dublin 8. ☎01 454 0044
One-year full-time course in counselling. Accredited by the National Council for Vocational Awards.

LSB College
6–9 Balfe Street
Dublin 2. ☎01 679 4844
BA in psycho-analytical studies (three years).

Marino Institute of Education
Griffith Avenue
Dublin 9. ☎01 833 5111
Diploma (one year), and certificate (one year) in

counselling skills.
Masters in counselling.

Northside Counselling
  Service
Coolock Development
  Centre
Bunratty Drive
Dublin 17. ☎01 848 4789

O'Halloran Education
  and Psychotherapy
12 Ballinclea Heights
Killiney, Co. Dublin
Diploma in humanistic
counselling (three years).

Rape Crisis Centre
70 Lower Leeson Street
Dublin 2. ☎01 661 0873
Diploma in sexual abuse
(two years).

St Vincent's Hospital
Elm Park, Dublin 4
☎01 269 4533
Diploma in group analytic
psychotherapy (four years).

The healing house
24 O'Connell Avenue
Berkeley Road
Dublin 7. ☎01 830 6413

The Tivoli Institute
24 Clarinda Park Estate
Dún Laoghaire
☎01 280 9178
Diploma and foundation
course in counselling.

Trinity College Dublin:

Dept. of Social Studies
☎01 702 1985
Diploma in counselling.

Dept. of Psychology
☎01 608 1886
Masters (two years) in
counselling psychology.

University College Dublin
Belfield, Dublin 4
☎01 706 7777

Dept. of Psychiatry
Master's in psychoanalytic
psychotherapy (two years).

Co. Galway
Centre for Biodynamic
  and Integrative Psy-
  chotherapy
Trácht Beach, Kinvara
☎091 37192
Foundation (one year),
certificate (three years), and
diploma (two years for
certificate holders) in bio-
dynamic and integrative
psychotherapy.

Institute of Biodynamic
  and Transpersonal
  Psychotherapy
85 Renmore Park
Galway. ☎091 638143/
  088 624023
One-year certificate, three-
year diploma in biodynamic
and transpersonal psycho-
therapy. Courses in Galway
and Dublin.

University College
  Galway
☎091 524 411
Introductory course in
psychology of counselling.

Co. Kildare
St Patrick's College
Maynooth. ☎01 628 5222
Courses at various centres
nationwide. Diploma (two
years), and certificate (one
year) in counselling skills.

Co. Limerick
Limerick Institute of
  Counselling and
  Psychotherapy
'Mignon', Corbally Road
Limerick. ☎061 347 506
Basic counselling skills.

Co. Louth
Dundalk Centre for
  Counselling
Oakdeane, 3 Seatown
Dundalk. ☎042 38333
Diploma in therapeutic
counselling (three years).

Co. Meath
Process Oriented
  Psychology, Ireland
c/o Bríd Commins
Sterling Cross
Dunboyne ☎01 825 1629
Four-day seminars held four
times yearly. Irish Certificate
in Process Work (three years
of study, supervision and
personal therapy).

Co. Wicklow
Amethyst
Curtlestown, Enniskerry
☎01 285 0976
Training courses and
workshops for helpers;
diploma in pre- and peri-
natal psychotherapy; basic
training in primal
integration and regression
therapy.

Cranio-sacral Therapy

The Cranio-sacral
  Educational Trust
29 Dollis Park
Finchley Central
London N3 1HJ, UK
☎0044 181 349 0297
Information on training.

The Karuna Institute
Natsworthy Manor
Widecombe-in-the-Moor
Newton Abbot
Devon TQ13 7TR, UK
☎0044 164 722457
Information on training.

Creative Therapies

Mary Roden
Arts Unlimited
66 Lower Baggot Street
Dublin 2. ☎01 287 2549
*Classes/workshops to
nurture our intuitive,
feeling and creative sides,
through creating images,
sculptures, writing, and
various creative arts.*

Crystal Healing

Terri Blanche
30 Sevenoaks, Frankfield
Douglas, Cork
☎021 891 527
and
Odyssey Healing Centre
15 Wicklow Street
Dublin 2. ☎01 677 1021
*Eight-week courses in
Dublin, Cork, Limerick,
Navan, Dundalk, Kildare.
How to identify different
crystals, properties of
crystals, how to use and
programme crystals,
information on chakras,
guided meditations.*

Jacquie Burgess
☎01 496 1316 *or*
0503 51057
*Workshops in Dublin,
Carlow and other venues.*

Cutting the Ties

Most practitioners have
studied in a related
area, such as counsel-
ling, spiritual healing,
meditation, hypnother-
apy or dream interpre-
tation. For information
on workshops in
Ireland, please contact:

Eunice Borland
31 Rahene Park, Bray
Co. Wicklow. ☎01 286 2688

UK
Jean Ralli
14 Oxford Square
London W2
☎0044 171 723 3757

US
Phyllis Krystal
PO Box 6061355
Sherman Oaks, CA 91473
Fax: 001 310 471 0126
*Information on all
workshops*

Energy Healing

Tony Quinn Centres:

Co. Armagh
Yvonne Sherry
41 Upper English St
Armagh
☎08 01861 525 742

Co. Cork
Imelda Farrell
20 Academy Street
Cork. ☎021 276 364

Co. Dublin
Aideen Cowman
9–11 Grafton Street
Dublin 2
☎01 671 2788/830 4211
or
66 Eccles Street, Dublin 7
☎01 830 4211/ 830 3717

Christine Kelly
98 Lower George's St
Dún Laoghaire
☎01 280 9891

Rita Kelly
2 Wynnfield Road
Rathmines, Dublin 6
☎01 497 4234

St Stephen's Green
Centre
Dublin 2. ☎01 478 5404

Co. Fermanagh
Yvonne Sherry
Aisling Centre
Darling St, Enniskillen
☎08 01861 525742
Weds/Fri 7.30 p.m.

Co. Galway
Eyre Square Shopping
Centre
Galway. ☎091 564 865

Victoria Hotel
Eyre Square, Galway
☎01 830 4211
Mon/Thurs 6 & 7.30 p.m.

Co. Kildare
Paul Doyle
Basin Street, Naas
☎01 830 4211
Tues/Fri 8 p.m.

Co. Louth
Georgina Dolan
18 Jocelyn Street
Dundalk. ☎042 38097

Faith Healing

There is no formal
training to become a
faith healer, nor is there
any professional body
of faith healers.

Family Therapy

The Clanwilliam
Institute
18 Clanwilliam Terrace
Grand Canal Quay
Dublin 2.
☎01 676 1363/676 2881
*One-year foundation
course for professional
training in family therapy,*

plus a three-year part-time certificate course in systemic family therapy. Courses aimed at professionals in health, social services, education and related disciplines. Three-year course includes study of family and marital therapy, mediation, sex therapy, child-centred approaches, ethical and political issues, gender and justice, family of origin and use of genograms. Supervision is also provided for trainee therapists. On successful completion of the three-year course, the therapist can apply for registration with the Family Therapy Association of Ireland.

Gestalt

Chrysalis
Donard, Co. Wicklow
☎045 404713
Residential course

Irish Gestalt Centre
136 Tonlegee Road
Raheny, Dublin 5
May Grills
☎01 847 2242
Four-year training in gestalt. Also a one-year personal development programme for people interested in self-awareness and personal growth and who can benefit from using gestalt skills in their lives and workplace. One-year course includes three residential courses, adding up to eighteen full days. Training involves working

at a deep level with small groups. Meditation, contact through awareness, grounding, body-work and dream work explored during introductory year, which is a prerequisite for the full gestalt psychotherapy training.

O'Halloran Education
   and Psychotherapy
12 Ballinclea Heights
Killiney
Introduction to gestalt therapy (one year).

University College Cork
☎021 296 871/903 000
Post-graduate higher diploma in gestalt therapy.

Herbalism

There is no professional training as yet in herbalism in Ireland.

The National Institute of Medical Herbalists
56 Longbrook Street
Exeter EX4 6AH, UK
☎0044 1392 426 022
Four-year training course, full-time or part-time. Subjects include anatomy and physiology, pathology, clinical diagnostic skills and training in basic medical procedures, training in identification, preparation, properties and medicinal qualities of plants, pharmacology, biochemistry, psychiatry, geriatrics, and gynaecology. Over 500 hours of clinical training required. All members adhere to a strict code of ethics.

See Traditional Chinese Medicine for information on training courses in Traditional Chinese Herbal Medicine.

Holotropic

For information about Grof Holotropic Breathwork training, contact:

Grof Transpersonal
   Training Inc.
20 Sunnyside Ave.
A-314 Mill Valley
CA 94941
☎001 415 383 8779

Individual workshops can be arranged by request. For one-day and residential workshops in Ireland, contact the following:

Jean Farrell
☎098 25162

Catriona Jackson
☎01 280 2523

Elis Clare Lynch O'Connor
☎01 285 9637

Margaret McQuaid
☎042 40069

Transpersonal Psycho-
   therapy Group
59 Waterloo Lane
Dublin 4. ☎01 668 5282

Home Births

There are seven midwifery training schools (within hospitals) in Ireland. Students will have already completed three years' general nursing training. Midwifery is a

further two years.
Public health nurses
must be registered
midwives. There is no
practical domiciliary
midwifery module.

Homoeopathy

Co. Dublin
Hahnemann School of
  Homoeopathic Medicine
29/30 Dame Street
Dublin 2. ☎01 679 4208
Three-year course.

Irish School of
  Homoeopathy
47 Ratoath Estate, Cabra
Dublin 7. ☎01 868 2581
*Four-year part-time
course in homoeopathic
studies and practice. The
licentiate of the school is
recognised by the Irish
Society of Homoeopaths.
Classes held in Milltown.*

Co. Galway
The Burren School of
  Homoeopathy
c/o The Old Fever
  Hospital
Lavalley, Gort
☎091 631 668/637 382
Four-year course.

Hypnotherapy

Irish Institute of Coun-
  selling and Hypno-
  therapy (IICH)
118 Stillorgan Road
Dublin 4. ☎01 260 0118
*Certificate (two days) and
diploma (two years) in
counselling, hypnother-
apy and NLP, accredited
by American Institute of
Hypno-Therapy (AIH).*

Irish School of Ethical
  and Analytical Hypno-
  therapy (ISEAH)
Therapy House
6 Tuckey Street, Cork
☎021 273 575
*Diploma in hypnotherapy
psychotherapy can be
studied by distance learning. Advanced diploma
awarded to those who
have passed first diploma
course, attended practical
training workshops of at
least 120 hours, com-
pleted required assign-
ments, and undergone
eight sessions of hypno-
analysis with a qualified
hypnotherapist. Work-
shops at Griffith College,
Dublin, and Therapy
House, Cork. Graduates
can apply for membership
of Irish Association of
Hypno-analysts (IAH).*

Indian Head Massage

Co. Dublin
Miriam Brady
7 York Ave., Rathmines
Dublin 6. ☎01 496 7605
Workshops.

Celtic Healing and
  Natural Health Clinic
117–119 Ranelagh
Dublin 6. ☎01 491 0689

Complementary
  Healing Centre
91 Terenure Rd North
Dublin 6. ☎01 492 9077
Workshops.

Complementary
  Healing Therapies
136 New Road, Cabra
Dublin 7. ☎01 868 1110

Harvest Moon Centre
24 Lower Baggot Street
Dublin 2. ☎01 662 7556
Workshops.

The House of Astrology
  at Temple Bar
9 Parliament Street
Dublin 2. ☎01 679 404
Workshops.

Siobhan Kennedy
West Wood Club
Leopardstown
  Racecourse
Dublin 18
☎01 289 5665/289 2399
Workshops.

Seamus Lynch
☎01 284 6073
Workshops.

Co. Wicklow
Avon Park
Glendalough Road
Rathdrum. ☎0404 46610
Workshops.

JoJo Loftus
Royal Hotel, Bray
☎01 282 9530/286 2935
Workshops.

Iridology

International
  Association of
  Clinical Iridologists
853 Finchley Road
London NW11 8LX, UK
Information on iridology.

Kinesiology

Co. Dublin
Association of System-
  atic Kinesiology
c/o Siobhan Barnes
48 Percy Place, Ballsbridge
Dublin 4. ☎01 660 2806
Foundation classes in

basic applied kinesiology ('Balanced Health'). Also two-year professional diploma course.

Beaumont Institute of Complementary Therapies
Beaumont Convent
Beaumont Road
Dublin 9
Sr Brega. ☎01 836 8363
Courses in Touch for Health, educational kinesiology and a one-year diploma course in holistic kinesiology.

The healing house
24 O'Connell Avenue
Berkeley Road
Dublin 7. ☎01 8306413
Workshops.

Massage

Only included are courses of at least three months' duration, or which lead to a professional qualification. For membership information or referral to a therapist, contact:

Irish Massage
Therapists Association
Cathie Hogan, PRO
☎01 668 9242
Francis Daly, Secretary
☎045 52557

Co. Antrim
Lifespring Centre
111 Cliftonville Road
Belfast, BT14 6JQ
☎08 01232 753 658
Classes held in Belfast and Cork. Massage practitioner diploma course.

Roberta Mechan
College of Beauty
17 Castle Arcade
Belfast BT1 5DG
☎08 01232 664960
ITEC diploma in massage.

Co. Cork
College of Commerce
Morrison's Island, Cork
☎021 270 777
ITEC diploma in massage.

Cork College of Beauty
Therapy
Queens Old Castle
Cork. ☎021 275 741
ITEC diploma in massage.

Nicola Darrell
The Evergreen Clinic
79 Evergreen Road
Cork. ☎021 966 209
ITEC diploma in massage.

Co. Derry
Owen Donnelly
Holywell Trust
10–12 Bishops Street
Derry BT48 6PW
☎08 01504 261941
ITEC diploma in massage.

Co. Dublin
Academy International
48 Upr Drumcondra Rd
Dublin 9. ☎01 836 8201
Rosemary Campbell
ITEC diploma in massage.

Ann Weeks Beauty
School LTD
75 Waterloo Road
Dublin 4. ☎01 668 9231
ITEC diploma in massage.

Aspens Beauty Clinic
and College
83 Lower Camden St
Dublin 2. ☎01 475 1079
ITEC diploma in massage.

Celtic Healing and
Natural Health Clinic
117–119 Ranelagh
Dublin 6. ☎01 491 0689
Healing massage; introduction to holistic massage.

Complementary
Healing Therapies
136 New Cabra Road
Dublin 7. ☎01 868 1110
ITEC diploma in holistic massage.

Bronwyn Conroy
40 Grafton Street
Dublin 2. ☎01 677 9184
ITEC diploma in body massage.

Coogan-Bergin Clinic
and College
Glendenning House
6 Wicklow Street
Dublin 2. ☎01 679 4387
ITEC diploma in body massage.

Crumlin College of
Business and Technical
Studies
Crumlin Road
Dublin 12. ☎01 454 0662
ITEC diploma in massage.

Donnybrook Medical
Centre
6 Main Street, Donnybrook
Dublin 4. ☎01 269 6588
ITEC diplomas in holistic massage and sports massage.

Dublin School of Sports
Massage
NCEHS
16A St Joseph's Parade
Dublin 7. ☎01 830 8757
One-year certificate in sports massage.

Galligan Beauty Group
12 Hume Street
Dublin 2. ☎01 661 1122
ITEC diploma.

Holistic Healing Centre
38 Dame Street
Dublin 2. ☎01 671 0813
ITEC diploma in massage.

Holistic School of
  Reflexology and Massage
2 Laurel Park
Clondalkin, Dublin 22
☎01 459 2460
ITEC diploma in massage.

Irish Association of
  Holistic Medicine
66 Eccles Street, Dublin 7
☎01 830 7191/ 671 2791
Diploma in ki massage.

Irish Health Culture
  Association
66 Eccles Street, Dublin 7
☎01 830 4078/830 4474
*Diploma in ki massage
therapy (one year); certificate
in massage therapy (City and
Guilds of London Institute).*

Massage Ireland
Avoca Road, Blackrock
or
Ballsbridge, Dublin 4
☎01 668 9242
Cathie Hogan
ITEC diploma in massage.

MELT, Temple Bar
  Natural Healing Centre
2 Temple Lane South
Dublin 2. ☎01 679 8786

Moytura Healing Centre
2 Lower Glenageary Rd
Dún Laoghaire
☎01 285 4005
Healing massage diploma.

Natural Living Centre
Walmer Hse, Station Rd
Raheny, Dublin 5
☎01 832 7859/832 7861
*ITEC diploma in holistic
massage. Also successful
graduates eligible for*

*membership of Irish
Massage Therapists
Association (IMTA).*

Sallynoggin Senior College
Pearse St, Sallynoggin
☎01 285 2997
ITEC diploma in massage.

Senior College Dún
  Laoghaire
Eblana Avenue
Dún Laoghaire
☎01 280 0385
*Certificate in massage
(one year).*

Co. Galway
American Holistic
  Institute of Ireland
73 Claremont
Circular Road, Galway
☎091 529 807
*Diploma in therapeutic
massage.*

Galligan College of Beauty
Lismoyle House
St Augustine Street
Galway. ☎091 565 628
ITEC diploma in massage.

Georgina's College of
  Beauty
37 Shop Street, Galway
☎091 564 796
ITEC diploma in massage.

Co. Kerry
FÁS Training and Em-
  ployment Authority
Monavalley, Tralee
☎066 22155/25617
ITEC diploma in massage.

Co. Kildare
Frances Daly
Sports Therapy Clinic
Ard Lynn, Mountrice
Monasterevin
☎045 525 579
ITEC diploma in massage.

Co. Kilkenny
Judith Ashton
Powerswood
Thomastown
☎056 24928
ITEC diploma in massage.

Kilkenny School of
  Beauty Therapy
4 Patrick Street, Kilkenny
☎056 61891
ITEC diploma in massage.

Co. Limerick
Galligan College of Beauty
123 O'Connell Street
Limerick. ☎061 410628
ITEC diploma in massage.

Co. Louth
Marygold School
90 Bridge Street
Dundalk. ☎042 32154
ITEC diploma in massage.

Mrs Scappaticci-Morris
Williamstown House
Castlebellingham
Dundalk. ☎042 72235
ITEC diploma in massage.

Co. Mayo
FÁS (Donegal) Manage-
  ment Consultants Ltd.
Treedull, Claremorris
☎094 84224/84334
ITEC diploma in massage.

Co. Monaghan
Olivia Keenan Beauty
  Salon
22/24 Glaslough Street
Monaghan. ☎047 83320
ITEC diploma in massage.

Co. Waterford
Central Technical Institute
Parnell Square
Waterford. ☎051 874 053
ITEC diploma in massage.

Further information available from:

The Irish Massage Therapy Association
c/o Oaklands
Ballsbridge, Dublin 4
☎01 668 9242

ITEC: International Therapy Examination Council
James House
Oakelbrook Mill
Newent, GL18 1HD, UK
☎0044 1531 821875

Co. Wicklow
Shirley Price International College of Aromatherapy
PO Box 16, Wicklow
☎0404 47319
Diploma in aromatherapy massage.

Metamorphosis

Co. Cork
Fermoy Natural Health and Chiropody Centre
Abbey House
2 Abbey Street
Fermoy. ☎025 32966
Information on courses.

Eithne O'Mahony
Metamorphosis Ireland
'Shiloh', Clondulane
Fermoy. ☎025 31525
Information on courses.

Movement and Dance Therapy

Co. Dublin
Joan Davis
'The Studio'
Rere 330, Harold's Cross Rd
Dublin 6. ☎01 287 6986
Information on workshops.

Co. Wicklow
Ann O'Hanlon/ Antoinette Spillane
Chrysalis, Donard
☎045 404 713/01 295 3882
Two-year course in 'dancing the rainbow' — combines movement and dance, yoga, voice work, music and colour therapy as a form of expression and healing. Workshops at Chrysalis and other venues including Dublin, Blessington and Naas. Training directed at those who wish to facilitate similar workshops.

UK
Hertfordshire College of Art and Design
7 Hatfield Road
St Albans, Herts.
Courses in dance movement therapy, art and drama therapy training at post-graduate diploma and MA levels.

Laban Centre
Laurie Grove, New Cross
London SE14 6NW
Courses for graduates in dance, physical education or social sciences with proven interest and training in movement or dance form and experience in caring services.

US
Antioch/New UK Graduate School
103 Roxbury Street
Keene, NH 03431

Hahnemann University
230N Broad Street
Philadelphia, PA 19102

Hunter College
425 E 25th Street
New York 10010

New York University
35W 4th Street, Ed 675
New York 10003

Pratt Institute
East Building
200 Willoughby Ave.
Brooklyn, NY 11205

UCLA
405 Hilgard Avenue
Los Angeles, CA 90024

Muscle Effect Therapy

Bobby MacLaughlin
33 Wellington Lane
Dublin 4. ☎01 668 0316
Information on workshops.

Neuro Linguistic Programming

Irish Institute of Counselling and Hypnotherapy (IICH)
118 Stillorgan Road
Dublin 4. ☎01 260 0118
Foundation skills certificate in NLP (two 2-day modules). Courses at St Michael's Hospital, Dún Laoghaire.

Irish School of Ethical and Analytical Hypnotherapy (ISEAH)
Therapy House
6 Tuckey Street, Cork
☎021 273 575
Includes a section on NLP in its hypno-analysis diploma courses.

Life Changes
Unit One, Blackrock
  Centre
Blackrock, Co. Dublin
☎01 278 0093
*Certification in NLP and
time-line therapy (four
modules), governed by
American Board of NLP
(ABNLP), and Time Line
Therapy Association,
Honolulu, Hawaii.*

Aidan Maloney
Centre for Creative
  Change
14 Upper Clanbrassil St
Dublin 8. ☎01 453 8356

NLP Ireland
c/o Ken Bowbrick
13 Abbeyvale Drive
Swords, Co. Dublin
☎01 840 7718
*Workshops in strategies
and techniques of NLP*

For information on
training abroad, contact:

USA
Richard Bandler &
  Associates
13223 Black Mountain
  Road # 1-429
San Diego, CA 92129

Grinder, De Lozier &
  Associates
200 7th Ave., Suite 100
Santa Cruz, CA 95062

UK
The NLP Training
  Programme
22 Upper Tooting Park
London SW17 7SR

PACE Ltd
86 South Hill Park
London NW3 2SN

Nutrition

Co. Cork
Coláiste Stiofáin Naofa
College of Further
  Education
Tramore Road, Cork
☎021 961 020
ITEC diploma in nutrition.

Co. Dublin
Donnybrook Medical
  Centre
6 Main Street, Donnybrook
Dublin 4. ☎01 269 6588
ITEC diploma in nutrition.

Dublin Institute of
  Technology (DIT)
Kevin Street, Dublin 8
☎01 402 3000
*Degree (four and a half years,
full-time) or diploma in
human nutrition and dietetics
awarded jointly with Trinity
College. Graduates of degree
course eligible for state
registration in Dietetics (UK)
and for membership of Irish
Nutrition and Dietician's
Institute (INDI). Also post-
graduate diploma in food
science (two years part-time
or one year full-time), which
includes food chemistry,
microbiology, and human
nutrition.*

Faculty of Agriculture
UCD, Belfield, Dublin 4
☎01 706 7777/7193/4
*Degree (four years) in
agricultural science with a
specialisation in food
science. Includes a study of
food microbiology,
nutrition, food chemistry,
ingredients, food process-
ing and manufacturing.*

Irish Health Culture
  Association
66 Eccles Street, Dublin 7
☎01 830 4078/830 4474
Diploma in holistic dietetics.

Massage Ireland
Ballsbridge, Dublin 4 *or*
Avoca Road, Blackrock
Cathie Hogan
☎01 668 9242
ITEC diploma in nutrition

Natural Living Centre
Walmer Hse, Station Rd
Raheny, Dublin 5
☎01 832 7859
ITEC diploma in nutrition.

Teach Bán
6 Parnell Rd, Harold's Cross
Dublin 6. ☎01 454 3943
*Wholefood cookery course
(eight sessions) to help create
nutritionally balanced meals
using wholefoods.*

Co. Louth
Marygold School
90 Bridge Street
Dundalk. ☎042 32154
ITEC diploma in nutrition.

Osteopathy

No professional train-
ing in osteopathy in
Ireland. For information
on UK courses, contact:

Osteopathic Informa-
  tion Service
PO Box 2074, Reading
Berkshire RGI 4YR
☎0044 1734 512 501

The Irish Osteopathic
  Association (IOA)
c/o 17 Windsor Terrace
Portobello, Dublin 8
☎01 473 0828
Insists on minimum

*standards for its members
— the successful comple-
tion of a recognised
course in osteopathy
(three to four years full-
time, or five to six years
part-time study). Those
already qualified as medical doctors, physiothera-
pists etc. can apply for
membership having
completed a recognised
course in osteopathy of
eighteen months to two
years in duration.*

Psychodrama

Newtown House Centre
Doneraile, Co. Cork
Catherine Murray
☎022 24117
*Four to five years, part-
time. Training is residential — 600 hours: semi-
nars, skill development
sessions, experiential
sessions with process re-
view learning and direct-
ing supervised practice;
therapy 300 hours;
psychiatric placement 100
hours; clinical group 200
hours — trainee must set
up and run a psychodrama
group; supervision 80
hours; external training
250 hours. Diploma
awarded on fulfilment of
above, writing a thesis,
and a practicum. Gradu-
ates eligible for
accreditation and
registration with British
Psychodrama Association,
and the UK Council for
Psychotherapy, with three
months' practice.*

Psychosynthesis

Institute of Psychosyn-
 thesis and Trans-
 personal Theory
Eckhart Hse, 19 Clyde Rd
Dublin 4. ☎01 668 4687
*Four-year training pro-
gramme for those who
wish to use psychosyn-
thesis, or practise as
psychosynthesis thera-
pists. Year 1: a study of
the theory and practice of
psychosynthesis;
examines personal and
spiritual psychosynthesis.
Year 2: focuses on daily
life as spiritual practice;
explores relationship
between personal self and
transpersonal self.
Admission to Years 3 and
4 available to students
thought suitable after first
two years. Years 3 and 4
allow students to deepen
their study of psychosyn-
thesis as a transpersonal
theory and to learn the
methodologies to practise
it in their work. Weekend,
evening, morning and
week-long workshops.
Attendance at two week-
end workshops in
meditation a prerequisite
for attendance at all other
courses.*

Reality Therapy

Institute for Reality
 Therapy in Ireland
c/o Eileen Hearne
24 Glendown Court
Templeogue, Dublin 6W
☎01 456 2216 *or*

c/o Brian Lennon
6 Red Island, Skerries
Co. Dublin. ☎01 849 1906
*Courses throughout the
year at various locations.
Five modules must be
completed before certifi-
cation is conferred. Basic
practicum module: five-
day intensive week,
during which students
attend workshops and
submit case studies.
Advanced practicum
module: further five-day
intensive week, including
attendance at workshops
and submission of case
studies. Certification
module: five-day week
where students present a
project on some aspect of
reality therapy.*

The healing house
24 O'Connell Avenue
Berkeley Road
Dublin 7. ☎01 830 6413

Rebirthing

The Association of Irish
 Rebirthers (AIR)
c/o Catherine Dowling
33 Inchicore Road
Dublin 8. ☎01 453 3166
*Registration body for
rebirthers in Ireland,
affiliated to the International Breathwork Foun-
dation. Accredits courses
and is currently associated
with two-year professional
diploma course run by
Stephen Gregory.
Recommends that any
rebirther course should
deal with conception and
birth, early childhood,*

human development, self-responsibility and the creative power of thought, self-esteem, relationships, types of breathing, the client-rebirther relationship, counselling skills and the practice of rebirthing.

The Association of
  Rebirther Trainers
  International (ARTI)
Rere No. 4 Crofton Tce
Dún Laoghaire
Patsy Brennan
☎01 284 1660
Nine-month training course for one weekend a month. Tuition includes the art and science of rebirthing, understanding conception, delivery, birth and childhood, recognising and changing relationship patterns, different kinds of breathing, birth types, the concept of physical immortality, and philosophy of rebirthing. Students must do ten sessions each with a male and a female rebirther, and do their own rebirthing regularly, and must obtain testimonials from five people whom they have facilitated in the rebirthing process. At least 85 per cent of the board must vote in favour of accepting a member. Ongoing training is necessary for continued membership.

Healing Arts Centre
  International
46 Walnut Rise
Drumcondra, Dublin 9
☎01 837 0832 *or*
088 274 9701

Reflexology

Only included are courses of at least three months' duration, or which lead to a professional qualification.

Co. Antrim
Lifespring Centre
111 Cliftonville Road
Belfast BT14 6JQ
☎08 01232 753 658
Reflexology practitioner diploma course.

Co. Cork
Cork College of Beauty
  Therapy
Queens Old Castle
Cork. ☎021 275 741
ITEC diploma in reflexology.

Johanna Gubbay
The Old Forge, Ahiohill
Enniskeane. ☎023 39250
ITEC diploma in reflexology.

Irish Institute of
  Natural Therapy
Croghta Park
Glasheen Road, Cork
☎021 964 313
Diploma in reflexology

Co. Down
International Institute
  of Reflexology
Lr Catherine St, Newry
☎08 01693 62567/848 904
International diploma

Co. Dublin
Academy International
48 Upr Drumcondra Rd
Dublin 9. ☎01 836 8201
Rosemary Campbell
ITEC diploma in reflexology.

Beaumont Institute of
  Complementary
  Therapies
Beaumont Convent
Beaumont Rd, Dublin 9
Sr Brega ☎01 836 8363
One-year course.

Celtic Healing and
  Natural Health Clinic
117–119 Ranelagh
Dublin 6. ☎01 491 0689
Introduction to reflexology

Complementary
  Healing Therapies
136 New Cabra Road
Dublin 7. ☎01 868 1110
Diploma (nine months).

Coogan-Bergin College
  of Beauty Therapy
Glendenning House
6 Wicklow Street
Dublin 2. ☎01 679 4387
ITEC diploma in reflexology.

Donnybrook Medical
  Centre
6 Main St, Donnybrook
Dublin 4. ☎01 269 6588
ITEC diploma in reflexology.

Galligan Beauty Group
12 Hume Street
Dublin 2. ☎01 661 1122
ITEC diploma in reflexology.

Holistic Healing Centre
38 Dame Street
Dublin 2. ☎01 671 0813
Diploma in reflexology.

Holistic School of
  Reflexology & Massage
2 Laurel Park
Clondalkin, Dublin 22
Olive Gentleman
☎01 459 2460
ITEC diploma in reflexology (one-year); fulfils requirements for membership of Irish Reflexologists Institute (IRI).

International Institute
of Reflexology
105 Carrick Court
Portmarnock
☎01 846 1514
Mary Canavan
*Diploma in original
Ingham method of Reflex-
ology(fifteen months).*

Mary Anderson
Healing Centre
13 Trafalgar Terrace
Monkstown
☎01 280 3635
*International diploma in
reflexology; successful
graduates eligible for
membership of the
International Federation of
Reflexologists.*

Massage Ireland
Avoca Road, Blackrock
or
Ballsbridge, Dublin 4
☎01 668 9242
Cathie Hogan
Diploma in reflexology.

Natural Living Centre
Walmer Hse, Station Rd
Raheny, Dublin 5
☎01 832 7859/832 7861
*ITEC diploma, plus mem-
bership of the Association of
Reflexologists (AOR).*

Portobello School
Rere 40 Lr Dominick St
Dublin 1. ☎01 872 1277
ITEC certificate (one year).

Senior College Dún
Laoghaire
Eblana Avenue
Dún Laoghaire
☎01 280 0385
*Confederation of Inter-
national Beauty Therapy
and Cosmetology*

*(CIBTAC) certificate in
reflexology (one year).*

Co. Galway
Susan Coen-Cantrell
College of Beauty
Therapy
Coen House, Salthill
Galway. ☎091 23296
ITEC diploma in reflexology.

Galligan College of
Beauty
Lismoyle House
St Augustine Street
Galway. ☎091 565 628
ITEC diploma in reflexology.

Co. Limerick
Foxall College of
Beauty Therapy
136 O'Connell Street
Limerick. ☎061 410 996
ITEC diploma in reflexology.

Galligan College of
Beauty
123 O'Connell Street
Limerick. ☎061 410628
ITEC diploma in reflexology.

Co. Tyrone
Chrysalis School of
Reflexology
14 Central Avenue
Cookstown
Sheila Nugent
☎08 016487 63664
*Diploma course in
reflexology in Belfast,
Derry, Enniskillen,
Cookstown & Republic.*

Reiki

There are four reiki
degrees: (1) empowerment
in which students connect
with the reiki energy
within and around them,
and learn to balance their

own energy; once the
twelve basic hand
positions are learnt, they
assist each other in the
healing process; (2) three
keys (symbols) are opened
within each student — first
allows for a greater
amount of energy to be
channelled and for a
greater sense of the power
within, second allows
students to tap into
universal consciousness,
and the third allows them
to go beyond the physical
limitations of time and
space to promote absentee
healing; (3) empowerment
in which the master key is
introduced, allowing stu-
dents to effect a shift of
consciousness in them-
selves; (4) students learn to
empower and teach others.
Training consists of
working with teacher,
learning what to teach,
empowerment on all levels
and assisting students in
their knowledge of reiki.
    Workshops for first three
degrees normally held
over a weekend, with a
support and feedback
evening after three weeks.
Fourth degree is taught
over one to three years.

Co. Cork
Carmel Long
Cork. ☎021 371 377

Co. Down
Peter Shields
House, 230 Scabo Road
Newtownards BT23 4SJ
☎08 01247 826474

Co. Dublin

Celtic Healing and
   Natural Health Clinic
117–119 Ranelagh
Dublin 6. ☎01 491 0689

Cocoon Reiki Centre
c/o Ann Faherty
20 Woodside
Windgate Road, Howth
☎01 832 1255

Complementary
   Healing Centre
91 Terenure Rd North
Terenure, Dublin 6
☎01 492 9077

Complementary
   Healing Therapies
136 New Cabra Road
Dublin 7. ☎01 868 1110

Cathleen Dillon
☎01 832 3894

Hands of Light
   Institute of Healing
160 Pembroke Road
Dublin 4. ☎01 668 1809

Healing Arts Centre
   International
46 Walnut Rise
Drumcondra, Dublin 9
Angela Gorman
☎01 837 0832/088 274 970
Workshops and seminars.

MELT, Temple Bar
   Natural Healing Centre
2 Temple Lane South
Dublin 2. ☎01 679 8786

Mary Roden
66 Lower Baggot Street
Dublin 2. ☎0404 61248

The healing house
24 O'Connell Avenue
Berkeley Road
Dublin 7. ☎01 830 6413

Co. Galway

Plexus Bio-Energy (Irl) Ltd.
Lismoyle House
Merchant's Road
Galway. ☎091 568 855

Co. Louth

Iomlánú
Roden Place, Dundalk
☎042 32804/27253

Co. Sligo

Rainbow's End Healing
   Centre
Castlebaldwin
☎071 65728

Co. Wicklow

Chrysalis, Donard
☎045 404713

Rolfing

Patricia Keane
Greenhills, Walkinstown
Dublin 12. ☎01 456 9501
Information on rolfing.

SHEN®

Training takes place in
three phases: (1) funda-
mental techniques (ten
days); (2) certified
practitioner internship
where trainees are
supervised at work
(two years); and (3)
ongoing education.

American Holistic
   Institute of Ireland
73 Claremont
Circular Road, Galway
☎091 25941/01 848 1852
*Classes held in Dublin,
Waterford, Cork,
Limerick and Galway.*

Shen Tao
Acupressure

Shen Tao Practitioners
   Association (SPA)
c/o Judith Hoad
Room for Healing
Inver, Co. Donegal
☎073 36406
*Workshops: 'Wandering
Through the Weeds'
(medicinal and nutritional
values of wild plants),
'Balanced Birthing' (Shen
Tao Acupressure in
pregnancy, birth and early
infancy), and 'Therapeutic
Loving Care' (for carers of
elderly, disabled or sick).*

Shiatsu

The Shiatsu Society of
   Ireland
c/o Patricia O'Hanlon
12 The Cove, Malahide
Co. Dublin. ☎01 845 3647
*Applicants for member-
ship must have completed
500 hours of study with
recognised teachers, over
three years, and a year of
professional practice.
Other subjects covered
include anatomy and
physiology, nutrition and
home remedies.*

Spiritual Healing

The National Federa-
   tion of Spiritual
   Healers (NFSH)
Old Manor Farm Studio
Church Street
Sudbury-on-Thames
Middlesex TW16 6RG, UK
☎0044 1932 783 164
Training for those seeking

to develop their healing ability. Two-year probationary period under supervision of a full member, plus attendance at four weekend workshops and weekly attendance at a probationer's spiritual healing group required for full membership of NFSH. Applicants must obtain testimonials from four people who have benefited from spiritual healing as channelled by them, and two full members must testify on behalf of the applicant.

The Irish Spiritual Centre
30–31 Wicklow Street
Dublin 2. ☎01 671 5106
Information on the NFSH and spiritual healing.

The healing house
24 O'Connell Avenue
Berkeley Road
Dublin 7. ☎01 830 6413
Courses in spiritual healing.

T'ai Chi Chuan

Information available from the following:

Celtic Healing and
Natural Health Clinic
117–119 Ranelagh
Dublin 6. ☎01 491 0689

Complementary
Healing Centre
91 Terenure Rd North
Dublin 6. ☎01 492 9077

International Taoist Society
☎01 855 7699

Natural Living Centre
Walmer Hse, Station Rd
Raheny, Dublin 5
☎01 832 7859/832 7861

The School of T'ai Chi
Chuan
c/o 10 Winon Avenue
Rathgar, Dublin 6
☎01 269 5281
Beginners and advanced courses at Haddington Road, Dublin 4. Arica courses also offered, including Chua Ka (self-massage).

T'ai Chi Chuan and
Qigong Training Centre
Parnell Square
Dublin 1. ☎01 284 2662

T'ai Chi Chuan
Association
c/o St Andrew's
Resource Centre
114–116 Pearse Street
Dublin 2. ☎01 677 1930
Also yoga, meditation and martial arts.

T'ai Chi Energy Centre
Milltown Park
Sandford Rd, Ranelagh
Dublin 6. ☎01 496 1533
Qi Gong classes also held.

Traditional Chinese Medicine

It is essential that practitioners have undergone a recognised training course, and have taken out private insurance.

Co. Cork
Irish Institute of
Natural Therapy
Croghta Park
Glasheen Road, Cork
☎021 964 313
Diploma courses in acupuncture.

Co. Dublin
Acupuncture Foundation
Dominick Court
41 Lower Dominick St
Dublin 1
☎01 873 3199/662 3525
Licentiate diploma course (three years, part-time); classes held in Milltown Park College. Courses linked to the Nanjing University of Traditional Chinese Medicine.

Chinese Medicine &
Acupuncture Centre
Milltown Park
Dublin 6. ☎01 496 1533

The Irish College of
Traditional Chinese
Medicine
100 Marlborough Road
Donnybrook, Dublin 4
☎01 496 7830
Licentiate in Traditional Chinese Medicine (three years).

The healing house
24 O'Connell Avenue
Berkeley Road
Dublin 7. ☎01 830 6413

Co. Galway
The College of Integrative Acupuncture
6 St Brendan's Road
Woodquay, Galway
☎091 561 676
Three years.

The European College
of Traditional
Chinese Medicine
34 Upper Abbeygate St
Galway. ☎091 567 416
Two years.

Co. Limerick
The European College
 of Traditional
 Chinese Medicine
☎029 60461
Two years.

Vega Test

Noma (Complex
 Homoeopathy Ltd.)
Unit 3
1–16 Hollybrook Road
Upper Shirley
Southampton SO16 6RB
UK. ☎0044 1703 770 513
*All practitioners must
have a medical or
paramedical qualification.
Training consists of a
basic training day, plus
an advanced training day.
Only practitioners with
the Noma qualification
are sanctioned to pur-
chase a vega machine.*

Clinic Support Services
78 Walkinstown Road
Dublin 12. ☎01 460 0203
*Noma representative in
Ireland.*

Voice Therapy

For information on
workshops, contact:
Kalichi. ☎01 497 3097

Chrysalis
Donard
Co. Wicklow
☎045 404 713

Joan Davis (Movement
 and dance)
'The Studio', Rere 330
Harold's Cross Road
Dublin 6. ☎01 287 6986

Yoga

Celtic Healing and
 Natural Health Clinic
117–119 Ranelagh
Dublin 6. ☎01 491 0689

Dublin Yoga Centre
19 Upper Mount Street
Dublin 2. ☎01 284 3445
Information on yoga.

The Holistic Health
 Centre
197 Lower Kimmage Rd
Dublin 6w. ☎01 492 9279

Irish Association of
 Holistic Medicine
9–11 Grafton Street
Dublin 2. ☎01 671 2788
Diploma in yoga.

The Irish Health
 Culture Association
66 Eccles Street
Dublin 7. ☎01 830 3717
*One-year yoga teachers
diploma course*

Irish Yoga Association
108 Lower Kimmage
 Road
Harold's Cross
Dublin 6w
☎01 492 9213
*Classes, workshops,
seminars and teacher-
training.*

MELT, Temple Bar
 Natural Healing
 Centre
2 Temple Lane
Dublin 2. ☎01 679 8786
*Information on yoga and
training in polarity yoga.*

Zero Balancing

Seamus Lynch
☎01 284 6073
Information.

Freda Roche
The Family and
 Counselling Centre
46 Elmwood Avenue
Ranelagh, Dublin 6
☎01 497 1188/497 1722
Information.

Acupuncture

see *Traditional Chinese Medicine*

Alexander Technique

Co. Antrim
Kate Kelly m.s.t.a.t.
Crescent Arts Centre
University Road, Belfast
☎08 01662 242338

Co. Cork
Rosemary Moone
101 Evergreen Road
Cork. ☎021 316723 *or*

The Natural Healing Centre
Thompson House
MacCurtain Street
Cork. ☎021 501600

Jerilyn Scott
Pigges Eye, Colla
South Schull. ☎028 28429

Co. Down
Nicola Brown
152 High St, Holywood
☎08 01662 423976

Co. Dublin
Mary Derbyshire
6 St Kevin's Park, Dartry
Dublin 6. ☎01 497 9762

Frank Kennedy
35 Callary Road
Mount Merrion
☎01 288 2446

Karin O'Flanagan
54 Mountjoy Sq. West
Dublin 1. ☎01 878 7778

Co. Galway
Kate Kelly m.s.t.a.t.
Spinners, Treanlaur
Maree, Oranmore
☎091 794028

Anthroposophy

CAMPHILL COMMUNITIES
Co. Down
Glencraig, Craigavad
Holywood BT18 0DB
☎08 01232 423 396

Mourne Grange
169 Newry Road
Kilkeel, BT34 4EX
☎08 016937 60100

Co. Kildare
The Bridge
Main Street, Kilcullen
☎045 481 597

Dunshane House
Brannockstown
☎045 483 628

Co. Kilkenny
Ballytobin, Callan
☎056 25114

Jerpoint House & Barn
Thomastown
☎056 24844

Kyle, Coolagh, Calan
☎056 25737

The Watergarder
Ladywell Street
Thomastown
☎056 24690

Co. Tipperary
Temple Michael
Grangemockler
Carrick-on-Suir
☎051 647202

Co. Tyrone
Clanabogan
Drudgeon Road
Clanabogan, Omagh
BT78 1TJ
☎08 01662 256 111

Co. Wexford
Duffcarrig, Gorey
☎055 25116

SCHOOLS
Co. Clare
Cooleenbridge School
Raheen Rd, Tuamgraney
Scariff. ☎061 921 494

Co. Dublin
The Dublin Rudolf
  Steiner School
28 Maxwell Rd, Rathmines
Dublin 6. ☎01 496 0525

Aromatherapy

For a list of members of
Irish and International
Aromatherapy
Association, contact
IIAA, Roscore, Bluebell
Tullamore, Co. Offaly

Co. Antrim
A. Arnold
66 Glenhugh Road
Ahoghill
☎08 01266 878 448

Aroma Care Plus
4 Windslow Court
Carrickfergus
Serena Sheppard SRN SCM
☎08 01960 36 610

Aromaticity
21 Knockhill Pk, Belfast
Penny Kennedy BA
  ICHT IIHHT
☎08 01232 656 109

The Beauty Booth
39 Main St, Broughshane
☎08 01266 862 477

Bodycare, 1st Floor
9 Governor's Place
Carrickfergus
☎08 01960 361 012

Lorna Chesney
120 Fenaghy Road
Cullybackey
☎08 01266 880 766

The House of Beauty
6A Mount Merrion Ave.
Rosetta, Belfast
☎08 01232 492 315

I.D. Aromatics
Belfast. ☎08 01232 739 390

Ivanhoe Clinic
35 Belfast Road, Antrim
☎08 01849 467 929

Lifespring Centre
111 Cliftonville Road
Belfast BT14 6JQ
Mary Grant Assoc.
☎08 01232 753 658

Patricia McDaniel MRQA
15 Cliftondene Gardens
Belfast BT14 7PS
☎08 01232 716 676

Ana M. Salcedo RGN
MIFHB
8 Glendhu Manor
Garnerville Rd, Belfast
☎08 01232 761 365

Co. Carlow
Always Natural
Kellistown, Carlow
☎0503 48657

Co. Clare
Body Beautiful
Moore Street, Kilrush
☎065 52266

Complexions Electrolysis
& Beauty Salon
44 Abbey Street, Ennis
☎065 29805

Lisdoonvarna Spa Wells
& Health Centre
Lisdoonvarna
☎065 74023

Luisne Health Centre
Ballyvaughan Craft Centre
Ballyvaughan
☎065 77177

Sláinte Aromatherapy
Clinic
Sláinte Car Park
Abbey Street, Ennis
Noelette Keane RGN
☎065 42019

Co. Cork
Eileen Ahern
34 Prince's Street, Cork
☎021 272 650

Beauty Regain
33 Grand Parade, Cork
☎021 277 181

The Bridge Clinic
2nd Floor, 8 Bridge Street
Cork. ☎021 551 263

Mary Collins, ICNHS
(Dip) Aroma Member
of IIAA and IFR
104 Oliver Plunkett St
Cork. ☎021 274 130

Noelle Corcoran
97 Palmbury Orchard
Tather, Cork

Anne Cronin
13 Uam Var Avenue
Bishopstown

Eileen Doody LLSA
MIIAA
Bridge Clinic
8 Bridge Street, Cork
☎021 551 263

Douglas Court Tan and
Beauty Salon
Douglas Court
Shopping Centre
☎021 893 733

Evergreen Centre for
the Study of Natural
Medicine
79 Evergreen Rd, Cork
Nicola Darrell BScHons
MIFA MIAA ITEC/
Carmel O'Sullivan
MIIAA LLSA
☎021 966 209

Jacinta Fitzgibbon
IMTA ITEC
Killowen, Enniskeane
☎021 338170

Melissa Hickey
Railway Cottage
Rockfort, Innishannon

Helen Holden Dip NTM,
ITEC ISPA M.AIR
Heathercroft
1 Castle Close Crescent
Blarney. ☎021 385 708

Theresa Hosford
Leylandii, Ardmore
Passage West

Noreen Hunt
9 Westbury Grove, Wilton

Inner Healing Centre
46 Sheares Street, Cork
☎021 278 243

LSA Ireland
Evergreen Centre for
the Study of Natural
Medicine
79 Evergreen Rd, Cork
☎021 966 209

Anne Lyons
Main Street, Millstreet

Mary C. McCarthy
IMTA, ITEC
Orchard Grove
Western Rd, Clonakilty

Paula Meehan
17 Nutley Avenue
Mahon, Blackrock

Monkstown
Aromatherapy
Parkgarriff Cottage
Monkstown
Linda Walsh LLSA MIIAA
☎021 841 793

Elizabeth Murphy
Fitzgerald House
74 Grand Parade, Cork
☎021 272 100

Natural Healing Centre
Thompson House
McCurtain Street
☎021 501 600

Natural Therapy Centre
Main Street, Macroom
Denise Moloney NTC
ITEC ISPA
☎026 41916

Noelle's Beauty Salon
36 Lakeview Lane
Mahon. ☎021 357 940

Margaret O'Callaghan
3 Gordon Villas, Monkstown

Colm O'Flynn
10 Douglas Hall Lawn
Well Road, Cork

Catherine O'Leary
29 Delfern Grove
Maryborough, Douglas

Sheila O'Shea
71 Arbour Heights
Waterpark, Carrigaline

Carmel O'Sullivan
c/o Douglas
Chiropractic Clinic
Broadvale, Maryborough

Elizabeth O'Sullivan ITEC
51 Pic-Du-Jer Park
Ballinlough. ☎021 294 830

Noelle Perrott
36 Lakeview Lawn
Blackrock, Cork

Julie Reed MFPHYS
Dip. Aromatherapy
The Square, Skibbereen
☎028 22 424

Mary Uí Chonchúir
Dromanallaigh
Ballingeary. ☎026 47 202

Linda Walsh
Parkgarrif Cottage
Monkstown

Co. Donegal
Britton's Beauty Centre
Main Street, Donegal
☎073 22656

Mary Boyle-O'Brien
Dungloe. ☎075 21011

Co. Down
Geraldine Bailie
Ballynester House
Cardy Road, Greyabbey
☎08 012477 88386

Florence Budd Health
& Beauty Clinic
Old Stone House
101 Main Street
Moira. ☎08 01846 613 147

Yvonne Gibson
2 Meetinghouse Lane
Newtownards
☎08 01247 810 928

Impact Health, Beauty
& Aromatherapy
50a Main St, Ballynahinch
☎08 01238 563 222

Moonstone
39 Church Rd, Holywood
☎08 01232 422 625

Natural Therapy Clinic
25 Bingham Street
Bangor. ☎08 01247 464 847

Co. Dublin
Academy International
48 Upr Drumcondra Rd
Dublin 9. ☎01 836 8201

Aromatherapy Beauty
Clinic
12 Wicklow Street
Dublin 2. ☎01 677 0512

Aromatherapy Centre
1d Brighton Road
Dublin 18. ☎01 289 8699

The Aromatherapy Clinic
Lower Camden Street
Dublin 2. ☎01 475 2323

The Aromatherapy Clinic
Foxrock, Dublin 18
☎01 289 8145

Aromatherapy Clinic
and New Age Shop
30/31 Wicklow Street
☎01 670 5216

Beauty &
Aromatherapy Clinic
70 Wellington Road
Ballsbridge, Dublin 4
☎01 660 0510

The Beauty Store
Frascati Centre
Blackrock. ☎01 283 6594

Business Therapeutic
Enterprise
Aromatherapy
5 Main Street, Dundrum
Dublin 14. ☎088 641 621

Maria Cassidy IMTA ITEC
Dundrum, Dublin 14
☎01 298 2565

John Caviston IMTA
ITEC MCS Ch
57a Glasthule Road
Sandycove. ☎01 284 5287

Peter Christian
Templeogue, Dublin 16
☎01 494 5493

Majella Conway
6 Clifton Terrace
Monkstown. ☎01 280 5506

Crystal Mystique
Unit 4, Townyard Lane
Malahide. ☎01 845 5599

Donnybrook Medical
Centre
6 Main St, Donnybrook
Dublin 4
Patricia McWilliams
ITEC/Audrey Ross
ITEC
☎01 269 6588

Drumcondra Health
Clinic
11 Sion Hill Road
Drumcondra
Dublin 9. ☎01 837 8310

Finishing Touches
1st floor
15 Upper Baggot Street
Dublin 4. ☎01 660 5348

Fortfield Pharmacy
48 Fortfield Park
Dublin 6W. ☎01 490 0789

Galligan Beauty Group
12 Hume Street
Dublin 2. ☎01 661 1122
or
109 Grafton Street
Dublin 2. ☎01 671 1843

Greenlea Pharmacy
116 Greenlea Road
Terenure, Dublin 6W
☎01 490 9273

Healthy Alternatives
Loughlinstown Leisure
Centre
Loughlinstown Drive
Dún Laoghaire
☎088 658 622

Heather Marsh (Ire) Ltd
120 Lr Kilmacud Rd
Stillorgan. ☎01 278 3043

Cathie Hogan IMTA
Sandymount
☎01 668 9242

Holistic Healing Centre
38 Dame Street
Dublin 2. ☎01 671 0813

The Holistic Health
Centre
197 Lr Kimmage Road
Dublin 6w. ☎01 492 9279

Home-A-Therapy Clinic
Griffith College
South Circular Road
Dublin 8. ☎088 623 266

Siobhan Kennedy
Arom. Dip, IMTA
West Wood Club
Leopardstown Race-
course, Foxrock
Dublin 18. ☎01 289 5665

Nuala Kiernan
22 Treesdale, Stillorgan Rd
☎01 283 5648

Patricia Langley IMTA
Dublin 14/16
☎01 298 0597/493 1050

The Living Space
u1 Blackrock Shopping
Centre, Blackrock
☎01 278 0093

Vincent McCabe IFA
ICM (Appr) ITEC
CIBTAC
Dublin 5. ☎01 839 2133

Laura McCormack
IMTA
9 Grange Park, Raheny
Dublin 5. ☎01 848 1939

Anne McDevitt DRE
BCAA
13 Wicklow Street
Dublin 2. ☎01 677 7962

Ethna McQuillan MIRI
ITEC
140 Foxfield Grove
Raheny, Dublin 5
☎01 831 2008

Stephanie Mahon/Ferga
McNamara IMTA
28 Havelock Square
Sandymount, Dublin 4
☎01 668 6460

MELT, Temple Bar Natural
Healing Centre
2 Temple Lane South
Dublin 2. ☎01 679 8786

The Natural Health
Clinic
Mews, 154 Leinster Rd
Rathmines, Dublin 6
☎01 496 1316

Natural Solutions
6 Clifton Terrace
Monkstown
☎01 280 5506

The Natural Therapy &
Beauty Clinic
Coolmine Sports Complex
Clonsilla, Dublin 15
☎01 820 7172

Orlagh O'Brien ITEC
SPA Dip
8 Dunmore Park
Ballymount, Dublin 24
☎01 452 4306

Therese O'Brien ITEC
45 Bulfin Road, Inchicore
Dublin 8. ☎01 454 0709

Elizabeth O'Neill
Walkinstown
Osteopathy Clinic
18 Cromwellsfort Road
Dublin 12. ☎01 450 4438

Pure Nature Aromatics
7 Cookstown Square
Belgard Road
Dublin 24. ☎01 451 0733

Quintessence MIIAA
89 Morehampton Road
Donnybrook, Dublin 4
☎01 660 8408

Mary Regan IMTA
47 Heatherview Lawn
Aylesbury, Tallaght
☎01 451 4915

Reynolds Pharmacy
42 Manor Road
Palmerstown, Dublin 20
☎01 626 4574

Shannon's Way
Malahide. ☎01 845 5459

Catherine Tindal
Churchtown, Dublin 14
☎01 298 4852

Co. Galway
Aromatherapy Health
& Beauty Clinic
1st Floor, 21 Eyre Square
Galway. ☎091 562 597

Carolyn's Beauty Salon
21 Sea Road, Galway
☎091 587 738

Martin Daly Ki Massage
Knocknacarra, Galway
☎091 528 982

Evergreen Healthfoods
19 Galway S.C.
Headford Road, Galway
☎091 564 550 *or*
High Street, Galway
☎091 564 215

Georgina's Skin Care
Clinic
37 Shop Street, Galway
☎091 564 796

Mary Irwin Dip. Arom.
Reflex
1A San Antonio Park
Salthill. ☎091 526 880

Evelyn Kitt
Kiniska, Claregalway
☎091 798 485

Bernie McInerney
21 Eyre Square (1st floor)
Galway. ☎091 562 597

Monica Maloney
Moycullen, Galway
☎091 555 144

O'Brien's Ltd
11 Henry Street, Galway
☎091 582 479

Co. Kerry
The Fragrant Haven
5 Charles Street
Listowel. ☎068 22970

Denise Hussey
Kiltormey, Lixnaw

Margot A. Keeman
Portre, Mill Road
Killarney. ☎064 36648

Áine McKivergan
Oakpark Medical Centre
Oakpark, Tralee
☎066 26255

Co. Kildare
Anne O'Neill
Maynooth Mall
Main Street, Maynooth
☎01 628 9395

Co. Kilkenny
Maura Murphy
Buruchurch, Cuffes Grange
☎056 29040

Transformations
Unit 7 Kilkenny
Shopping Arcade
High Street, Kilkenny
☎056 52688

Co. Limerick
Breda Berkery SRN RM
CST
23 Willow Park, Raheen
☎061 304 955

Marion Fenton SRN Lic
TCM
5 Alphonsus Terrace
Quin Street, Limerick
☎061 417 781

M. McElduff Lic Ac
MAIC IHCA Dip TCM
Limerick. ☎061 227 601

Natural Harmony ITEC
& CIBTAC Qualified
26 William Street
Limerick. ☎061 419 455

J. O'Connell SRN Mem
Inst PB Hons Dip Paris
18 Upper Mallow St
Limerick. ☎061 413 528

Ada Quillinan
Sarsfield Street
Kilmallock. ☎063 98966

Serenity
26 High Street, Limerick
☎061 419 569

Touch Of Class
U3 Belfield House
Ennis Road, Limerick
☎061 325 005

Co. Longford
Longford Beauty Clinic
Dublin Street, Longford
☎043 45590

Co. Louth
Marygold
Aromatherapy Clinic
90 Bridge Street
Dundalk. ☎042 32154

New Faces Beauty
Clinic
2 Dublin Street, Dundalk
☎042 31313

Totally-You
29 Stockwell Street
Drogheda. ☎041 39220

Co. Mayo
The Aromatherapy &
Beauty Clinic
Main Street, Kiltimagh
☎094 81092

Bellederma
Cornmarket, Ballinrobe
☎092 42000

Tir na nÓg Holistic
Beauty Centre
The Square, Claremorris
☎094 62678

Co. Monaghan
Well Being
71 Glaslough Street
Monaghan. ☎047 84299

Co. Offaly
Jennifer Spollen
Hophill Avenue
Tullamore. ☎0506 22666

Co. Roscommon
Mary O'Hara RGN
Castle Street, Roscommon
☎0903 26041

Co. Tipperary
Liz Fenton League
Marlfield Rd, Clonmel

Marie Foley
35 Summerhill Drive
Clonmel

Co. Tyrone
Barbara's Health &
Beauty Salon
31 Carland Road
Dungannon
☎08 01868 752 262

Co. Waterford
June Finn
9 Pinewood Avenue
Hillview, Waterford

Co. Westmeath
Thomas Mannion
20 Willow Drive
Athlone. ☎0902 78766

Britta Stewart
U17 Mullingar
Enterprise Centre
Mullingar. ☎044 43444

Totally-You
Austin Friar Street
Mullingar. ☎044 49585

Co. Wexford
Ena Dunne
Grove Cottage
Borovale, Enniscorthy

The Quay Pharmacy
3 Donovan's Wharf
Crescent Quay
Wexford. ☎053 2 29 22

Kathryn Redmond ITEC
The Beauty and
Aromatherapy Salon
28 Lower Henrietta St
Wexford. ☎053 22527

Hatti Thompson
Talbot Hotel Leisure
Complex
Wexford. ☎051 422 566

Co. Wicklow
Aaron Holistics
Rere 5 Duncairn Lane
Bray. ☎01 286 2899

Atlantic Aromatics
9 Ardee Street, Bray
☎01 286 5399

Bomar Ltd.
Mail Order Service
Kilcoole. ☎01 287 5110
Fax: 01 287 6717

Holistic Options
3 Sydenham Mews
Bray. ☎01 286 6084

Lady Greystones
Church Rd, Greystones
☎01 287 2311

JoJo Loftus
Royal Hotel Bray
☎01 276 1206/282 9530

Mary O'Neill Beauty Clinic
Butler House
Main Street, Arklow
☎0402 32143

Shirley Price Aroma-
therapy College
Natural Therapy Centre
PO Box 16, Wicklow
☎0404 47319

Aromatology

Evergreen Clinic of
Natural Medicine
79 Evergreen Road, Cork
Nicola Darrell
☎021 966 209

Art Therapy

The following can be
contacted by writing to:

The Irish Association of
Drama, Art and
Music Therapists
PO Box 4176, Dublin 1

Co. Clare
Leslie Wiggins

Co. Cork
Carol Hardie

Co. Dublin
Suzie Cahn

Daniel Cullen
Dublin 6

Diane Da Cruz
Dublin 5

Gerri Geoghegan
Dublin 6

Deirdre Horgan
Dublin 14

Maeve Keane
Swords

Bernadette McLeavey
Ballybrack

Mary McMahon
Dublin 13

Lisa Moran
Dublin 7

Máire Muldowney
Dublin 14

Liam Plant
Dublin 6

Pamela Whitaker
Dublin 9

Marja Wilmer
Dublin 4

Co. Wicklow
Suzie Cahn

Northern Ireland
Alice McLaughlin

Aura Soma

Co. Cork
Gert-Jan Brockman
Beara Circle
Castletownbere

Co. Dublin
Patricia Dempsey
8 Montrose Court
Artane, Dublin 5

Thilde Devlin
59 Park Avenue
Castleknock, Dublin 15

Patricia Fleming
13 Milltown Grove
Churchtown, Dublin 14

Raymond Glennon
37 Sutton Park
Dublin 13

Nuala Kiernan
22 Treesdale. Stillorgan Rd
☎01 283 5648

Valerie Mitchell
129 Mangerton Road
Drimnagh, Dublin 12
☎01 455 1729

Cathleen Morley Stratford
Barnhill Road, Dalkey

Phillipa Quilligan
Fairwinds, Strand Road
Sutton, Dublin 13

Gerlinde Steinle
Ananda
23 Priory Avenue
Blackrock

Mary Varilly
7 Lawnswood Park
Stillorgan

Gertrude Walsh
Ranelagh, Dublin 6
☎01 496 4616

Mary Watkins
14 Shanliss Way, Santry

Co. Kerry
Eileen Quinlan
Irremore, Listowel

Co. Kilkenny
Carmel Russell
Fernhill
Dunningstown

Co. Limerick
Limerick Natural
   Healing Centre
64 Catherine Street
Limerick
John Quinlivan
☎061 400431

Co. Louth
May Coyle
Bellurgan, Dundalk

Co. Mayo
Joan Judge
14 the Harbour
Westport. ☎098 27127

Bach Flower Remedies

Co. Cork
Beara Circle
Castletownbere
Ulla Kinon. ☎027 70744

Hannah O'Brien MIRI
Inchnagree, Buttevant
☎022 24286

Co. Derry
Attracta Marla Bradley
15 Belvedere Park
Foyle Springs, Derry

Nancy Hynes
23 Glen Road, Derry

Co. Dublin
Angelina Kelly
20 Forest Park
Kingswood Estate
Dublin 24. ☎01 451 9283

Co. Roscommon
Philomena Collins
Ballinagare, Castlerea

Co. Wexford
Laurence Maher
2 Mount Ross, New Ross
☎051 425 721

Co. Sligo
Nora Bourke
17 Rosehill, Sligo

Janet Duffill
Kiltykene, Grange
Co. Sligo. ☎071 63973

Bio-energy

Co. Clare
Michael O'Doherty
Lower Market Street
Ennis. ☎065 41844

Co. Cork
Plexus Bio-energy
Douglas Hall Mews
Douglas
Mary Ring
☎021 364 048

Co. Dublin
Bio-energy Therapist
4 Abbeyfield, Killester
Dublin 5. ☎01 831 0544

A. Hughes BSc Lic TCM
1 Leopardstown Drive
Stillorgan. ☎01 288 0352

Co. Galway
Patrick and Bernie
  Glennon
The Beeches
Kilconnell, Ballinsloe
☎0905 86800

Plexus European
  Institute of Bio-energy
Lismoyle House
Merchant's Road
Galway. ☎091 568 855

Co. Limerick
Ada Quillinan
Sarsfield Street
Kilmallock. ☎063 98966

Co. Mayo
Martin Byrne
T/A Plexus Bio Energy
  (Irl) Ltd
James Street
Claremorris. ☎094 62333

Plexus European
  Institute of Bio-
  energy
Enterprise House
Aiden Street, Kiltimagh
☎094 81494

Co. Wicklow
Plexus Bio-energy and
  Therapeutic Massage
Glencarrig, Eden Road
Greystones. ☎01 287 5416

Biofeedback

Joan Fitzpatrick Dip COT
61 Kerrymount Rise
Dublin 18. ☎01 289 3060

Ann Gallagher
20 Heathfield Road
Dublin 6. ☎01 490 5378

Body Harmony

Assumpta Byrne
The Banks, Manor Kilbride
☎01 458 2407

Brenda Doherty
☎01 677 1021

The Holistic Health
  Centre
197 Lr Kimmage Road
Dublin 6w. ☎01 492 9279

Rosemary Khelifa
☎01 833 0656

Nuala Lavelle
☎01 490 0017

Chiropractic

For a list of members of
the Chiropractic
Association of Ireland,
contact ☎01 833 4026

Co. Antrim
Ballyclare Chiropractic
  Clinic
53–55 Main St, Ballyclare
☎08 01960 324880

Ballymena Chiropractic
  Clinic
1 Henry Street, Ballymena
☎08 01266 655755

Ballymoney
  Chiropractic Clinic
51a Queen St, Ballymoney
☎08 012656 66667

Belfast Chiropractic Clinic
228 Ormeau Road
Belfast BT7 2FZ
Roy J. Hamley D.C., Dip.
  Biomech./Anne
  Matthews BSc Hons
  DC/Robert Hilary Lic
  Ac BSc (Chiro)/
  Annette O'Neill BSc
  (Chiro) DC
☎08 01232 641111/
693150

Cregagh Chiropractic
  Clinic
162 Upper Knockbreda Rd
Belfast. ☎08 01232 402266

Glengormley
  Chiropractic Clinic
57 Ballyclare Road
Glengormley
☎08 01232 848938

Lisburn Chiropractic Clinic
28a Bachelors Walk
Lisburn
☎08 01846 665405

Dr C. Perks M Chiroprac./
  Dr M. Flanagan BApp Sc
  (Chiro)
122E Upper Lisburn Rd
Finaghy. ☎08 01232 604292

Co. Armagh
Craigavon Chiropractic
  Clinic
25 High Street, Lurgan
☎08 01762 349495

Co. Clare
Patricia McFadden
CPMCA
23 Limerick Road
Ennis ☎065 24845

Co. Cork
Dr Virginia Cantillon/
  Dr Ivan Dunne
2A Harley Court
Whiteoaks, Wilton
☎021 342 933

Douglas Chiropractic
  Clinic
Broadale
Maryborough Hill, Douglas
Mary Lavin SRN MCSCHI/
  Dr Leon Taylor
☎021 363 312

Kilworth Chiropractic
  Clinic
The Market House
Kilworth Village
Drs Maria Blumenthal/
  Mark Broe/Wendy
  Cole/James Cosgrave
☎025 27436

Riverside Chiropractic
Clinic
Unit 9, Penrose Wharf
Penrose Quay, Cork
Dr James Cosgrave
☎021 551 747

Dr Billy Tague
Raleigh Lodge
Macroom. ☎026 42116

Leon Taylor
92 Belgard Downs
Douglas. ☎021 895 088

Co. Derry
Clarendon Chiropractic
Clinic
5 Clarendon Street
Derry. ☎08 01504 373822

Claudy Chiropractic Clinic
522 Glenshane Road
Claudy. ☎08 01504 338748

Coleraine Chiropractic
Clinic
10 Lodge Rd, Coleraine
☎08 01265 328157

Foyle Chiropractic Clinic
2 Spencer House
18–22 Spencer Road
Derry. ☎08 01504 43991

Magherafelt
Chiropractic Clinic
4 Hospital Rd, Magherafelt
☎08 01648 34676

Co. Donegal
Letterkenny
Chiropractic Clinic
Glencar Road
Letterkenny. ☎074 25207

Co. Down
Ards Chiropractic Clinic
69 Frances Street
Newtownards BT23 7DX
Robert Hilary BSc
(Chiro) D.C. Lic AC
☎08 01247 826696

Bangor Chiropractic
Clinic
186 Rathgael Rd, Bangor
☎08 01247 275556

Dr Andrew J. Noble
Chiropractic Clinic
19 Hamilton Road
Bangor, BT20 4LL
☎08 01247 471200

Dr C. Perks M. Chiroprac./
Dr M. Flanagan BApp Sc
(Chiro)
The Mall, Newry
☎08 01693 66166

Pringle Chiropractic
The Kensington Suite
Church View, Holywood
Dr Paul Pringle, D.C.
(USA) FIACA, Doctor
of Chiropractic (USA)
☎08 01232 423 232

Co. Dublin
Back to Health
Chiropractic Clinic
Unit 84, Omni Park S.C.
Swords Road, Santry
Dublin 9
Dr Brenda Bower
☎01 862 1188

Dr Chris Barnett
Unit 6 Drogheda Mall
Finglas, Dublin 11
☎01 834 0182

Dr Clive Dennis
58 Main Street
Swords ☎01 840 3305
or 088 601 466

Dr Clive Dennis
12 Clarinda Park
Dún Laoghaire
☎01 280 0488
or 088 508 885

Dr Owen Dennis
126 Clontarf Road
Dublin 3. ☎01 833 6198

Dr Owen Dennis
1 Lr Rathmines Road
Rathmines, Dublin 6
Freefone ☎ 1800 44 74 47
or ☎01 491 0448/
088 593 737

Dr Robert Finley
Newtownpark Avenue
Blackrock. ☎01 288 2801
or 01 283 5957

Dr Linda Finley-McKenna
4 Belgrave Road
Rathmines, Dublin 6
☎01 497 0174

Dr J.J. Gilmore
12 Clarinda Park Nth
Dún Laoghaire
☎01 280 0488

Dr Rory Hayes
5 Vergemount
Clonskeagh, Dublin 6
☎01 269 6380

Dr Bill Hodges
12 Clarinda Park
Dún Laoghaire
☎01 280 0488
or ☎088 508 885

Dr Robert McCleary
126 Clontarf Road
Dublin 3. ☎01 833 6198
or 29 Phibsboro Road
Dublin 11. ☎01 830 5358

Dr Hagen McQuaid
58 Main Street, Swords
☎01 840 3305
or ☎088 601 466
also 1 Lr Rathmines Rd
Rathmines, Dublin 6
Freefone 1800 44 74 47
or ☎01 491 0448
or ☎088 593 737

MELT, Temple Bar
Natural Healing Centre
2 Temple Lane South
Dublin 2. ☎01 679 8786

Dr Aidan Mitchell
125 St Helen's Road
Booterstown
☎01 278 2483

Dr Thomas Moore
   MBBCH DIP M.S Med
115 Haddington Road
Dublin 4. ☎01 660 8416

Dr Richard Power
26 Fitzwilliam Square
Dublin 2. ☎01 676 3036

Dr Brett Stevens
126 Clontarf Road
Dublin 3. ☎01 833 4026

Swords Chiropractic
58 Main Street, Swords
☎01 840 3305

Dr Carl Tijerina
Raheny Chiropractic Clinic
Walmer House
Station Road, Raheny
Dublin 5. ☎01 832 7859

Fergal Tobin MBAAC
9 The Castlelands
Rathfarnham, Dublin 14
☎01 490 0530

Turner Clinic of
   Alternative Medicine
Cluain Árd
Dublin Road, Stillorgan
Dr Ronald J. Turner AC
☎01 288 4327

Sean Wall
12 Clarinda Park North
Dún Laoghaire
☎01 280 0488

Dr John Walshe
133 Walkinstown Road
Dublin 12
☎01 456 4804 *and*
58 Morehampton Road
Dublin 4. ☎01 660 9012

Dr Peter Wass
126 Clontarf Road
Dublin 3. ☎01 833 6183

Glen Watkins
Lough Bawn
Newtownpark Avenue
Blackrock. ☎01 288 2801

Co. Fermanagh
Enniskillen
   Chiropractic Clinic
22 New Street
Enniskillen, BT74 6AH
J.O. Pedersen D.C.
☎08 01365 325774

Co. Galway
Dr Cleo A. Bludworth
   DCDICS
Roscam, Merlin Park
Galway. ☎091 751 858

Clinic of Complementary
   and Natural Medicine
Forster Street, Galway
Dr Hussain Bhatti
☎091 568 804

The Galway
   Chiropractic Clinic
Estelle, Tuam Road
Dr Simon Coad/
   Charles Sawyer
☎091 755 205

Dr Laurel A. Martin
The Farm, Williamstown
Castlerea Post Office
☎0907 43235

Co. Kerry
Dr Regina Cantillon
Ivy Terrace, Prince's St
Tralee. ☎066 23876

Dr Billy Tague
1 St Anne's Road
Killarney. ☎064 36835

Co. Kildare
Naas Chiropractic Clinic
4 New Row, Naas
Dr Clive Dennis/Dr
   Monty Nighswonger
☎045 876 355

Dr Linda Finley-McKenna
Dublin Road, Maynooth
☎01 628 5962

Co. Kilkenny
Kilkenny Chiropractic
   Clinic
U1 Priory House
Dean Street, Kilkenny
Dr Mary Sheedy
☎056 51959

Co. Limerick
A.C.T. Centre
64 Catherine Street
Limerick
Dr John Le Boeuf D.C.
☎061 419 920

Dr Jess Lawrence D.C.
Summerhill
Old Cratloe Road
Limerick. ☎061 327 716

Co. Louth
Dr Chase Riley
28 Fair Street, Drogheda
☎041 30599 *and*
Unit 1, 86 Clanbrassil St
Dundalk ☎042 28699

Co. Mayo
Dr Charles Jenkins
Foxford Road, Ballina
☎096 70664

Co. Tipperary
Dr Rory Hayes
66 Liberty Square
Thurles. ☎0504 22250

Dr Jess Lawrence D.C.
Portroe, Nenagh
☎067 2 33 44

Dr Noel Ryan
51 Queen Street
Clonmel. ☎051 85548

Dr Dan Sullivan
38 Cherrymount
Clonmel. ☎052 26855

Co. Tyrone
Cookstown Chiropractic
35 Molesworth Street
Cookstown
☎08 016487 66454

Dungannon
  Chiropractic Clinic
7 Ranfurley Road
Dungannon
☎08 01868 753663

Co. Waterford
Airmount Chiropractic
  Clinics
Rocklands, Gracedieu
Waterford
Dr Noel T. Ryan
☎051 855 481

Waterford Chiropractic
  Clinic
38/39 Patrick Street
Waterford
Soren/Lotte O'Neill
☎051 843 157

Co. Westmeath
Mullingar
  Chiropractors Clinic
60 Austin Friars Street
Mullingar
Dr Owen Dennis/
  Dr Rory Murphy
☎044 48374

Riley Chiropractic
  Clinic
Rocklong House
Baylough, Athlone
Chase Riley/Dr Felix S.
  Paterek
☎0902 93160

Dr Carl Tijerina
Newbury Hotel
Dominick Street
Mullingar. ☎044 42888

Co. Wexford
Airmount Chiropractic
  Clinic
Killanick, Wexford
Dr Noel T Ryan
☎053 58107/051 85548

Co. Wicklow
Dr Rory Hayes
Ship Shape, Mall Centre
Main Street, Wicklow
☎0404 69267

Paul Noone
2 Triton House
The Harbour, Greystones
☎01 287 5944

Fiona Sheperd MC MCA
79 Castle Street, Bray
☎01 286 6611

Colour Therapy

Co. Antrim
Lifespring Centre
111 Cliftonville Road
Belfast BT14 6JQ
☎08 01232 753 658

Co. Dublin
Mary Stewart Carroll
Tallaght
☎01 4513364/4901750

Nuala Kiernan
22 Treesdale
Stillorgan Road
☎01 283 5648

The Natural Living
  Centre
Walmer House
Raheny, Dublin 5
☎01 832 7859/832 7861

Co. Limerick
Limerick Natural
  Healing Centre
64 Catherine Street
Limerick
John Quinlivan
☎061 400 431

Counselling and Psychotherapy

For a list of members of
the Irish Association of
Counselling and
Therapy (numbering
over 1,100) or for
referrals, contact:

The Irish Association of
  Counselling and
  Therapy (IACT)
8 Cumberland Street
Dún Laoghaire
Co. Dublin
☎01 230 0061

For a referral list of
members of the Irish
Council for
Psychotherapy, contact:

The Irish Council for
  Psychotherapy
17 Dame Court
Dublin 2. ☎01 679 4055

For a referral list of
therapists with an Irish
Institute of Counselling
& Hypnotherapy
diploma, contact:

Irish Institute of
  Counselling and
  Hypnotherapy
118 Stillorgan Road
Dublin 4. ☎01 260 0118
*List is updated in June of
each year.*

COUNSELLING/
PSYCHOTHERAPY
SERVICES

Co. Antrim
Absolute Stress
  Management
3 Botanic Avenue
Belfast
☎08 01232 434 991

Anchor Counselling
179 Holywood Road
Belfast
☎08 01232 650 690

Belfast Counselling and
  Training Centre
40 Victoria Square
Belfast
☎08 01232 242 597

Belfast Counselling
  Group, Ardoyne
  Women's Centre
32 Castlereagh Street
Belfast BT5 4NH
Margaret Radford BA
  BSc(Hons) Dip Couns
☎08 01232 461 481

Belfast Rape Crisis
  Centre
29 Donegall Street
☎08 01232 321 830

Avril Brown
113 University Street
Belfast
☎08 01232 312 942

Christine Christie BSc
110A University Street
Belfast BT7 1HH
☎08 01232 664 691 *and*
320 318

Contact Youth
2A Ribble Street, Belfast
☎08 01232 456 654 *or*
457 848

Barbara Corkey
163 University Street
Belfast. ☎08 01232 313 281

Department of
  Psychotherapy
100 King's Road, Belfast
☎08 01232 401 141

Epic
33a Woodvale Road
Belfast. ☎08 01232 748 922
or 351 908

Mary Grant Associates
Lifespring Centre
111 Cliftonville Road
Belfast BT14 6JQ
☎08 01232 753658

Carol Horner
21 Wandsworth Road
Belfast BT4 3LS
☎08 01232 653 651

Institute for Coun-
  selling & Personal
  Development
20–24 York St, Belfast
☎08 01232 330 996

Lifespring Centre
111 Cliftonville Road
Belfast BT14 6JQ
☎08 01232 753658

London Institute of
  Stress Management
336 Lisburn Rd, Belfast
☎08 01232 663 414 *or*
663 425

Eolath Magee BACAcc.
5 Victoria Road, Belfast
☎08 01232 421 678

The NEXUS Institute
119 University Street
Belfast BT7 1HP
☎08 01232 326 803

Quo Vadis Counselling
  Consultancy
539 Lisburn Road
Belfast BT9 7GQ
☎08 01232 665 502

Rape Crisis Centre
☎08 01232 249 696

Shankill Stress Group
Unit 22
Argyle Business Centre
39 North Howard Street
Belfast
☎08 01232 231 900

South Belfast Coun-
  selling Psychology
92–94 Lisburn Road
Anne Kelly BA Hons
  (Psych) CQSW
☎08 01232 491 759

Stepping Stone
123 Cavehill Road
Belfast BT15 5BJ
Lorraine Dell BSc.
  Hons Dip. Couns.
☎08 01232 777 378

Twin Spires
  Counselling Facility
Curran House
155 Northumberland St
Belfast. ☎08 01232 326 575

University Street
  Counselling Services
110a University Street
Belfast. ☎08 01232 320 218

YouthLine
2a Ribble Street, Belfast
☎08 01232 456 654

Co. Armagh
Foundation Ministries
The Pastoral Centre
35 Charlemont Gardens
Armagh. ☎08 01861 525 282

The NEXUS Institute
☎08 01762 350 588

Stepping Stone
333 Westacres
Drumgor, Criagavon
☎08 01762 343 287

Co. Carlow
Ionad Falláin
Myshall. ☎0503 57810

Anne Nolan MIACT
24 Burrin Street, Carlow
☎0503 42039

Solace
Dublin Street, Carlow
☎0503 30611

Co. Clare
Dominic Considine Dip CH; NLP Pract
Ennis. ☎065 28356

Liz Moorcroft, Dip. Couns. London CSCT
5 Springfield Court
Ennis. ☎065 23306

Co. Cork
Aids Alliance Cork
16 Peter's Street, Cork
☎021 275 837
Helpline: ☎021 276 676

Anthropos Centre
40 South Mall, Cork
☎021 278 591

Beara Circle Ltd
Castletownbere
Patricia Farrell/
Dr Martin Guggenheim/
Marianne Wagner
☎027 70744

Bettina Berger DRS
Donour West
Castlefreke, Clonakilty
☎023 40897

John Colly
5 North Main Street
Bandon. ☎023 41075

Counselling Centre
7 Fr Mathew Street
Cork. ☎021 273 995

Counselling and Psychotherapy
6 Sydney Place
Wellington Road, Cork
☎021 507 247

Cura (Cork) Pregnancy Counselling Service
34 Paul Street, Cork
☎021 277 544

Freda Emery BA, MSc (Psych.)
40B Pope's Quay, Cork
☎021 508 854

Anthony Fryer
Cush Grange
☎024 94530

Sr Mary Keenan
3 College View
Old Youghal Road
Cork. ☎021 364 177

Brenda Kelly BA HDE D.Psych. (UCD) MIACT
Montenotte, Cork
☎021 551 484

Dr Cormac Lankford MA Psychol.
71 Wilton Court, Cork
☎021 343 942 *and*
Waterfall, Cork
☎021 341 032

Carmel Long
Carrigaline, Cork
☎021 371 377

Joan Long
1 Rose Arden
Sunday's Well Road
Cork. ☎021 210 266

Fergus Lyons BSc D.Psych. MIAH
Kanturk. ☎087 460 465

Catherine Murray MIACT MUCKP MBPA
Newtown Hse Centre
Doneraile. ☎022 24117

Ray O'Connor
1 Rose Arden
Sunday's Well Road
Cork. ☎021 210 288

Anne O'Mahoney BA (Psych) MCoun.
Emmet House
Emmet Place, Cork
☎021 27 80 09

Martin Philpott MA HDCG Reg Psychol AFPs SI
The Medi Centre
Denney's Cross, Cork
☎021 343 791

Thelma Strickland Dip CH
☎021 292 749

Steps (ISPCC) Youth Advice & Counselling
12 Mary Street, Cork
☎021 318 600

Co. Derry
C.A.L.M.S. Stress Centre
32 Shipquay Street
Derry
☎08 01504 268 698

Cura — Derry
☎08 01504 268 467

Mid-Ulster Counselling & Therapy Service
6 Castledawson Road
Magherafelt *and*
10 Main St, Tobermore
Maghera
☎08 01648 45757

The NEXUS Institute
☎08 01504 260 566

Co. Donegal
Tír Chonaill Consultation & Therapy Practice
Glencar Scotch
Letterkenny
☎074 26405

Women's Aid Donegal Resource Centre
Letterkenny
☎074 26267

Co. Down
The Counselling Centre
36 Hamilton Road
Bangor
☎08 01247 274 664

Jim Hall Psychotherapist MMedSc(Phy) PGDipG & C CQS W Dip SW
2 Trummery Lane, Moira
☎08 01846 611068

Dr Ian Hanley,
BSc(Hon), MSc, PhD
7 Lynnehurst Drive
Comber. ☎08 01247 873 644

Mercy Counselling Unit
Catherine St, Newry
☎08 01693 250 529

Co. Dublin
Abba-Imma Centre
55 Main Street
Rathfarnham, Dublin 14
☎01 492 5757

Accept Counselling
Training
Blackrock. ☎01 280 0280

Acorn Centre
Portmarnock
Teresa Kavanagh BA
M.Psych Sc.
☎01 846 0390

Acorn Clinic
17 The Oaks
Upper Churchtown Rd
Dublin 14. ☎01 296 1551

Adult Child Institute
26 Anne Devlin Park
Dublin 14
☎01 494 4222/287 4804

Aisling Psychotherapy
Marlborough Road
Dublin 4. ☎01 497 6140

Albany Clinic
Lr Fitzwilliam St, Dublin 2
Mary O'Conor IACT
Accred. Dip PST
☎01 661 2222

Albany Psychological
Services
Clifton Court
Lr Fitzwilliam St, Dublin 2
Máiread Ryan BA Dip Psych
☎01 661 4828

Alfa Advisory &
Counselling Services
☎01 288 0222

Alisar Counselling
Ranelagh Court
Chelmsford Road
Dublin 6. ☎01 491 0187

Amethyst Centre
28 Beechcourt, Killiney
☎01 285 0976

Arduna Counselling &
Psychotherapy Centre
55 Clontarf Road
Dublin 3. ☎01 833 2733

Ark Counselling
86 St Begnet's Villas
Dalkey. Neal Keyes
☎01 284 8766

Mary & Hugh Arthurs
22 de Courcey Square
Glasnevin, Dublin 9
☎01 830 2187

Asklepios
Psychotherapy Centre
36 Balally Park. Dublin 16

Anthony Wilson MPhil,
Dip J Psychol Dip J
Psychotherapy FAPI
MEAP MEAC
MIITD/Sandra
Wilson Dip J Psychol
Dip J Psychotherapy
FAPI MIACT MEAP
MEAC
☎01 294 0601

Ashroy Counselling &
Hypnotherapy
22 Rathgar Avenue
Dublin 6
Frank McArdle MIACT
NCP (UK) Hyp Dip C
☎01 492 1793

Awakenings
Ranelagh, Dublin 6
Dr Bernard Stein MB
MMedSc (Psych)
☎01 492 0122

Aware Administration
147 Phibsoro Road
Dublin 7 ☎01 830 8449

Aware Help Line
☎01 679 1711

Pauline Beegan
110 Rock Road
Booterstown
☎01 288 2749

Belgrave Centre for
Counselling and
Psychotherapy
3 Charleston Rd, Rathmines
Dublin 6. ☎01 497 5666

Carl Berkeley MIACT
24 Terenure Road East
Rathgar, Dublin 6
☎01 490 9088

Noreen Bermingham
BA HDip Ed Dip C.G
MIACT
Milverton, Skerries
☎01 849 1658

Body Positive
53 Parnell Square West
Dublin 1. ☎01 872 0554

Kathleen Bolger Dip CH
Ballsbridge, Dublin 4
☎01 269 5383

Margaret Boland RGN
MEd (Human Relations)
MIACT
5 Cross Guns Quay
Phibsboro, Dublin 7
☎01 830 2545

Fierman Bolt M.SocSc/
Barbara Kohnstamm
5 Tivoli Terrace East
Dún Laoghaire
☎01 280 3789

Sean M. Bourke MIACT
MCHPC
54 Vernon Avenue
Clontarf, Dublin 3
☎01 833 6648

Eileen Boyle MIACT
57 Upr Grand Canal St
Dublin 4 ☎01 660 4574

Richard Boyle Dip CH
    M Pract NLP
Dartmouth Road
Dublin 6. ☎01 668 4480

Kay Branigan Dip CH
    NLP Pract
15 Kempton Avenue
Navan Road, Dublin 7
☎01 838 1912

Mary Brophy
66 Monkstown Road
Monkstown
☎01 284 3693

Paddy Browne IACT
    Accord
15 Riverside Crescent
Clonshaugh, Dublin 17
☎01 847 1669

Elvera Butler MA Dip.
    Hyp. M Prac NLP
77 Haddington Road
Dublin 4. ☎01 660 1578

Marie Campion Dip.
    CH, NLP Pract
    MAED (NY)
6 Marino Mart
Fairview, Dublin 3
☎01 833 3126

Mary Cantwell-Lynch
☎01 288 0222

Caring Solutions
    Counselling
Walkinstown
Dublin 12. ☎01 459 0551

Noel Carroll Dip CH
Clondalkin, Dublin 22
☎01 457 1924

Susan Cassidy
16 Main Street
Lucan. ☎01 628 3431

Paola Catizone Dip
    CH, Dip IYA
22B Ormond Road
Rathmines, Dublin 6
☎01 497 3215

Centre Care
1a Cathedral Street
Dublin 1
☎01 872 6775/874 6915

Centre for Creative
    Change
14 Upper Clanbrassil St
Dublin 8. ☎01 453 8356

Cherish
2 Lr Pembroke Street
Dublin 2. ☎01 668 2744

Christian Counselling
    Service
95 Sandyford Road
Dundrum, Dublin 14
☎01 295 0670

Ciaran Counselling &
    Healing Practice
4 Trimleston Road
Booterstown
☎01 269 1492

Clanwilliam Institute
18 Clanwilliam Terrace
Grand Canal Quay
Dublin 2. ☎01 676 1363

Helena Coghlan Dip
    Group Analysis
    MIACT
41 Lower Baggot Street
Dublin 2
☎01 660 9490

Catherine Collins ITEC
    MSRI LT Phys
136 New Cabra Road
Dublin 7. ☎01 868 1110

Dr Sean Collins BA
    (Psych) DCH M Pract
    NLP
32 Dawson Street
Dublin 2. ☎01 283 1000

Dr Maureen Concannon
    Dip. Psych. PhD
St Stephen's Green
Dublin 2. ☎01 475 1710

Connect Assocs.
Lonsdale House
Avoca Avenue
Blackrock. ☎01 288 4155

Lucy Costigan RT
    (Cert), Maynooth
    Dip. in Counselling,
    MIAH, Adv Dip in
    Clinical Hypnosis,
    Healer Mem (NFSH)
Irish Spiritual Centre
30–31 Wicklow Street
Dublin 2. ☎053 22923
*Holds sessions at the Irish
Spiritual Centre. Please
phone her Wexford
number for appointments.*

Counselling Direct
    (Ireland) Ltd
23 Sth Frederick Street
Dublin 2. ☎01 679 9638

Counselling for Eating
    Disorders
6 Marino Mart
Dublin 3. ☎01 833 3126

Ann Cox
3 Brookville Pk, Artane
Dublin 5. ☎01 831 2889

Brigid Coyle
100 St Lawrence Road
Dublin 3. ☎01 833 2479

Creative Counselling
    Centre
82 Upper George's St
Dún Laoghaire
☎01 280 2523

Dialogue Centre
69 Whitworth Road
Dublin 9. ☎01 830 9384

Margaret Dillane
Dublin 12. ☎01 455 1882

Rhoda Draper BA (Psych)
Dip CH, M Pract NLP
118 Stillorgan Road
Dublin 4. ☎01 260 0118

John Drum Counselling
Service
147 Lr Drumcondra Rd
Dublin 9. ☎01 837 6690

Dublin Counselling &
Therapy Centre
41 Upper Gardiner St
Dublin 1. ☎01 878 8236

John Duffy BA MSc
Medical Centre
Manor Mall Swords
☎01 840 1666

Dundrum Counselling
& Psychotherapy
4 Ashgrove Terrace
Dundrum, Dublin 16
☎01 296 2115

F.A. Dwyer
M.Sc.Counsl. Psych
49 Meadowbank
Bushy Park Road
Rathgar, Dublin 6
☎01 490 1058

Maeve Farrell Dip
Couns TCD MIACT
11 Hillcourt Park
Glenageary. ☎01 285 8324

Vivian Farrell Dip CH
Lucan. ☎01 624 1084

Adrian Farrelly Dip CH
21 Vernon Avenue
Clontarf, Dublin 3
☎01 833 1712

Ria Farren Dip CH
32 Ardagh Avenue
Blackrock ☎01 288 6764

Terry Ferris Dip CH
Rathfarnham
Dublin 14
☎01 837 7626

Kay Ferriter MSocSc
24 Hamilton Street
Dublin 8. ☎01 454 2140

Mark Fielding Dip CH
Churchtown, Dublin 14
☎01 296 1551

Siobhan Fielding
Churchtown, Dublin 14
☎01 296 1551

Joan Foran
331 Orwell Park Glen
Templeogue, Dublin 6w
☎01 450 7424

Una Gallagher Dip CH
Dip Addiction Studies
Lucan. ☎01 624 0076

Rita Gerrard RN DHyp
Adv DHyp DCS
16 Pine Valley Drive
Dublin 16. ☎01 493 9024

Iris Greene FRCOG MST
Glankeen
9 Sth Richmond Avenue
Dublin 6. ☎01 496 6961

Stuart Greene
☎01 450 9596

The Greenlea Clinic
118 Greenlea Road
Terenure, Dublin 6w
Diane Hayes MSc Dip
C.Psych
☎01 490 8979

Patrick Griffin BA Psych.
MSc Couns. Psych.
4 Charleville Road
Phibsboro, Dublin 7
☎01 838 0979

Group Analytic Practice
Global House
29 Lower Abbey Street
Dublin 1. ☎01 878 6486

Tim Hannan
11 Laurencebrook
Chapelizod, Dublin 20
☎01 623 3490

Isobel Haugh Dip.
Psych. Relationship
MIACT
6 Haddington Terrace
Dún Laoghaire
☎01 280 7117

Diane Hayes M.Sc. Psych
118 Greenlea Road
Terenure, Dublin 6W
☎01 490 8979

Terence Herron BA
CCDC (Hazelden)
MIACT
Lr Albert Rd, Sandycove

The Holistic Health
Centre
197 Lr Kimmage Road
Dublin 7. ☎01 492 9279

Celia Homan BA MIACT
Ballinclea Road
Killiney. ☎01 285 4717

Incare
32 Parnell Square
Dublin 1. ☎01 872 2419

Institute of Psychosocial
Medicine
2 Eden Park, Dún Laoghaire
☎01 280 0084

The Irish Institute for
Integrated
Psychotherapy
26 Longford Terrace
Monkstown
Patrick & Inger Nolan
☎01 280 9313

Irish Psycho-Analytical
Association
2 Belgrave Terrace
Monkstown
☎01 280 1869/496 7288
also 832 7111

Athene Keating MSc
Dip. Psych.
Monkstown. ☎01 285 2029

Dr Tom Kelly MB Dip.
Human Sexuality
67 Pembroke Road
Dublin 4. ☎01 283 1276

Patricia Kennedy MA
Psychol MIACT
3 Charleston Road
Dublin 6. ☎01 497 5666

Gerald Kenny
40 Ballymun Road
Dublin 9. ☎01 836 0669

Neal Keyes
86 St Begnet's Villas
Dalkey. ☎01 284 8766

Sheila Killoran-Gannon
BA Dip. Psychotherapy
MIACT
43 Belgrave Square West
Rathmines, Dublin 6
☎01 496 0545

Kilmacud Medical
Centre, St Luke's
Lower Kilmacud Road
Stillorgan
Eimear Burke BA MSc
☎01 288 1473

Norman Levine
7 Flemingstown Park
Churchtown, Dublin 14
☎01 298 4709

Life Pregnancy
Counselling Service
29 Dame Street
Dublin 2. ☎01 679 8989

Lucan Counselling Services
12a Lower Main Street
Lucan, Dublin 24
☎01 820 6597

Sarah MacAuley BA
55 Philipsburgh Ave.
Fairview, Dublin 3
☎01 837 0158

James McCabe
93 Grove Park
Dublin 6. ☎01 497 1745

Catherine McCann
MIACT
42 Donnybrook Manor
Belmont Avenue
Dublin 4. ☎01 283 8711

Áine McCarthy BASMT
Accred, MIACT
Howth Road, Raheny
Dublin 5. ☎01 831 8313

Paul McKeever
10 Prospect Road
Dublin 9
☎01 830 4371/830 3214

Fionnuala MacLiam
Dip B Psych
24 Belgrave Rd, Rathmines
Dublin 6. ☎01 497 3498

Brian McNamee MSc CAS
31 Taney Avenue
Dublin 14. ☎01 296 0773

Dr Anjm Madani MBBCH
Leonard's House
Leonard's Corner
Dublin 8. ☎01 453 2816

Patricia Malone
Dundrum, Dublin 14
☎01 298 9552

Cora Marshall MIACT
331 Orwell Park Glen
Templeogue, Dublin 6w
☎01 452 0941

Regina Martin RPN BA
MA Dip. Couns.
51 Northumberland Rd
Dublin 4. ☎01 667 2781

Pauline Meek
52 Dargle Road
Hollypark, Blackrock
☎01 289 6435

Joan Melvin-Perrem
108 Westbury, Stillorgan
☎01 283 2940

Milltown Counselling
Centre
Rowan Hall, Milltown
Dublin 6. ☎01 283 8248

Alan Mooney MIACT
MIAHIP
14 Upper Clanbrassil St
Dublin 8. ☎01 453 8356

Brendan Murphy Dip.
Psych, MPsychSc
(Psycho) MIACT
377 Clontarf Road
Dublin 3. ☎01 833 1758

Natural Health Clinic
The Mews
154 Leinster Road
Rathmines, Dublin 6
Maeve Halpin/
Bobbie Sparrow
☎01 496 1316

Paul Neiland Dip CH
Rathmines, Dublin 6
☎01 496 1316

New Day Counselling
Centre
Meath Street, Dublin 8
☎01 454 7050

New Perspectives
20 Main Street, Bray
☎01 287 3468

Newlands Institute for
Counselling
2 Monastery Road
Clondalkin, Dublin 22
☎01 459 4573

Jacinta Nolan BA MA
M. Psych Sc.
46 Woodley Park
Dublin 14
☎01 298 4356

Northside Counselling
Glasnevin, Dublin 9
☎01 830 2187

Northside Counselling
  Service
Greencastle Road
Dublin 5. ☎01 848 4789

Gay O'Brien BA Psych
  MEd Psych Science
1 Auburn Road
Castleknock, Dublin 15
☎01 821 7548

Áine O'Connor (Primal
  Janovian Psychotherapy,
  Existential — UK)
Donnybrook, Dublin 4
☎01 668 3123

Catherine O'Dea Dip.
  Psychotherapy MIACT
Eglinton House
Eglinton Terrace
Dundrum, Dublin 14
☎01 298 6204

Margot O'Donovan MA
  Dip Psychotherapy
5 Sycamore Walk
The Park, Dublin 18
☎01 284 9605

A.A. O'Driscoll Dip.
  Psych. Dip. Couns
69 Sweetmount Avenue
Dundrum, Dublin 14
☎01 298 3442

Alan O'Dwyer MIACT
26 Anne Devlin Park
Rathfarnham, Dublin 14
☎01 494 4222

Odyssey Healing
  Centre
15A Wicklow St, Dublin 2
Lesley Shoemaker MSc Ph
☎01 677 1021

Magda O'Farrell Dip.
  Psychotherapy
Springfield Lodge
Ballybride Road
Rathmichael
☎01 282 2893

Gill O'Halloran CQSW
  MIACT/Mike
  O'Halloran MA (Couns)
  MIACT
71 Monkstown Avenue
Monkstown. ☎01 280 5140

Omega Counselling
  Services
39 Wyteleaf Grove
Raheny, Dublin 5
☎01 848 6291

Terry O'Sullivan
98 Lr Churchtown Rd
Dublin 14. ☎01 296 1548

Liam Plant, Art
  Psychotherapist
91 Terenure Road North
Terenure, Dublin 6
☎01 492 9077

Practical Stress
  Management Ltd
Halcon House
Glenageary Office Park
☎01 285 0300

Professional
  Counselling Services
206 Moyville
Rathfarnham, Dublin 16
☎01 494 5818

Rape Crisis Centre
70 Lower Leeson Street
Dublin 2
(24 Hour) ☎01 661 4911
Counselling Line:
  ☎1800 77 88 88

Stephanie Regan
17 Main Street, Raheny
Dublin 5. ☎01 831 4812

Jocelyn Reilly DHP MIAH
1 Coast Road, Baldoyle
Dublin 13. ☎01 832 6758

Rock Road Psycho-
  therapy Centre
110 Rock Rd, Booterstown
☎01 288 2749

Dermot Rooney
  Psychotherapist
55 Clontarf Road
Dublin 3. ☎01 833 2733

Dr Eamonn Ryan
  G MRC Psych
7 Dartry Road
Dublin 6. ☎01 497 9807

Martin Ryan Dip CH
Glasnevin, Dublin 9
☎01 860 0078

Liz Ryan-Laragy
Clontarf, Dublin 3
☎01 853 0765

Saint Francis Therapy
  Centre
65 Crumlin Road
Dublin 12.
☎01 454 0559

Sue Saunders BSc MIACT
4 Trimleston Road
Booterstown
☎01 269 1492

Sensory Communications
6 Lakelands Close
Stillorgan
☎01 288 9355

J. Silver
Dublin. ☎087 445 516

Noeleen Slattery DAc
  PHyp. NCP
Main Street, Rathcoole
☎01 458 9672

Southside Counselling
  Service
Dublin 14. ☎01 298 3535

Stauros Foundation
1 Maywood Drive
Dublin 5. ☎01 831 5385

Dr B.M.B. Stein M.Med
  Sc (Psych)
Ranelagh, Dublin 6
☎01 492 0122

Steps Youth Advice &
  Counselling Service
4 Eustace Street
Dublin 2. ☎01 670 7690

Patricia Stewart BA
  (Psychol) MA
81 Monkstown Road
Monkstown
☎01 280 9565

The Stress Clinic
13 Upper Fitzwilliam St
Dublin 2. ☎01 661 1223

Tivoli Institute
24 Clarinda Park East
Dún Laoghaire
☎01 280 9178

Deborah Troop Reg.
  MICP MIACT
31 Castle Park
Monkstown
☎01 280 6321

Turning Point
23 Crofton Road
Dún Laoghaire
☎01 280 7888

Alec Watson
5 Mariner's Lane
Dún Laoghaire
☎01 280 5974

Patricia Watson BA Dip
  Psychotherapy
29 Balkhill Road
Howth, Dublin 13
☎01 832 2472

The Well Woman
  Centre
73 Lower Leeson Street
Dublin 2. ☎01 661 0083

Colm Wells Counselling
15 Riversdale Green
Dublin 22. ☎01 457 7417

W.O.V.E.
24 O'Connell Avenue
Dublin 7 ☎01 830 0153

Jenny Wright Dip CH,
  NLP Pract
Kilmacud
☎01 288 9355

Co. Galway
Aids Help West
Oznam House
St Augustine Street
Galway. ☎091 566 266

Brothers of Charity
10 Church Hill
Ballinasloe
☎0905 43687

M. F. Chambers
Gort Road, Loughrea
☎091 84 24 10

Mary Deneny
6 Francis St, Galway
☎088 624 023

Galway M.A.B.S. Ltd
Augustine House
St Augustine Street
☎091 569 349

Diarmuid Lavelle BA,
  Dip CH
Canavan House
Nuns Island, Galway
☎091 569 770

Edel Moylan BA MSc IACT
Drinagh
3 The Mass Path
Newcastle, Galway
☎091 525 283

Michael Mullally
Abbey House,
25 Upr Abbeygate St
Galway. ☎091 568 449

North Galway MABS Ltd
Social Services Centre
Dublin Road, Tuam
☎093 24421

Daniel Tanguay BA Litt
Spinners, Treannlaur
Maree, Oranmore
☎091 794 028

John P. Walls
Caherogan Athenry
☎091 844 196

Norman Warden
Knocan an Bhodaigh
Furbo, Galway
☎091 591 443

Dr Harvey Wasserman
Arch Tack Room
Flood Street, Galway
☎091 566 712

Co. Kerry
A. Kelliher
4 Cedar Court
Ashleigh Downes
Tralee. ☎066 20142

Kerry Counselling Service
Lr Liss, Cahirciveen
☎066 73095

Kerry Rape Crisis Centre
11 Denny Street, Tralee
☎066 23122

Killarney Counselling
  Service
Franciscan Friary
Killarney. ☎064 36416

Val & Tony McGinley
9 Westcourt, Tralee
☎066 24694

Mary Kate McMahon
  BA (Psych), Dip CH
Tralee. ☎066 56374

Ray O'Connor
Flat 1 Oakpark Cottage
Tralee. ☎066 29878

P.J. O'Neill
2 Denny Street, Tralee
☎066 20121

Desmond Quirke Dip CH
Tralee. ☎066 30293

Co. Kildare
Avision Counselling &
  Psychotherapy Services
Maynooth. ☎01 628 5353

Anne Ahern
1 Liffey Lawns
Clane. ☎045 868 751

Declan Burke Dip CH
16 Kerdiff Park, Naas
☎045 875 790

Angela Carr Dip CH,
NLP Pract
Kilcock. ☎01 628 4578

Adrian C. Doyle MIAHM
St David's Castle, Naas
☎045 874 350

Dúile Counselling Centre
Celbridge
Mary Lalor Reg FTNI IACT
☎01 627 3909

Gillford D'Souza MSc
Couns
Beaufield, Maynooth
☎01 628 5353

Lifestream Counselling
& Psychotherapy
Straffan Road, Maynooth
M. Dennison BSocSc
CQSW Dip Coun
☎01 628 9939

Co. Kilkenny
Teresa Foley Dip CH,
NLP Pract
Kilkenny. ☎056 65226

Rape Crisis Centre
(Carlow & Kilkenny)
5 Dean Street, Kilkenny
☎056 51555/1800 478478

South Leinster Rape
Crisis Centre
James Street House
Kilkenny ☎056 51950

Co. Limerick
Alcoholic Counselling
Service
Br Stephen Russell Hse
Mulgrave Street
Limerick. ☎061 310 303

Alternative Medicine
Clinic
40 William St, Limerick
Vincent L. Power MD
(MA) MS MBCMA
☎061 418 383

C.A.R.I. Foundation
2 Garryowen Road
St John's, Limerick
☎061 413 331

Marion Fenton SRN Lic
TCM
5 Alphonsus Terrace
Quin Street, Limerick
☎061 417 781

Ann Hamilton
40 Shannamore Park
Clareview. ☎061 327 717

Michael Hughes DHP
MIAH
Elm Park, Clarina
☎061 355 365

Eileen Lee RSM, M.Ed,
MSW, CSW
Mount St Vincent
O'Connell Avenue
Limerick. ☎061 314 576

Derry O'Malley Dip CH,
Lic Acu, MRTCMI
34 Catherine Street
Limerick ☎061 317 670

Rape Crisis Centre
17 Upper Mallow St
Limerick
☎1800 31 15 11

Co. Louth
Acorn Counselling
Wellington Quay
Drogheda
☎041 27489/51276

Áit Na Daoine
Muirhevnamore
Dundalk. ☎042 26645

Joan Clinton BA(Psych)
MSc(Psych)
Park Court, Park Street
Dundalk. ☎042 30172

Dundalk Centre For
Counselling
3 Seatown Place
Dundalk. ☎042 38333

Dundalk Christian
Counselling Centre
Ardee Terrace, Dundalk
☎042 27094

Patrick Griffin
Greenvale House
Ardee. ☎041 53297

Iomlánú Centre for Healing
& Creative Living
5 Roden Place
Dundalk. ☎042 32804

Lifestream Counselling
& Psychotherapy
Community Services
Centre
Fair Street, Drogheda
☎041 42810

Lifestream Counselling
& Psychotherapy
c/o CIC Clanbrassil St
Dundalk. ☎042 27823

Progressive
Hypnotherapy Clinic
Dundalk. ☎042 31206

Co. Mayo
Kilfinan Women's Centre
Moygownagh, Ballina
☎096 31900

Mayo Rape Crisis Centre
Ellison Street, Castlebar
☎094 25657

Co. Meath
Counselling Consultants
College Hill House
Braystown, Slane
☎041 24781

Co. Monaghan
Lifestream Counselling
 & Psychotherapy
Main Street, Castleblayney
☎042 49189

Co. Offaly
Thomas O'Connor Dip
 CH, Dip HH Mass.
73 Greenwood Park
Edenderry
☎0405 3 13 46

Tullamore Rape Crisis
 Centre
Bolger House
Patrick St, Tullamore
☎0506 22500

Co. Roscommon
Roscommon Support
 Group
Resource Centre
Derrane
☎0903 25852

Co. Sligo
Frances McArdle
Keely, Drumcliff
☎071 63694

Rape Crisis Centre
The Manse, Wine Street
Sligo. ☎071 71188

Co. Tipperary
Clonmel Rape Crisis
 Centre
20 Mary Street, Clonmel
☎052 27677/1800 340340

Knockanrawley
 Resource Centre
Tipperary Town
☎062 52688

Anne McKee
Lisgarode, Kilruane
Nenagh. ☎067 32871

Libby McManus BA
Rosemary Square
Roscrea. ☎0505 21222

Gerard Myers
40 Kenyon Street
Nenagh. ☎067 33280

Co. Tyrone
St Anne's Pastoral Centre
Newtownkennedy St
Strabane
☎08 01504 884 938

Tara Counselling &
 Personal Development
 Centre
11 Holmview Terrace
Omagh
☎08 01662 250 024

Co. Waterford
E.A.P. Institute
143 Barrack Street
Waterford. ☎051 855 733

D. Graham. D.Psy
 D.Hyp DHC MIAH
Clinic, Main Street
Tramore. ☎051 386 651

Anne Howard MIACT
Tramore. ☎051 38 11 80

Phyllis Lea Dip CH
Tramore. ☎051 390 625

Oasis House
72 Morrisson's Road
Waterford. ☎051 370 367

Maura O'Meara Med.,
 MSc DAC
20 Lr Alphonsus Road
Newtown. ☎051 877 050

Mary Murphy
Coolhull, Duncormick
☎051 561 132

Waterford Rape Crisis
 Centre
2A Waterside, Waterford
☎051 873 362 *or*
1800 29 62 96

Co. Westmeath
Oliver Gallagher Dip CH
Mullingar. ☎044 41315

Lifestream Counselling
 & Psychotherapy
Parish Ctre, Bishopsgate St
Mullingar. ☎044 40871

Co. Wexford
Lucy Costigan RT (Cert),
 Maynooth Dip. in
 Counselling, MIAH, Adv
 Dip in Clinical Hypnosis,
 Healer Mem (NFSH)
Wexford. ☎053 22923

ISPCC Steps
40 Abbey Street
Wexford ☎053 23864

Alice McLoughlin IACT
 IAAAC MA Couns. &
 Human Relations
☎053 37412

Oasis Counselling
 Service MIACT
Creagh, Gorey. ☎055 21591

Tony O'Neill
Klaradine, The Cools
Barntown. ☎053 34513

Wexford Rape Crisis Centre
Clifford Street, Wexford
☎053 22722

Co. Wicklow
Assumpta Byrne
The Banks, Manor Kilbride
☎01 458 2407

Patricia Cameron
76 Beachdale, Kilcoole
☎01 287 5330

Chrysalis Centre
Donard. ☎045 404 713

Emily Counselling Centre
2 Emily Hse, Trafalgar Rd
Greystones. ☎01 287 3764

Holistic Therapy Clinic
Bray
Massan Ghorbani Dip
 CH CHHS
☎01 286 4085

Mary Johnson MIACT
St George's, Herbert Rd
Bray. ☎01 287 1257

New Perspectives
20 Main Street, Bray
☎01 287 3468

Maura O'Toole Dip CH
Manor Kilbride
Blessington. ☎01 458 2314

Aurelie Silverlock Dip CH
20 Main Street, Bray
☎01 287 3468

MARITAL/RELATIONSHIP
COUNSELLING

Co. Antrim
Accord Catholic Marriage
  Counselling Service
Kenbaan
13 Broughshane Road
Ballymena
☎08 01266 44072 *and*
Cana House
56 Lisburn Rd, Belfast
☎08 01232 233 002 *and*
Curran House
Twin Spires Centre
155 Northumberland St
Belfast. ☎08 01232 339 944

Jackie Graham BSSc
  Cert C.C Relate
1 Cranmore Park
Belfast. ☎08 01232 662 942

Relate
Station Road, Antrim
☎08 01849 464 931 *and*
76 Dublin Road, Belfast
☎08 01232 323454

Co. Armagh
Accord Catholic Marriage
  Counselling Service
1 Tavanagh Avenue
Portadown
☎08 01762 334 781

Co. Carlow
Accord Catholic Marriage
  Counselling Service
St Catherine's Commu-
  nity Service Centre
St Joseph's Rd, Carlow
☎0503 31354

Co. Cavan
Accord Catholic Marriage
  Counselling Service
Cana Hse, Farnham St
Cavan. ☎049 31378

Co. Clare
Accord Catholic Marriage
  Counselling Service
Clarcare Harmony Row
Ennis. ☎065 24297

Co. Cork
Accord Catholic Marriage
  Counselling Service
Parish Centre, Cobh
☎021 813 095 *and*
Family Centre, Fermoy
☎025 32249 *and*
Monument Hill, Fermoy
☎025 31899 *and*
Parish Centre, Mallow
☎022 20276

Cork Marriage
  Counselling Centre
34 Paul Street, Cork
☎021 275 678
Bantry. ☎027 50272
Skibbereen. ☎028 22564

Counselling &
  Mediation Services
16 Academy Street
Cork. ☎021 271 606 *and*
6 Sidney Place
Wellington Road, Cork
☎021 507 247

Colum Layton
1 Park Villas, Victoria Rd
Cork. ☎021 313 129

Marriage Counselling
23 Tuckey Street, Cork
☎021 277 906

Dr Gillian Moore-
  Groarke BA (Hons)
  PhD NUI AFP PsIR
Cork. ☎021 343 073

Co. Derry
Accord Catholic Marriage
  Counselling Service
164 Bishop Street, Derry
☎08 01504 362 475 *and*
159 Glen Road, Maghera
☎08 01648 42983

Relate
4–6 Strand Road, Derry
☎08 01504 371 502

Co. Down
Accord Catholic Marriage
  Counselling Service
32 English Street
Downpatrick
☎08 01396 613 435 *and*
Cana House
4 Trevor Hill, Newry
☎08 01693 63577

Co. Dublin
Accord Catholic Marriage
  Counselling Service
39 Harcourt Street
Dublin 2. ☎01 478 0866
and
Central Office
All Hallows
Gracepark Road
Dublin 9. ☎01 837 1151
and
Unit 23 Ballymun S. C.
Ballymun, Dublin 9
☎01 862 1508 *and*
Accord House
Church Avenue
Blanchardstown
Dublin 15
☎01 820 1044 *and*

St Kevin's
Monastery Road
Clondalkin, Dublin 22
☎01 459 3467 *and*
7 Eblana Avenue
Dún Laoghaire
☎01 280 1682 *and*
71 Griffith Ave., Marino
Dublin 9. ☎01 833 8631
and
15 Dalymount
Phibsborough, Dublin 7
☎01 868 0028/868 0053
and
Seatown Road, Swords
☎01 840 4550 *and*
The Square, Tallaght
☎01 459 0337 *and*
265 Templeogue Road
Templeogue, Dublin 6w
☎01 490 8739

Accord Pre-Marriage
   Course
Mount Argus, Dublin 6
☎01 492 3165
also ☎01 478 4400

Belgrave Marriage
   Counselling Service
3 Charleston Road
Rathmines, Dublin 6
☎01 497 5666

Clanwilliam Institute
19 Clanwilliam Terrace
Grand Canal Quay
Dublin 2. ☎01 676 1363

Carroll Kelly
Milltown, Dublin 6
☎01 283 8248

Patricia Kennedy BA MA
   Reg Psychol, PsSI
3 Charleston Road
Dublin 6. ☎01 497 5666

Marriage Counselling
   Service
24 Grafton Street
Dublin 2. ☎01 872 0341

Newlands Institute for
   Counselling
2 Monastery Road
Clondalkin, Dublin 22
☎01 459 4573

Premarriage Courses &
   Marriage Guidance
16 Nth Gt George's St
Dublin 1. ☎01 878 6156

Co. Fermanagh
Accord Catholic Marriage
   Counselling Service
Aisling Centre
37 Darling St, Enniskillen
☎08 01365 325 696

Co. Galway
Accord Catholic Marriage
   Counselling Service
Social Service Centre
Brackernagh, Ballinasloe
☎0905 43573 *and*
Árus De Bruen
Newtownsmyth
Galway. ☎091 562 331
and
Cathedral Terrace
Tuam. ☎093 24900

Galway Marriage Tribunal
7 Waterside, Woodquay
Galway. ☎091 565 179

Co. Kerry
Accord Catholic Marriage
   Counselling Service
Pastoral Centre
Rock Road, Killarney
☎064 32644 *and*
St Johns Pastoral Centre
Castle Street, Tralee
☎066 20 94/22280

Co. Kildare
Accord Catholic Marriage
   Counselling Service
Parish Centre
Station Rd, Newbridge
☎045 431 695

Clane Counselling
1 Liffey Lawns, Clane
☎045 868 751

Lifestream Marriage
   Counselling
Straffan Road
Maynooth. ☎01 628 9939

Co. Kilkenny
Accord Catholic Marriage
   Counselling Service
St Mary's Centre
James' Street, Kilkenny
☎056 22674

Co. Laois
Accord Catholic Marriage
   Counselling Service
St Joseph's
Dublin Road
Portlaoise. ☎0502 21142

Co. Limerick
Accord Catholic Marriage
   Counselling Service
66 O'Connell Street
Limerick. ☎061 313 287
and
Parish Centre
Newcastlewest
☎069 61000

Co. Longford
Accord Catholic Marriage
   Counselling Service
Family Centre
St Mel's Rd, Longford
☎043 47222

Co. Louth
Accord Catholic Marriage
   Counselling Service
Verona, Crosslanes
Drogheda. ☎041 29614
and
Roden Place, Dundalk
☎042 31731

Co. Mayo
Accord Catholic Marriage
  Counselling Service
Pastoral Centre
Cathedral Grounds
Ballina. ☎096 21478 *and*
Family Centre
Castle Street, Castlebar
☎094 25900 *and*
Charlestown
☎094 54317

Co. Meath
Accord Catholic Marriage
  Counselling Service
CYWS Hall, Navan
☎046 23146

Co. Monaghan
Accord Catholic Marriage
  Counselling Service
St MacArtan's College
Monaghan. ☎047 83359

Co. Offaly
Accord Catholic Marriage
  Counselling Service
St Brigid's Place
Tullamore. ☎0506 41831

Co. Roscommon
Accord Catholic Marriage
  Counselling Service
St Coman's Club
Abbey St, Roscommon
☎0903 26619

The Family Institute
Ballaghaderreen
☎0907 61000

Co. Tipperary
Accord Catholic Marriage
  Counselling Service
Pastoral Centre
Irishtown, Clonmel
☎052 24144 *and*
Accord House
Cathedral St., Thurles
☎0504 22279 *and*

Loretta House
Kenyon Street, Nenagh
☎067 34300 *and*
Social Service Centre
St Michael's Street
Tipperary. ☎062 33330

Co. Tyrone
Accord Catholic Marriage
  Counselling Service
Pastoral Centre
48 Brook Street, Omagh
☎08 01662 242 439

Professional
  Counselling Centre
Tullycall House
10 Tullycall Road
Cookstown
☎08 016487 61158

Co. Waterford
Accord Catholic Marriage
  Counselling Service
4 George's Street
Waterford
☎051 878 333

Co. Westmeath
Accord Catholic Marriage
  Counselling Service
Alverna, Northgate St
Athlone. ☎0902 75491
and
Mullingar Social
  Service Centre
☎044 48707

Co. Wexford
Accord Catholic Marriage
  Counselling Service
St Brigid's Centre
Roches Road, Wexford
☎053 23086

Co. Wicklow
Accord Catholic Marriage
  Counselling Service
New Street, Wicklow
☎0404 67119

BEREAVEMENT
COUNSELLING

Co. Derry
Cruse Bereavement Care
9 Crawford Square
Derry
☎08 01504 262 941

Cruse Bereavement Care
Citizens Advice Bureau
43 Queen Street
Magherafelt
☎08 01648 301 808

Co. Antrim
Cruse Bereavement Care
Room 31, Spruce House
Braid Valley Hospital
Cushendall Road
Ballymena
☎08 01266 630 900

Cruse Bereavement Care
Robinson Memorial
  Hospital
Newal Rd, Ballymoney
☎08 012656 66686

Cruse Bereavement Care
Knockbracken
  Healthcare Park
Saintfield Road, Belfast
☎08 01232 792 419

Cruse Bereavement Care
50 University Street
Belfast
☎08 01232 232 695

Co. Carlow
Bereavement
  Counselling Service
Carlow. ☎0503 40977

Co. Down
Cruse Bereavement Care
Unit 55
4 Balloo Avenue
Balloo Industrial Estate
Bangor
☎08 01247 272 444

Co. Dublin
Bereavement
  Counselling Service
Dublin Street, Baldoyle
☎01 839 1766 *and*
St Anne's, Dawson St
☎01 676 7727
also at:
Baldoyle
☎01 832 1367
Ballyboden
☎01 494 4966
Dundrum/Phibsborough
☎01 839 1766
Raheny. ☎01 831 3700
Rialto. ☎01 453 9020

Co. Fermanagh
Cruse Bereavement Care
Aisling Centre
Darling St, Enniskillen
☎08 01365 322 844

Co. Kildare
Bereavement
  Counselling Service
Newbridge
☎045 433 563

Co. Tyrone
Cruse Bereavement Care
4b Dungannon St, Moy
☎08 01868 784 004

Cruse Bereavement Care
Riverside House
County Hospital
Woodvale Avenue
Omagh
☎08 01662 244 414

Cranio-sacral Therapy

Co. Dublin
Joan Davis
'The Studio'
Rere 330
Harold's Cross Road
Dublin 6. ☎01 287 6986

Ann Gill
☎01 845 0698

The Healing Place
61 St Assam's Park
Raheny, Dublin 5
☎01 848 4270 *or*
087 461 853

MELT, Temple Bar
  Natural Healing Centre
2 Temple Lane
Dublin 2. ☎01 679 8786

Áine O'Connor
Donnybrook, Dublin 4
☎01 668 3123

Co. Wicklow
Mary O'Brien DO
41 Glenthorn, Bray
☎01 286 2054

Creative Therapy

Co. Dublin
Kiltalown House
  Creativity Centre
Blessington Road
Jobstown, Tallaght
Dublin 24. ☎01 452 2466

Mary Roden
66 Lower Baggot Street
Dublin 2. ☎01 287 2549

Co. Wicklow
Arts Unlimited
4 Carrig Villas
Killincarrig, Greystones
Mary Roden
☎01 287 2549.

Crystal Healing

Co. Carlow
Jacquie Burgesse
Slaney Hse, Barrack St
Tullow. ☎0503 51057

Co. Cavan
Christine McGuinness
Upper Main Street
Cavan. ☎049 61019

Co. Cork
Terri Blanche
30 Sevenoaks
Frankfield
Douglas. ☎021 891 527

Inner Healing Centre
46 Sheares Street, Cork
☎021 278 243

Co. Dublin
Terri Blanche
16B Clonskeagh Road
Ranelagh, Dublin 6
☎01 269 8217 *and*
Odyssey Healing
  Centre
15 Wicklow Street
Dublin 2. ☎01 677 1021

Crystal Mystique
Unit 4 Townyard Lane
Malahide. ☎01 845 5599

The Natural Health
  Clinic
The Mews
154 Leinster Road
Rathmines, Dublin 6
Jacquie Burgesse
☎01 496 1316

Cutting the Ties

Co. Clare
Zahid Abdullah
136 Finian Park
Shannon. ☎061 363 347

Co. Dublin
Sarah Branagan
Irish Spiritual Centre
30/31 Wicklow Street
Dublin 2.☎01 670 7034

The College of
  Metaphysicians
Park Centre
120 Sundrive Road
Dublin 12
Jay Silver. ☎087 445 516

George Rhattigan
7 The Drive
Kingswood Heights
Tallaght, Dublin 24
☎01 452 2722

Drama Therapy

The following can be contacted by writing to:

The Irish Association of
Drama, Art and
Music Therapists
PO Box 4176, Dublin 1.

Co. Dublin
Ann Cole, Dublin 4

Martina Dunne
Rathcoole

Damien McCormack
Dublin 15

Katie Woolett
Dublin 4

Co. Longford
Angela Bracken

Co. Sligo
Bernadine McManus

Northern Ireland
Janet O'Hagan

Energy Healing

Co. Limerick
Limerick Natural
 Healing Centre
64 Catherine Street
Limerick
John Quinlivan
☎061 400431

TONY QUINN CENTRES

Co. Armagh
Yvonne Sherry
41 Upper English St
Armagh
☎08 01861 525 742

Co. Cork
Imelda Farrell
20 Academy Street
Cork. ☎021 276364

Co. Dublin
Aideen Cowman
9–11 Grafton Street
Dublin 2
☎01 671 2788/830 4211
and
66 Eccles Street
Dublin 7
☎01 830 4211/830 3717

Christine Kelly
96 Lr George's Street
Dún Laoghaire
☎01 280 9891

Rita Kelly
2 Wynnfield Road
Rathmines, Dublin 6
☎01 497 4234

Co. Fermanagh
Yvonne Sherry
Aisling Centre
Darling Street
Enniskillen
☎08 01861 525 742

Co. Galway
Victoria Hotel
Eyre Square, Galway
☎01 830 4211

Co. Kildare
Paul Doyle
Basin Street, Naas
☎01 830 4211

Co. Louth
Georgina Dolan
18 Jocelyn Street
Dundalk. ☎042 38097

Faith Healing

As there is no professional
body of faith healers, it is
not possible to publish a full

list of faith healers. The
following are available
for appointments:

Co. Carlow
Dan O'Neill
Hollybrook, Myshall
☎0503 57636

Co. Wexford
Paddy Murphy
8 Bosheen Road
New Ross, Co. Wexford
☎051 21236

Family Therapy

For a list of members of the
Family Therapy Association
of Ireland contact Ann
Daly, ☎01 679 4055

Co. Dublin
Clanwilliam Institute
19 Clanwilliam Terrace
Grand Canal Quay
Dublin 2. ☎01 676 1363

Family Therapy &
 Counselling Centre
46 Lr Elmwood Avenue
Ranelagh, Dublin 6
☎01 497 1188/497 1722

Pauline Meek
52 Dargle Rd, Hollypark
Blackrock. ☎01 289 6435

Co. Kilkenny
Friary Court Family
 Therapy Service
Friary Street, Kilkenny
☎056 61602

Co. Laois
Family Group Help Line
87 Marian Place
Portlaoise. ☎0502 60479

Co. Tipperary
Anne McKee
Lisarode, Kilruane
Nenagh. ☎067 32871

Gestalt

Co. Cork

Freda Creedon
Demesne, Dunmanway
☎023 45361

Fiona Devlin
6 Sydney Place
Wellington Road, Cork
☎021 507 247

Frank Dorr
Cork Social and Health
   Project
Grattan Street, Cork

Carmel Hamill/
   Máiréad Lindon
1 Ballinure Crescent
Mahon. ☎021 358 372

Eileen Harrington
11 Derrynane Road
Turner's Cross
☎021 962 198

Eileen Lynch
5 Kilbarry Cottages
Dublin Hill, Cork
☎021 305 945/273 088

Derry Mohally
22 Glendale Rd, Glasheen

Brenda Perrem
3 Sydenham Terrace
Monkstown. ☎021 842 087

Sue Stevens
Foilnamuck, Ballydehob
☎028 37264

Ronnie Swain
Dept of Applied Psychology
University College Cork

George Wallace
5 Castle Close
Ferney Road, Mahon
☎021 358 206

Co. Donegal

Janet Gaynor
5 Tara Court, Letterkenny
☎074 24730

Dan McCarthy
3 Knocknamona Park
Letterkenny. ☎074 22774

Maura McNally
Dromore, Mount Charles
☎073 21506/35411

Co. Dublin

Dundrum Gestalt Centre
Dundrum Road
Dublin 14. ☎01 296 2015

Emma Foy
The Mews, Summerhill Hse
Marino Avenue West
Killiney. ☎01 284 0501

Brian Howlett
1B Belfield Court
Donnybrook, Dublin 4
☎01 283 8233

Ann Kavanagh
100 Martello Court
Portmarnock
☎01 847 2242

Sarah Kay
2 Longwood Avenue
South Circular Road
Dublin 8. ☎01 453 0344

Derry McDermott
56 Monastery Drive
Clondalkin, Dublin 22
☎01 459 3191

Mary O'Halloran
10 Woodcliff Heights
Howth. ☎01 832 5004

Joan O'Leary
5 Abbey Street, Howth
☎01 839 0437

Mary Prenderville
Grange Cottage
Kilbride, Dublin 15
☎01 825 6599

Muireann Quinn
34 Ben Éadair Road
Dublin 7. ☎01 838 4688

Karen Shorten
28 Parkwood Grove
Aylesbury, Tallaght
Dublin 24. ☎01 451 4637

Co. Limerick

Declan Aherne
3 Stradbally North
Castleconnell, Limerick
☎061 202 332/377 485

Tom Geary
23 The Moorings
Westbury, Corbally
☎061 340 826

Teresa Moloney
Aherina, Kilmore

Mag Tierney
Kilmoremoy, Friarstown
Ballyclough. ☎061 229 143

Co. Wexford

Susan Mooney Duggan
Dunmoy, Kylerue
Ballyanne, New Ross
☎051 21278

Herbalism

For a full listing of medical
herbalists, contact the
National Institute of
Medical Herbalists (MH)
at ☎0044 1392 426 022

Co. Antrim

Belfast Chinese Medical
   Clinic
80 Upper Lisburn Road
Belfast BT10 0AD
☎08 01232 600 600

Co. Clare

Carole Guyett MH
The Lodge, Feakle
☎061 924 268

Clare de Freitas MH
Santa, Belvar Cross
Sixmilebridge
☎061 367 073

Co. Cork
Beara Circle
Castletownbere
Ulla Kinon. ☎027 70744

Evergreen Clinic of
  Natural Medicine
79 Evergreen Rd, Cork
Kevin Orbell-McSean MH
☎021 966 209

Juliet Fishbourne MH
5 Montpellier Terrace
Wellington Road, Cork
☎021 507 246

Jackie Kilbryde MH
Cooragurteen, Ballydehob

Margaret Kruijswijk
Mourneabbey, Mallow
☎022 29102

John Twomey
Main St, Carrigtwohill
☎021 883 800

White Hall Products Ltd
Church Cross
☎028 38117

Co. Derry
Derry City Clinic of
  Herbal Medicine
18A Queen Street
Derry BT48 7EF
David Foley MH
☎08 01504 271 500

Co. Donegal
Jamshid Hashemi-Zadeh
  MH
23 Whitehorn Park
Gortlee Rd, Letterkenny
☎074 27164

Co. Down
Vivien. E. Bell MH, Ir.
Rockfield, 89A Carnreagh
Hillsborough BT26 6LJ
☎08 01846 683 390

Co. Dublin
Chinese Natural Health
  Centre
80 Aungier Street
Dublin 2. ☎01 475 6974

Fitzwilliam Acupuncture
  & Herbal Clinic
77 Lower Leeson Street
Dublin 2
Dr M.S. Khan MBBS C
  AC China
☎01 676 4912

A. Hughes BSc Lic TCM
1 Leopardstown Drive
Dublin. ☎01 288 0352

Helen McCormack MH
186 Philipsburgh Ave.
Marino, Dublin 3
☎01 836 8965

Cathryn Morley
31 Wicklow Street
Dublin 2
☎01 671 3467/679 1846

The Natural Health Clinic
Mews, 154 Leinster Rd
Rathmines, Dublin 6
☎01 496 1316

The Natural Living
  Centre
Walmer Hse, Station Rd
Raheny, Dublin 5
Helen McCormack
☎01 832 7859

Natures Way Dublin Ltd
115 St Stephen's Green
  Shopping Centre
Dublin 2. ☎01 478 0165

E. Nielsen
Castlefield, Monastery Rd
Dublin 22. ☎01 459 3058

Nicholas Power Lic Ac
  D Ac
50 Sandycove Road
Dún Laoghaire
☎01 280 3505

Co. Galway
Linda Heffernan Lic Ac
6 St Brendan's Road
Woodquay, Galway
☎091 561 676

Co. Kerry
Mega Herb Store Ltd
Wholesale Chinese
  Herb Prescriptions
38 New Street, Killarney
☎064 35995

Co. Limerick
Alternative Medicine
  Clinic
40 William St, Limerick
Vincent L. Power MD
  (MA) MS, MBCMA
☎061 418 383

Cherryfield Clinic of
  Herbal Medicine
Ballysimon Rd, Limerick
☎061 415 588

Eats of Eden
Henry St–Shannon St
Limerick. ☎061 419 400

Co. Louth
Herbalwise
Rockmarshall, Jenkinstown
Dundalk. ☎042 76163

Co. Meath
Sean Boylan/Mary Hutton/
  Martin O'Reagan
Edenmore, Dunboyne
☎01 825 5250

Co. Roscommon
Áine Molloy MH
Tinecarra, Boyle

Co. Tipperary
Christine Maxwell
Dulcamara, Modeshill
Mullinahone
☎052 53256

Co. Tyrone
Cookstown Clinic of
  Herbal Medicine
4 Fairnhill Road
Cookstown BT80 8AG
Robert Elliot MH
☎08 016487 61661

Co. Wicklow
The Herbal and
  Homoeopathic Clinic
Eagle Hse, Sidmonton Ave.
Bray. ☎01 286 6280

Holotropic

Co. Dublin
Dublin Counselling
  and Therapy Centre
41 Upper Gardiner St
Dublin 1. ☎01 878 8236

Co. Louth:
Dundalk Counselling
  Centre
Oakdeane, 3 Seatown
Dundalk. ☎042 38333

Home Births

The Home Birth Centre
keeps a current list of
midwives available to
attend home births. The
Centre is based in *Co.
Meath* (see below). The
regional contacts are
also listed below.

Co. Clare
Clare Sheehan
☎061 925 187

Co. Cork
Mary Horan. ☎021 874 135

Christina Nicholas
☎027 50003

Co. Donegal
Geraldine Leech-West
☎074 47116

Co. Galway
Margaret O'Riordan
☎091 85659

Co. Kerry
Theresa Murphy
☎066 26901

Co. Kilkenny
Phyllida Clarke
☎056 69109

Susie Long. ☎056 64510

Co. Leitrim
Ester Hoad
Cloonboney, Mohill

Co. Meath
The Home Birth Centre
Langford Cottages
Summerhill
Monica O'Connor
☎0405 57795

Carmel Duffy. ☎0405 55595

Linda Fitzpatrick
☎01 835 1630

Co. Offaly
Francis Heaney
☎044 23230

Co. Sligo
Deirdre Cox. ☎071 42367

Co. Tipperary
Joanne Berkery
☎067 38172

Carmel & Ger McEvoy
☎052 23135

Co. Waterford
Catherine Drea
☎051 96172

Co. Westmeath
Francis Heaney
☎044 23230

Co. Wexford
Frederike Fredericks
☎053 59218

Co. Wicklow
Judith Crowe
☎01 281 9515

MIDWIVES

The following are
available to facilitate
home births.

Co. Cork
Mary Cronin
Melifontstown, Kinsale
☎021 500 819

Juana Dunworth
27 Calderwood Court
Donnybrook, Douglas
☎021 363 712

Elke Hasner
Kilnarovanagh
Toames, Macroom
☎026 46312

Anita Kuishi
☎023 34862

Betty O'Toole
☎021 361016.

Co. Dublin
Ann Kelly
Temple Crescent
Blackrock. ☎284 5058

Margaret O'Riordan
54 Páirc na gCaor
Moycullen. ☎091 85659

Kate Spillane
78 Bayside Crescent
Sutton. ☎01 839 1158
Co. Galway

Co. Kerry
Ann Govan
18 Rock Road
Killarney. ☎064 32901

Co. Leitrim
Lesley Foley
Monien, Kinlough
☎072 41839

Co. Meath
Dolores Staunton
Khublai, Harristown
Kilcloon. ☎01 628 5302

Co. Wicklow
Bridget Cummings
Calva, Ballybawn
Enniskerry. ☎01 286 3501

Cliona McLoughlin
7 Greenpark Road
Bray. ☎01 286 6106

BIRTH POOLS
Co. Dublin
Anne and Mary Dunne
10 Carrrickhill Drive
Portmarnock
☎01 846 3130

Co. Wicklow
Judith Crowe
The Hermitage
Newtownmountkennedy
☎01 281 9515

Homoeopathy

For a list of registered
members of the Irish
Society of Homoeopaths
(IS Hom), contact:

The Irish Society of
Homoeopaths
☎01 278 3161

Co. Antrim
The Nature Nook
4 Victoria St, Ballymoney
☎08 012656 64178

Co. Clare
Franz Scholand
Caherbarnagh
Liscannor. ☎065 81563

Jane Tottenham
Bíseach Holistic Centre
Lysaght's Lane, Ennis
☎065 23890

Co. Cork
W.S. Allen
Lower Rathduff
Grenagh. ☎021 886 592

Beara Circle
Castletownbere
Ulla Kinon IS Hom
☎027 70744

Betic Holistic Healing
Centre
Knocknagallagh
Bandon. ☎023 43015

Cork Road Clinic
Carrigaline
Drs Sean & Mary Dunphy
☎021 371 177

Freedom Holistic Centre
Church Mews
Church Lane, Midleton
☎021 642 466

Lindsay Hickey
Mallow Cottage
Finaha, Castletownbere
☎027 70456

Angela Kearney IS Hom.
Knockeen, Toormore
Goleen. ☎028 35182

Margaret Kruijswijk
Mourneabbey, Mallow
☎022 29102

Natural Medicine
Clinic
Main Street, Carrigaline
Dr Jennifer Daly MB
MICGP Lic Ac MIRI
☎021 372 787

Hannah O'Brien MIRI
Inchnagree, Buttevant
☎022 24286

Sandra Tyrrell
Reentrisk, Allihies
Beara. ☎027 73080 *or*
11 Marlboro Street
Cork. ☎021 274 273

Dr Bastiaan Van Eynatten
5 Adelaide Terrace
Wellington Road, Cork
☎021 509 488

Co. Donegal
Hans Martin
Weitbrecht IS Hom
Letterbarrow
☎073 35319

Co. Dublin
Acupuncture &
Homoeopathic Clinic
Unit 6 Phibsboro S.C.
Dublin 7. ☎01 830 9551

Ruth Appleby DSH
RSHom IS Hom
168 Harold's Cross Rd
Dublin 6w. ☎01 491 0387

Frances Bowe IS Hom
66 Mount Anville Wood
Goatstown, Dublin 14
☎01 278 3161

Clinic of Wholistic
Medicine
50 Merrion Square
Dublin 2. ☎01 676 4640

Dr James A Dolan MB.
DOBS. DCH MF Hom
Suite 1B, Olympia House
62 Dame Street, Dublin 2
☎01 677 3591 *or*
191 Howth Rd, Killester
Dublin 5. ☎01 833 5962

Marie Doyle
The Harcourt Clinic
20Harcourt Street
Dublin 2. ☎01 475 7358

Farmer's Pharmacy
Unit 2, Dundrum S.C.
Dublin 14. ☎01 298 7337

Dr Brendan Fitzpatrick
MB MRCPI DCH DO
MF Hom
115 Morehampton Rd
Dublin 4. ☎01 269 7768

Dr Richard Fitzpatrick
LRCPI MICGP MF Hom
196 Upr Glenagerary Rd
☎01 285 4709

Dr Madeline Gordon
MF Hom
119 Meadow Grove
Dundrum, Dublin 16
☎01 298 6365

Hahnemann Institute
of Homoeopathy
29 Dame Street
Dublin 2. ☎01 679 4208

Declan Hammond
LCH IS Hom
73 The Rise, Mount Merrion
☎01 288 2422

Homoeopathic
Women's Clinic
Well Woman Centre
Bridget Cummings
☎01 661 0083/661 0086

A. Hughes BSc Lic TCM
1 Leopardstown Drive
Dublin. ☎01 288 0352

Irish Centre for
Homoeopathic Medicine
29 Dame Street
Dublin 2. ☎01 679 4208

Irish School of
Homoeopathy Clinic
Milltown Park
Sandford Road
Dublin 6. ☎01868 2581

Dr Brian Kennedy
MRCGP MF Hom
46 Lr Elmwood Avenue
Ranelagh, Dublin 6
☎01 496 6481

Dr Siobhán Kierans BAO
MICGP MF Hom
Level 3
Tallaght Medical Centre
The Square, Tallaght
Dublin 24. ☎01 459 0962

Joy Lennon
Ashfield, 66 Kincora Rd
Dublin 3. ☎01 833 4356

Anne McDevitt DRE
BCA A
13 Wicklow Street
Dublin 2 ☎01 677 7962

Dr Goodwin McDonnell
MB MB MLCOM MF
Hom
3 Upper Ely Place
Dublin 2. ☎01 661 6844

Deirdre Maguire Lis Hom
31 Hazelwood Court
Artane, Dublin 5
☎01 847 9422

MELT Temple Bar
Natural Healing
Centre
2 Temple Lane South
Dublin 2. ☎01 679 8786

Morehampton
Pharmacy
79 Morehampton Road
Dublin 4. ☎01 668 7103

Tom Murphy Lic ISH
16 Castleknock Rise
Dublin 15. ☎01 821 6856

Nelsons Homoeopathic
Pharmacy
15 Duke Street
Dublin 2. ☎01 679 0451

Dr Elizabeth Ogden
MICGP MF Hom
29 Pembroke Park
Dublin 4. ☎01 668 0342

Lloyd Smythe DSH,
BRCP (Hom)
29/30 Dame Street
Dublin 2. ☎01 679 4208

Turner Clinic of
Alternative Medicine
Dublin Road, Stillorgan
Dr Ronald J. Turner AC
☎01 288 4327

Co. Galway
Clinic of Complementary
& Natural Medicine
Kiltartan House
Forster Street, Galway
☎091 568 804

Clinic of Wholistic
Medicine
34 Upper Abbeygate St
Galway. ☎091 567 416

Dr Ray Doyle MB BAO
BcH MRCGP MF
Hom
33 Woodquay, Galway
☎091 562 165

Dr Annabel Duff MB
BcH BAO MF Hom
53 Winfield Gardens
Clybaun Road
Knocknacarra, Galway
☎091 528 878

Nuala Eising IS Hom
Kinvara. ☎091 37382

Nuala Hughes
Caherawoneen
Kinvara. ☎091 63 73 82

Lilian Van Eiken
Moycullen. ☎091 85810

Bray Williamson LBSH
Castlecreevy, Corrandulla
☎091 791 12

Co. Kerry
P.J. O'Neill
2 Denny Street, Tralee
☎066 20121

Pauline Tyndale
6 Manor Park, Tralee
☎066 26441

Co. Kildare
The Complementary
Medical Centre
Fairgreen, Naas
Françoise Drion
☎045 874 477

Co. Kilkenny
Sally Ardis
The Amcotts, Clonmore
Piltown. ☎051 643 371

Co. Limerick
Mary Dolan LCH
35 Shelbourne Park
Limerick. ☎061 453 890

Eoin MacMahon LCH
Clancy Strand, Ennis Rd
Limerick. ☎061 454 652

Ann Moore
14 Mulcair Road
Raheen. ☎061 229 079

New Vistas Healthcare Ltd
7 Plassey Technical Park
Limerick. ☎061 334 455

Co. Louth
Ollie Kelly IS Hom
32 Strand Street
Clogherhead. ☎041 22702

Co. Mayo
Stephen Blendall BA
RSHom
Community Centre
Ballina. ☎094 21672 *or*
3 Fortfield, Castlebar
☎094 21672

Health Food Centre
Ellison Street, Castlebar
☎094 21908

Willie Kirkman IS Hom.
Cloona, Westport
☎098 27722

Hans Weitbrecht
Tullynagrene
Letterbarrow
☎073 35319

Co. Offaly
Complementary Health
Centre
Patrick's Court
Tullamore . ☎0506 22417

Co. Roscommon
Anne Walker IS Hom
Carrigeen, Kilglass
☎078 37221

Co. Sligo
Dr Ray Doyle MB BAO
BcH MRCGP MF Hom
1 High Street, Sligo
☎071 46162

Co. Tipperary
Margaret Kenny
92 Connolly Street
Nenagh. ☎067 34677

Co. Tyrone
Dr Annabel Duff MB
BCh BAO MFHom
70 Urbal Road, Coagh
Cookstown
☎08 016487 37467

Co. Westmeath
Clinic of Wholistic
Medicine
Church Street, Athlone
☎0902 78750

Co. Wexford
Centre for Natural
Therapies
16 George's Street
Wexford. ☎053 21363

Co. Wicklow
Bray Holistic Health
Clinic
79 Castle Street, Bray
Linda Ronayne Lic ISH
☎01 286 6611

Ann Callaghan LCH ISHom
St George's
Herbert Road, Bray
☎01 281 8438/286 3222

The Herbal &
Homoeopathic Clinic
Eagle House
Sidmonton Avenue
Bray. ☎01 286 6280

Antoinette O'Connell IS Hom
Leabeg Cottage
Newcastle. ☎01 281 9705

OTHER USEFUL ADDRESSES
Homoeopathic
remedies and books are
available from:

Nelsons Homoeopathic
Pharmacy
15 Duke Street
Dublin 2. ☎01 679 0451

Hypnotherapy

For full lists of members
of the Irish Association of
Hypno-analysts (IAH),
the Council for Hypnotic
Psychotherapy and
Counselling (CHPC),
and the Irish Institute of
Counselling and Hypno-
therapy, contact the
organisations (numbers
and addresses listed in
Professional Associations
directory pp. 208–10).

Co. Antrim
Ballymena Hypnotherapy
45a Wellington Street
Ballymena
☎08 01266 49734

Belfast Hypnotherapy
37 Lisburn Road, Belfast
☎08 01232 333 303

Michael Gannon MIAH
312A Antrim Road
Glengormley
Newtownabbey
☎08 01232 838 024/
865 986

Edith McGreevy BSc DipSW
Dip Ther Hyp (N-SHAP)
238 Townhill Road
Portglenone BT44 8HA
☎08 012665 71625

Natural Solutions
Hypnotherapy Centre
Valley Business Centre
67 Church Road
Newtownabbey
☎08 01232 402 635

Neuro-Solutions
Ballymoney Enterprise
Centre
Garryduff Road
Ballymoney
☎08 012656 66133

Raymond Patton
MNCH (Acc) MIAH
20 Ladas Drive
Belfast BT6 9FS
☎08 01232 704 004

Thomas Power MIAH
125 Burnthill Road
Newtownabbey
☎08 01232 848 605

The Therapy Centre
MIAH
312A Antrim Road
Glengormley
☎08 01232 86986/838024

Pat Waterson MIAH
32 Fry's Road
Ballymena BT43 7EN
☎08 01266 41408

Co. Armagh
Tony Hamilton MIAH
8 Rosemount Avenue
Armagh BT60 1BB
☎08 01861 526 352

Portadown Stress
Management Clinic
21 The Green, Portadown
☎08 01762 362 040

Co. Clare
Samuel Merrigan
MIAH
104 Aidan Park, Shannon
☎062 360 832

Paudie O'Donoghue
MIAH
Lahinch Rd, Ennistymon
☎065 72883

Co. Cork
Richard Cooke MIAH
9 Crones Lawn Cottage
Evergreen Street, Cork
☎021 318 894

Choices Hypnotherapy
Clinic
Plunkett Chambers
Business Centre
21/23 Oliver Plunkett St
Cork
Tim O'Callaghan DHP,
MIAH
☎021 271 020

Cork Hypnotherapy
Clinic
Therapy House
6 Tuckey Street, Cork
Dr Joe Keaney MIAH
☎021 273 575

Jeanne Estella MIAH
Burgatia Road
Roscarbery. ☎023 48639

William J. Hammond
MIAH
Capri, Duntaheen Road
Fermoy. ☎025 534 418

Brenda Kelly BA HDE
DPsyc. UCD MIACT
Carrigaline
☎021 373 443 *and*
Drummond Falcon Hill
Lovers Walk, Cork
☎021 551 484

Martin Kiely AAPH
1 Windsor Place
St Luke's, Cork
☎021 344 199

Fergus Lyons BSc
DHyp MIAH
Kanturk. ☎087 460 465

Michael O'Donnell
MIAH
Apt 1, Ardbrack Heights
Kinsale. ☎088 534 418

Anthony O'Sullivan MIAH
Ardrach East, Bantry
☎027 66049

Thomas Ryan MIAH
Bawnmore, Ballygarvan
☎021 888 116

Elisabeth Stanton MIAH
13 Hazelwood Close
Glanmire. ☎021 821 870

George Treacy MIAH
Spindelwood
Knocknamullagh
Rochestown
☎021 841 298

Co. Derry
Richard Glenn DHP MIAH
26 Carlisle Road, Derry
☎08 01504 261767

Co. Donegal
Patrick J. McGettigan
MIAH
Fawns, Termon
Letterkenny
☎074 39327

New Beginnings
Hypnotherapy Clinic
Main Street, Killybegs
Mike Egan Adv Dip
Hyp. MIAH/
Noelline Egan MIAH
☎073 30311

Co. Down
Chris Cassidy DHP
NRAH MICR
15 Villa Grove, Warrenpoint
☎08 16937 52520

Róisín Coulter MIAH
St Clare's Convent
High Street, Newry
☎08 01693 250 272

Dr G. (Deena) M. Craig DHy FIHP. Acc.Hyp IIHHT
33 Church Street
Bangor BT20 3HX
☎08 01247 458 161

Elizabeth Cunningham MIAH
61 Point Road, Banbridge
☎08 018206 62890

Moira Hypnotherapy Centre
76 Main Street, Moira
☎08 01846 613 112

Co. Dublin
Abba-Imma Centre
55 Main St, Rathfarnham
Dublin 14. ☎01 492 5757

Acorn Clinic
17 The Oaks
Upper Churchtown Rd
Dublin 14. ☎01 296 1551
or 087 441 083

Albany Clinic
Lr Fitzwilliam Street
Dublin 2. ☎01 661 5656

Alisar Counselling
Ranelagh Court
Chelmsford Rd, Dublin 6
Ken Gregan DPsych DHyp MIAH
☎01 491 0187

Ashroy Counselling & Hypnotherapy
22 Rathgar Ave., Dublin 6
Frank McArdle MIACT NCP (UK) Hyp. Dip.C
☎01 492 1793

Sean M. Bourke Dip Hy Dip SocSc
54 Vernon Avenue
Clontarf, Dublin 3
☎01 833 6648

D. Bradshaw McD CH Psych
65 Hollybrook Rd, Clontarf
Dublin 3. ☎01 833 1976

Alistair Bredee Dip Hyp MIAH
6 Clifton Terrace
Monkstown. ☎01 280 5506

John Bree MIAP
2 Hillsbrook Drive
Perrystown, Dublin 12
☎01 456 2232

Elvera Butler MA Dip. Hyp. M Prac NLP
77 Haddington Road
Dublin 4. ☎01 660 1578

Nino Cafolla Dip. Hyp MNACHP
40 Bolton Street
Dublin 1. ☎01 872 6915

Centre for Creative Change
14 Upper Clanbrassil St
Dublin 8. Aidan Maloney
☎01 453 8356/295 0094

Pradeep Kumar Chadha MIAH
48 Upper Drumcondra Rd
Dublin 9. ☎01 857 1145

Brian Colbert MIAH
84 Sundrive Rd, Kimmage
Dublin 12. ☎01 492 1447

Catherine Collins ITEC MSRI LT Phys
136 New Cabra Road
Dublin 7. ☎01 868 1110

Dr Sean Collins BA Psych.
32 Dawson Street
Dublin 2. ☎01 670 9799

Lucy Costigan RT (Cert), Maynooth Dip. in Counselling, MIAH, Adv Dip in Clinical Hypnosis, Healer Mem (NFSH)
Irish Spiritual Centre
30–31 Wicklow Street
Dublin 2. ☎053 22923
Holds sessions at the Irish Spiritual Centre. Please

phone her Wexford number for appointments.

Colette Cunningham MIAH
171 Griffith Avenue
Drumcondra, Dublin 9
☎01 837 4742

Dublin Hypnotherapy Centre
52a Main Street, Swords
James Ronan MCHPC CHyp (UK)
☎01 840 4161/088 588 787

Seamus Farrell MIAH
15 Delaford Lawn
Templeogue, Dublin 6w
☎01 494 1422

Owen Fitzpatrick MIAH
446 Orwell Park Green
Templeogue, Dublin 6w
☎01 450 0122

Elizabeth Foxworth MNRH (UK) MIAH
69 Lower Baggot Street
Dublin 2. ☎01 662 5656/ 087 234 0169

Rita Gerard RN D.Hyp. Adv D.Hyp. DCS MIAH
16 Pine Valley Drive
Dublin 16. ☎01 493 9024

Paul Goldin
Knapton Court
York Rd, Dún Laoghaire
☎01 280 2797

Kenneth F. Gregan MIAH
19 Carleton Rd, Marino
Dublin 4. ☎01 833 4178

Mary Grogan MIAH
The Medical Centre
Omni Park SC, Santry
Dublin 9.
☎01 862 0200/842 5901

Sharon Grumley MIAH
The Lodge
1A Willow Terrace
Blackrock. ☎01 662 1265

Anthony Guy MIAH
48 Laurel Park
Clondalkin, Dublin 22
☎01 459 3249

Seamus Hayes MIAH
6 Seapark
Mount Prospect Avenue
Clontarf, Dublin 3
☎088 547 292

The Holistic Health Centre
197 Lr Kimmage Road
Dublin 6w. ☎01 492 9279

Raymond Lawlor
  MIAH
24 St Brendan's Cottages
Irishtown Road
Dublin 4. ☎01 668 5059

Norman Levine
7 Flemingstown Park
Churchtown
☎01 298 4709

Littledales Natural
  Health Centre
15 Wicklow St, Dublin 2
Brendan Quinn MIAH
☎01 677 1021

Frank McArdle Dip
  MIAC Acc Hyp
22 Rathgar Road
Dublin 6. ☎01 492 1793

Michael McHugh
  MIAH
15 Westbury Park
Westbury Court, Lucan
☎01 624 1035

Noel B. McMahon
  MIAH
25 Sweetmount Park
Dundrum, Dublin 14
☎01 298 5850

Therese McNamee
  MIAH
45 Dargle Wood
Knocklyon Road
Templeogue, Dublin 16
☎01 494 5835

Ethna McQuillan CHyp
140 Foxfield Grove
Raheny, Dublin 5
☎01 831 2008

Dr Anjum Madani MB
  BCh LRCP MISH
Leonard's House
Leonard's Corner
Dublin 8. ☎01 453 2816/
088 590 510

Aidan Maloney MA
  Dip Stats NLP Pract
33 Coolkill, Sandyford
☎01 295 0094

The Natural Health Clinic
Mews, 154 Leinster Rd
Rathmines, Dublin 6
☎01 496 1316

Natural Solutions
6 Clifton Terrace
Monkstown
☎01 280 5506

Kara Nugent MIAH
519 Blackhorse Avenue
Dublin 7. ☎01 843 6139

John O'Connor MIAH
28 Kilbarrack Road
Dublin 5. ☎01 832 2567

Sandra O'Hare MIAH
11 Connolly Gardens
Inchicore. ☎01 453 9720

Options Hypnotherapy
  Clinic
Healing Circle
10a Lr Camden Street
Dublin 2
J.A. Hickey MIAH
☎01 475 2323

Billy Powell MIAH
4 Hillside Gardens
Skerries. ☎01 849 2696

Jocelyn Reilly DHP MIAH
1 Coast Road, Baldoyle
Dublin 13. ☎01 832 6758

Tony Sadar AAPH
37 Woodlands Road
Johnstown, Dún Laoghaire
☎01 285 2271

Noeleen Slattery PHyp
3 Charleston Road
Rathmines, Dublin 6
☎01 497 5666 *or*
Main Street, Rathcoole
☎01 458 9672

Michael Walsh MIAH
25 Park Court
Glenageary Heights
☎01 285 6751

Maurice P. White
9 Whitehall Park
Whitehall Road
Dublin 12. ☎01 450 7429

Co. Galway
Clinic of Complementary
  and Natural Medicine
Forster Street, Galway
Dr Hussain Bhatti
☎091 568 804

Carol Cunningham-
  Fahey MIAH
Menlo Park, Menlo
Galway. ☎091 761 487

Peter Deegan MIAH
Partners Restaurant
Main Street, Kinvara
☎091 37587

Linda Keady MIAH
Ardrahan, Barratreena
☎091 635 225

Bernadette Kelly MIAH
Cnoc Mhuire
Caheronaun Rd, Loughrea
☎091 841 023

Diarmuid Lavelle BA Dip
Canavan House
Nuns Island, Galway
☎091 569 770

John McCarthy MIAH
The Presbytery
Roundstone. ☎095 35846

Co. Kerry
David A. Fitzgerald MIAH
Cordal East, Castleisland
☎066 41978

Yvonne Henry
Cappa, Brandon
Tralee. ☎066 38233

P.J. O'Neill MIAH
2 Denny Street, Tralee
☎066 20121

Co. Kildare
Anne and Thomas
  Ahern MIAH
Sliabh na mBan
Liffey Lawns, Clane
☎045 868 751

Adrian C. Doyle MIAH
St David's Castle, Naas
☎045 874 350

Dr J.S. Gibson FRCSI
St David's Castle, Naas
☎045 897 389

Joe Griffin BSc Psych
  Dip Hypn
30 Forest Park, Athy
☎0507 38663

Hypnotherapy Ethical
  and Analytical Clinic
Maynooth
Ruth Allen MIAH
☎01 629 1743

Michael McGuinness
  BEd, DHP, MIAH
☎01 628 9946

Maynooth Hypnotherapy
35 Newtown Court
Maynooth

Ruth Monahan MIAH
31 Moyglare Village
Maynooth

Terence O'Connor
  MIAH
42 Walled Garden
Castletown, Celbridge
☎01 627 3032

Co. Laois
Seamus Hyland
Rathmiles, Portarlington
☎0502 43546

Co. Leitrim
Chris Gavican MIAH
Cloonart, Ruskey
☎078 38063

Co. Limerick
Michael Hughes DHP
  MIAH
Elm Park, Clarina
☎061 355 365/087 526 399

Hypnotherapy Centre
62 Catherine Street
Limerick
Michael Payne MIAH
  DHP MISPH MAAEH
☎061 413 500

Derry O'Malley
34 Catherine Street
Limerick ☎061 317 670

Co. Longford
John Kenny MIAH
Barley Harbour
Newtowncashel
☎043 25227

Co. Louth
Dundalk Hypnotherapy
  Clinic
Deerpark Road
Ravensdale, Dundalk
Aidan Noone DHP MIAH
☎042 71980

Progressive
  Hypnotherapy Clinic
Dundalk
Oisín O'Hare MIAH
☎042 31406

Flora M. Smyth RGN
  MNSPH,
Drogheda. ☎041 36928

Co. Mayo
Caitriona Doyle MIAH
Clogher, Bohola
☎094 81462

Co. Meath
Patrick Fox AAPH
  NBHECF
Fox House, Bective
Navan. ☎046 22700

Francis Harris MIAH
Newstone, Drumconrath
Navan. ☎041 54429

Kieran Staunton MIAH
21 College Park
Dunshaughlin
☎01 825 9475

Mark Telford MIAH
22 Kells Road, Trim
☎046 37729

Jim Wall MIAH
Riverstown, Rathfeigh
Tara. ☎041 25696

Co. Monaghan
Martin Byrne MIAH
Sheetrim
Castleblayney
☎042 46925

Mary Flora MIAH
Corbeg, Silverstream
☎047 82809

Co. Roscommon
Joe Duffy MIAH
Cloverhill
Ballaghadereen
☎0907 60959

Regina Spellman
Finnerman MIAH
The Lawns, Deerpark
Boyle. ☎079 62641

Co. Sligo
Anthony J. Martin MIAH
Llewellyn
Rosses Point
☎071 77401

Sligo Hypnotherapy Clinic
Weston House
Union Street, Sligo
Ken Keane Dip. Hyp
  Adv Dip AH, MIAH
☎071 50255

Co. Tipperary
Mary Frances Griffin
  MIAH
Hills Lot, Cashel
☎062 62548

Kevin Keating MIAH
Clonagoose
Mullinahone
☎052 53169

Brendan Kerins MIAH
Dublin Road, Cahir
☎052 41353

Annette O'Brien-Fahey
  MIAH DHP
27 Willow Park
Clonmel. ☎052 27250

William T. Power MIAH
57 O'Connell Street
Clonmel. ☎052 22580

Co. Tyrone
Laurence McCann MIAH
1 Willowmount Park
Killybrack Rd, Omagh
☎08 01662 249 479

Co. Waterford
Dan Averdung ICNH
  BHHSA MIAH
Ferrybank, Waterford
☎051 841 627

George Goulding
  MIAH
19 Morley Terrace
Waterford. ☎051 52235

Dermot Graham MIAH
Main Street, Tramore
☎051 386 651

Psychotherapy &
  Hypnotherapy Clinic
Main Street, Tramore
D. Graham D.Psy
  D.Hyp. DHC MIAH
☎051 386 651

Damien Stones MIAH/
  Marian Stones MIAH
Hillcrest Grove
Butlerstown
☎051 378 588

Co. Westmeath
Marion Keaney MIAH
24 Newlands
Mullingar. ☎044 41628

Co. Wexford
Lucy Costigan RT
  (Cert), Maynooth
  Dip. in Counselling,
  MIAH, Adv Dip in
  Clinical Hypnosis,
  Healer Mem (NFSH)
Wexford. ☎053 22923

John Kelly MIAH
The Rookery
Camolin, Enniscorthy
☎054 83425

Michael Lalor MIAH
66 Fort Road, Gorey

Indian Head Massage

Co. Dublin
Miriam Brady ITEC
7 York Avenue
Rathmines, Dublin 6
☎01 496 7605.

Complementary
  Healing Centre
91 Terenure Rd North
Dublin 6. ☎01 492 9077

Harvest Moon Centre
24 Lower Baggot Street
Dublin 2. ☎01 662 7556

The Healing House
24 O'Connell Avenue
Berkeley Road
Dublin 7. ☎01 8306413

The House of Astrology
9 Parliament Street
Dublin 2. ☎01 6793404

West Wood Club
Leopardstown
  Racecourse
Dublin 18
Siobhan Kennedy
☎01 289 5665

Seamus Lynch
☎01 284 6073

Co. Kerry
Áine McKivergan
Oakpark Medical Centre
Oakpark, Tralee
☎066 26255

Co. Wicklow
Avon Park
Glendalough Road
Rathdrum. ☎0404 46610

Holistic Therapy Clinic
Bray
Massan Ghorbani
☎01 286 4085

JoJo Loftus
Royal Bray Hotel, Bray
☎01 282 9530

Iridology

Co. Cork
Beara Circle Ltd
Castletownbere
Ulla Kinon. ☎027 70744

Co. Dublin
MELT, The Temple Bar
Natural Healing
Centre
2 Temple Lane
Dublin 2. ☎01 679 8786

Co. Wexford
Centre for Nutritional
Therapies
16 George's Street
Wexford. ☎053 21363

Kinesiology

Nature's Way
New Life Foundation
of Ireland
Hebron Road, Kilkenny
☎056 65402

The following trained
with Nature's Way:

Co. Dublin
Joe Kevelighan
☎01 837 3479

Nuala Kilduff-Coade
☎01 628 6860

Caoimhe Purcell
☎01 497 2189

Mary Stewart Carroll
☎01 451 3364

Co. Cork
Eoin McCuirc &
Tonia Briones
☎021 293 978

For a list of applied
kinesiologists, contact:

The Association of
Systemic Kinesiology
c/o Siobhan Barnes
48 Percy Place
Ballsbridge, Dublin 4
☎01 660 2806

INDIVIDUALS
Co. Dublin
Deirdre Downs BSc HDip
☎01 286 8465

The Holistic Health Centre
197 Lr Kimmage Rd
Dublin 6w. ☎01 492 9279

Kinesiology Institute
84 Cappaghmore
Clondalkin, Dublin 22
Rísteard de Barra
☎01 457 1183

MELT, Temple Bar
Natural Healing Centre
2 Temple Lane South
Dublin 2. ☎01 679 8786

Natural Solutions
6 Clifton Terrace
Monkstown
☎01 280 5506

Co. Clare
Still Point
Barrack Street, Ennis
Richard Healy Lic Ac
RPN MBAcC
☎065 20454

Co. Cork
Freedom Holistic Centre
Church Lane, Midleton
☎021 642 466

Marriage Guidance
See Counselling

Massage Therapy

For lists of members of the
Irish Massage Therapists
Association (IMTA) and
the Irish Health Culture
Association (IHCA),
contact the organisations
(numbers and addresses
listed in Professional
Associations directory
pp. 208–10).

Co. Antrim
Brian & Helen McCrystal
SSPCPT SMD
Pentagon House
George Street, Ballymena
☎08 01266 49701

M. Nixon
358 Old Glenarm Road
Larne
☎08 01574 260 066

John Rock MIHCA
249 Antrim Road
Glengormley
Newtownabbey
☎08 01232 837 164

Co. Armagh
Mary Fagan MIHCA
123 Navan Street
Armagh BT60 4AX
☎08 01861 527923

Patricia Larmour
MIHCA
30 Lakeview Park
Craigavon BT654AJ
☎08 01762 322 906

Martina McGuigan
MIHCA
4 Douglas Row, Lislea
Armagh
☎08 01861 527 183

Kate Savage MIHCA
5 Newry Road
Newtownhamilton
☎08 01693 878 851

Co. Carlow
Josephine Donnelly
MIHCA
'The Rising Sun'
26 Mountain View
Pollerton, Carlow
☎0503 41878

Co. Cavan
Dolores Farrell MIHCA
Drumconnick, Cavan
☎049 31791

Mary Greaney MIHCA
'Troutbeck', Cullies
Cavan. ☎049 32236

Clare McGurk MIHCA
Main Street, Virginia
☎049 44143

Co. Clare
Ennis Fitness World
Mill Road, Ennis
☎065 20969

Health & Harmony
Tulla Business Centre
Main Street, Tulla
☎065 35196

The Health Haven
Lr Market St Car Park
Ennis. ☎065 40613

Lisdoonvarna Spa Wells
& Health Centre
Lisdoonvarna
☎065 74023

Co. Cork
Mary Allen MIHCA
32 Woodlands
Kerry Pike, Cork
☎021 872 322

Mary Barrett BSc, ITEC
4 Glendale Road
Glasheen, Cork *and*
Riverside Clinic
Unit 9 Penrose Wharf
Penrose Quay, Cork
☎021 551 747

Beara Circle
Castletownbere
Margaret Deas
☎027 70744

Kieran Corcoran IMTA
San Roja, Hawthorn Mews
Dublin Hill
☎021 301 935/
894 949/319069

Sarah Courtney ITEC
Ballineadig, Farran

Mary Cronin MIHCA
17 Uam Var Grove
Bishopstown
☎021 545 514

Evergreen Clinic of
Natural Medicine
79 Evergreen Rd, Cork
Nicola Darrell
☎021 966 209

Anne Fahy MIHCA
35 Clover Hill Estate
Blackrock. ☎021 357 328

Jacinta Fitzgibbon IMTA
Killowen, Enniskeane
☎021 338 170

Breda Galvin ITEC
26 Calderwood Court
Donnybrook, Douglas

May Grainger
10 Vicars Road, Togher
☎021 310 718

Carmel Greehy
MIHCA
Cullenagh, Fermoy
☎025 31320

Sandra Hodnett ITEC
2 Convent View
Strawberry Hill, Cork

Holistic Health Centre
'Ballyannon Court'
Coolbawn, Midleton
Mary Horan
☎021 874 135
Mary O'Farrell
☎021 632 937

Agnes Kelleher MIHCA
6 Mill Road, Youghal
☎024 93130
Carmel Long
Cork. ☎021 371 377

Mary Kiely IMTA
Alys Morrissey
Physiotherapy
Millerd Street, Cork
☎021 272 855

LSA Ireland
Evergreen Clinic of
Natural Medicine
79 Evergreen Road
Cork. ☎021 966 209

Claire McCarthy ITEC
Glencurragh Road
Skibbereen

Gretta McCarthy
MIHCA
81 Sandown
Grange Heights
Douglas. ☎021 362 011

Gus McCarthy MIHCA
Upper Ballinora
Waterfall. ☎021 874 859

Mary McCarthy IMTA
Orchard Grove
Western Rd, Clonakilty

Carmel Madigan
School Rd, Whitechurch
☎021 385 942

Monkstown Aromatherapy
Parkgarrif Cottages
Monkstown. ☎021 841 793

Dolores Moynihan
MIHCA
6 Beverley Drive
Milbourn, Bishopstown
☎021 344 937

Natural Healing Centre
Thompson House
McCurtain Street
☎021 501 6 00

Michael O'Connor
MIHCA
16 Riverview
Hazelwood Estate
Riverstown
☎021 866 338

Maeve O'Donovan
MIHCA
Barrack Street, Cork
☎021 316 339

Gwynne O'Kelly
MIHCA
'Kelmac'
88 Earlwood Estate
The Lough, Cork
☎021 962 656

Nuala O'Halloran
MIHCA
5 Glenthorn Drive
Dublin Hill, Cork
☎021 304 203

Anne Olney
24 Westbury Street
Wilton. ☎021 344 574

Jeremiah O'Sullivan
MIHCA
19 Shandon Street
Cork. ☎021 307 876

Nuala O'Sullivan
MIHCA
Vermont Hartlands Ave
The Lough, Cork
☎021 964415

Lesley Proctor MIHCA
Russell Hill, Upton
Innishannon
☎021 775 504

Brenda Ratcliffe
MIHCA
Upper Ballinora
Waterfall, Cork
☎021 874 859

Keshari Renwick ITEC
Greenhill House
Kinsale

Neil Sheehan ITEC
28 Rosewood Estate
Ballincolly

Noel Sullivan IMTA
Turk Head, Church Cross
Skibberreen. ☎028 38185

Co. Derry
Triona Sweeney
18a Queen Street
Derry. ☎08 01504 266 700

Marian Walker MIHCA
32 Pennyburn Court
Derry BT48 ORT
☎08 01504 372 798

Co. Donegal
Mary Boyle-O'Brien IMTA
Dunglor. ☎075 21011

Mary Kelly MIHCA
Hilltown, Buncrana
☎077 62484

Eileen McGonigle
MIHCA
412 O'Duignan Avenue
Donegal. ☎073 22646

Co. Down
Margaret Bennett
MIHCA
100 Longfield Road
Adanove, Mullaghbawn
Newry. ☎08 01693 888 660

Marie Douglas MIHCA
33B Church Street
Warrenpoint
☎08 01693 752931

Eileen Murtagh
MIHCA
102 Blayney Road
Crossmaglen
☎08 01693 861 572

Rose Reel MIHCA
116 Longfield Road
Mullaghbawn
Newry BT35 0QJ
☎08 01693 878 360

Co. Dublin
Deirdre Ahern MIHCA
7 Dixon Villas, Glasthule
☎01 280 9156

The Albany Clinic
Lr Fitzwilliam Street
Dublin 2
Jacqueline McDonnell
☎01 624 9048

Aromatherapy Beauty
Clinic
12 Wicklow Street
Dublin 2. ☎01 677 0512

Aura Ki Massage Clinic
Castle Shopping Centre
Swords
Luke Kelly MIHCA
☎01 840 2633

Kay Bannon MIHCA
43 Furry Park Road
Dublin 5. ☎01 833 5093

Patricia Bastick MIHCA
134 Glenview Park
Tallaght, Dublin 24
☎01 462 2029

Terri Blanche ITEC
16B Clonskeagh Road
Ranelagh, Dublin 6
☎01 269 8217

Helena Boland MIHCA
119 Watergate Estate
Tallaght, Dublin 24
☎01 459 8091

Mary Bolger MIHCA
5 McAuley Ave, Artane
Dublin 5. ☎01 832 7473

Patricia Bowler MIHCA
Ninth Lock Cottage
The Royal Canal
Dublin 11. ☎01 830 8001

Lorraine Brady MIHCA
14 Cedarwood Rise
Dublin 11. ☎01 834 8705

Marie Brennan MIHCA
18 Tonduff Close
Green Park, Walkinstown
Dublin 12. ☎01 451 3159

Michael Cantwell MIAHM
14 Lr Pembroke Street
Dublin 2. ☎01 661 6195

Geraldine Carroll MIHCA
76 Beaumont Avenue
Churchtown, Dublin 14
☎01 298 0604

Anne Carter MIHCA
Templeogue
Adelaide Rd, Dún Laoghaire
☎01 284 1602

Maria Cassidy IMTA
Dundrum, Dublin 14
☎01 298 2565

John Caviston IMTA
Sandycove Foot and
   Health Clinic
57a Glasthule Road
Sandycove. ☎01 284 5287

Kevin Clark ICR IMTA
Medical Clinic
Haddington Road
Dublin 4. ☎01 660 8416

Club 59 Health Studio
59 Jervis Lane, Dublin 1
☎01 872 7915 *or*
088 522 316

Maureen Coggins
   MIHCA
110 Stillorgan Wood
Stillorgan. ☎01 288 1110

Catherine Collins ITEC
   MSRI LT Phys
136 New Cabra Road
Dublin 7. ☎01 868 1110

Audrey Conalty
   MIHCA
60 Jamestown Road
Inchicore, Dublin 8
☎01 453 7766

Gertie Connell MIHCA
1 Cherryfield Close
Hartstown, Dublin 15
☎01 820 8788

Moya Connelly
   MIHCA
363 Navan Road
Dublin 7. ☎01 838 2547

Majella Conway
6 Clifton Terrace
Monkstown
☎01 280 5506

Katherine Cooke
5 The Crescent
Fairview, Dublin 3
☎01 833 7252

Catherine Cooney IMTA
Beaumont/Rathfarnham
☎01 837 6177

Margaret Cowman
   Darcy MIHCA
40 Strand Road, Baldoyle
Dublin 5. ☎01 832 2023

Gerard Cox MIHCA
79 Trimleston Park
Booterstown
☎01 269 1455

Lucia Creed MIHCA
16 Cremore, Templeogue
Dublin 16. ☎01 494 6867

Margaret Crehan
   MIHCA
1 Hainault Lawn
Foxrock, Dublin 18
☎01 289 4779

David Culhane MIHCA
14 Vernon Avenue
Clontarf, Dublin 3
☎01 833 4823

Rosemary Cullinan HHC
   Dip Remedial Massage
   MIHCA
Monkstown. ☎01 284 6482

Catherine Cummins
   MIHCA
12 Sheelin Avenue
Ballybrack. ☎01 272 0846

Grainne Davitt MIHCA
40 Donnybrook Manor
Belmont Avenue
Donnybrook, Dublin 4
☎01 283 8252

Maureen Dempsey
   MIAPT Ass
2 Parklands Rise
Maynooth. ☎01 629 0677

Ann Doherty MIHCA
311 Charlemont
Griffith Avenue
Dublin 9. ☎01 836 7379

Jenny Dolan MIHCA
7 Pinecourt
Newtownpark Avenue
Blackrock. ☎01 283 1188

Josephine Donnelly
26 Mountain View
Pollerton, Carlow
☎0503 41878

Donnybrook Medical
   Centre
6 Main St, Donnybrook
Dublin 4

Patricia McWilliams/
   Audrey Ross ITEC
☎01 269 6588

Deirdre Downs ITEC
   BSc HDip
☎01 286 8465

Dublin School of Sports
   Massage
16a St Joseph's Parade
Dublin 7. ☎01 830 7063

Bernadette Duff
   MIHCA
10 Ratra Park, Navan Rd
Dublin 7. ☎01 838 4772

Jacqueline Duffy
   MIHCA
Marino Park Avenue
Dublin 3. ☎087 497 650

Marcella Dunne
Medina, Thormanby Rd
Howth. ☎01 324 720h

Thérèse Ellis MIHCA
20 Coolgreena Road
Beaumont, Dublin 9
☎01 837 3297

Energy Massage Therapy
4 Wynnefield Road
Rathmines, Dublin 6
☎088 670 604

John Fallon MIHCA
22 Coolevin, Ballybrack
☎01 285 9973

Noreen Farrell MIHCA
Cherry Lodge
Berrysteed, Leeson Park
Dublin 6. ☎01 496 2784

Francis E. Finnegan
MIHCA
38 St Andrew's Park
Swords. ☎01 840 6193

Ita Fitzmahony MIHCA
21 Mask Green, Artane
Dublin 5. ☎01 831 5837

Nora Fitzpatrick
MIHCA
111 Sperrin Road
Drimnagh, Dublin 12
☎01 455 3617

Emer Fleming IMTA
Templeogue/Lucan
☎01 490 2950

Derek Franzoni
MIHCA
40 Carrigwood, Firhouse
Dublin 24. ☎01 493 8774

Janet Fry MIHCA
40\C Merchamp
Seafield Road East
Clontarf, Dublin 3
☎01 332 194

Sean George MIHCA
2 Beach Park, Portmarnock
☎01 846 0952

Catherine Gleeson
MIHCA
50 Seapark
Mount Prospect Avenue
Clontarf, Dublin 3
☎01 833 4025

Joan Gleeson DHPM
MIAHM
61 Seapark Drive
Clontarf, Dublin 3
☎01 833 1917

Angeline Grant MIHCA
18 Highfield Green
Highfield, Swords
☎01 840 7174

Amanda Halpin MIHCA
37 Traders Wharf
Ushers Quay, Dublin 8
☎01 672 9664

Teresa Harrington
MIHCA
1 Ballyowen Court
Ballyowen Park, Lucan
☎01 624 0695

Harvest Moon Centre
24 Lower Baggot Street
Dublin 2. ☎01 662 7556

Healing Hands
4 Shantalla Road
Dublin 9. ☎01 857 0495

Health & Beauty Clinic
Irish Life Mall
Talbot Street, Dublin 1
Karen Greene
☎01 874 5106

Ashlie Hill MIHCA
95 Allen Park Road
Stillorgan. ☎01 288 8796

Cathie Hogan IMTA
Sandymount
☎01 668 9242

Marita Hogan MIHCA
18 Carlisle Street
Dublin 8. ☎01 454 0283

Holistic Healing Centre
38 Dame Street
Dublin 2. ☎01 671 0813

The Holistic Health
Centre
197 Lr Kimmage Rd
Dublin 6w. ☎01 492 9279

Elizabeth Homan
MIHCA
6 Orchardstown Avenue
Rathfarnham, Dublin 14
☎01 494 3103

Home-A-Therapy Clinic
Griffith College
South Circular Road
Dublin 8. ☎088 623 266

Anthony Horrigan MIHCA
97 Philipsburgh Avenue
Fairview, Dublin 3
☎01 836 9216

Margaret Hyland IMTA
Stillorgan. ☎01 288 6105

Sheila Hyland IMTA
Mount Merrion
☎01 288 1165

Emer Ivory MIHCA
57 Corke Abbey
Woodbrook
☎01 282 1968

Declan Kavanagh
MIHCA
13 Belmont Park, Raheny
Dublin 5. ☎01 831 9909

Aisling Kelly IMTA
Malahide. ☎01 845 0059

Christine Kelly MIHCA
32 Beechwood Lawns
Killiney. ☎01 285 1667

Eileen Kelly IMTA
Templeogue
☎01 493 0904

Linda Keenan MIHCA
167 St Brigid's Grove
Killester, Dublin 5
☎01 832 8741

Jane Kennedy IMTA
Donnybrook, Dublin 4
☎088 272 4506

Siobhan Kennedy IMTA
West Wood Club
Leopardstown Racecourse
Foxrock, Dublin 18
☎01 289 5665

Ann Kenny IMTA
Sandymount
☎01 269 2346

Ki Massage Therapy
Clinic
Fairview, Dublin 3
Geraldine Molloy MIHCA
☎01 833 5903

Anne Kinsella MIHCA
18 Sherick Park, Swords
☎01 840 1061

Patricia Langley IMTA
Dublin 14/16
☎01 298 0597/493 1050

Siobhan Larkin IMTA
Blanchardstown
☎01 822 0018

Norah Lawlor MIHCA
50 Carleton Road
Marino, Dublin 3
☎01 833 4387

Deirdre Layzell IMTA
Ranelagh/Rathmines
☎01 491 0928

Marie McCluskey MIHCA
14 Furry Park Road
Killester, Dublin 5
☎01 833 7287

Annmarie McConnell
MIHCA
11 Effra Rd, Rathmines
Dublin 6. ☎01 497 8721

Laura McCormack IMTA
MIHCA
9 Grange Park, Raheny
Dublin 5. ☎01 491 0928

Louise McCormack
18 Sycamore Avenue
Castleknock, Dublin 15
☎01 820 0631

Anne McDevitt DRE BCAA
13 Wicklow Street
Dublin 2. ☎01 677 7962

Una McEvoy MIHCA
10 Park Drive Grove
Castleknock, Dublin 15
☎01 820 4029

Joseph McGuire
12 Grange Park View
Raheny, Dublin 5
☎01 848 4270

Patricia McKenna MIHCA
2 Bloomfield Avenue
South Circular Road
Dublin 8. ☎01 854 3319

Ferga McNamara IMTA
Havelock Sq., Sandymount
Dublin 4. ☎01 668 6460

Nora McNamara
MIHCA
354 Cashel Rd, Kimmage
Dublin 12. ☎01 490 8820

Una MacNamara
10 Melrose Court
Philipsburgh Avenue
Fairview, Dublin 3
☎01 836 7841

Nuala McNeeley
DHPM MIAHM
MIHCA
11 Westway Park
Blanchardstown
Dublin 15. ☎01 820 4125

Brendan Madden MIHCA
23 Cherbury Court
Booterstown Avenue
Blackrock. ☎01 288 3862

MELT, Temple Bar
Natural Healing Centre
2 Temple Lane South
Dublin 2. ☎01 679 8786

Emily Miggin AAD
CIBTAC
3 Lr Pembroke Street
Dublin 2. ☎01 662 1211

Cathryn Morley
31 Wicklow Street
Dublin 2. ☎01 671 3467

Dermot Morris MIHCA
12 Maywood Avenue
Raheny, Dublin 5
☎01 831 3153

Bernadette Mulhall
MIHCA
22 Wigan Road
Drumcondra, Dublin 9
☎01 830 5491

The Natural Health Clinic
154 Leinster Road
Rathmines
Stephanie Mahon
☎01 496 1316

Muriel F. Neville
MIHCA
108 Hampton Cove
Balbriggan. ☎01 841 1342

Florence Newman
MIHCA
44 Ailesbury Mews
Sidney Parade
Dublin 4. ☎01 269 3645

Ann O'Brien MIHCA
52 Ellesmere Avenue
North Circular Road
Dublin 7. ☎01 838 8820

Dymphna O'Brien
Dublin 6. ☎01 496 1267

Gertie O'Connell MIHCA
Phibsboro, Dublin 7 *and*
Hartstown, Dublin 15
☎01 820 8788

Eileen O'Connor
MIHCA
30 Kirwan Street
Dublin 7

Kay O'Connor MIHCA
30 Ashfield Drive
Kingswood, Dublin 22
☎01 451 8816

Máiread O'Connor
MIHCA
4 Radlett Grove
Portmarnock
☎01 846 0760

Mary O'Connor MIHCA
232 Griffith Avenue
Dublin 9. ☎01 837 8515

William O'Connor MIHCA
30 Kirwan St, Dublin 7

Rory O'Donoghue MIHCA
Sallypark Lodge
Ballycullen Road
Knocklyon, Dublin 16
☎01 493 3927

Dearbhla O'Dwyer MIHCA
114 Ashley Rise
Martello, Portmarnock
☎01 846 3352

Anne O'Loughlin MIHCA
Apt. 4, Salisbury
214 South Circular Road
Dublin 8. ☎01 454 4181

Ann O'Neill RGN MIHCA
'Saoirse'
17 Mt Pleasant Terrace
Ranalagh, Dublin 6
☎01 497 0774 *or*
Terenure, Dublin 6
☎01 492 9077

Jude O'Neill MIHCA
2 St Ignatius Road
Dublin 7. ☎01 830 0200

Anne O'Sullivan MIHCA
75 Palmerstown Avenue
Palmerstown, Dublin 20
☎01 626 0435

Alan Pelly MIHCA
7 Ardmore Park
Artane, Dublin 5
☎01 847 6440 *or*
Dundrum, Dublin 16
☎01 298 6428

Catherine Phelan ITEC
☎01 671 9874

Loraine Preston MIHCA
73 Innisfallen Parade
North Circular Road
Dublin 7. ☎01 830 4969

James Quirke MIHCA
25 Templemore Avenue
Rathgar, Dublin 6
☎01 497 3162

Mary Regan IMTA
47 Heather Lawn
Aylesbury, Tallaght
Dublin 24. ☎01 451 4915

Helen Reidy MIHCA
33 Binn Éadair View
Sutton, Dublin 13
☎01 839 2412/703 2399

The Relaxation Centre
86 Parnell Street
Dublin 1. ☎01 878 8420

Mary Rice
'Cleaghmore', Garristown
☎01 835 4542

Josephine Robbins MIHCA
125 St Maelruan's Park
Tallaght, Dublin 24
☎01 451 3179

Ephrem Santiago
DHPM MIAHM
91 Terenure Road North
Terenure, Dublin 6
☎01 492 9077

Shannon's Way
Malahide. ☎01 845 5459

Sun City
283 Harold's Cross Rd
Dublin 6W. ☎01 496 7349

Teresa's Inspiring
Living Health Shop
8 Main Street, Raheny
Dublin 5. ☎01 832 9464

Brian Timmons MIHCA
31 Llewllyn Lawn
Rathfarnham, Dublin 16
☎01 493 7150

Vivienne Tobin MIHCA
92 Wilfield Road
Dublin 4. ☎01 283 8550

Tony Quinn Health Centres
66 Eccles St, Dublin 7
☎01 830 4211 *and*
2 Wynnefield Road
Rathmines, Dublin 6
☎01 497 4234 *and*

96 Lr George's Street
Dún Laoghaire
☎01 280 9891 *and*
10/11 Grafton Street
Dublin 2. ☎01 671 2788

Eugene Traynor MIHCA
31 Claddagh Road
Dublin 10. ☎01 626 9383

Irene Tucker-
Cunningham MIHCA
58A Road 'M'
Stonebridge, Clonsilla
Dublin 15. ☎01 838 3222

Marie Tully
Dublin 6. ☎01 497 9505/
088 594 040

John Wall MIHCA
21 Ferrycarrig Road
Coolock, Dublin 17
☎01 847 8505

Sylvia Wall MIHCA
6 The View, Woodpark
Ballinteer, Dublin 16
☎01 295 1242

Gertrude Walsh ITEC
Ranelagh, Dublin 6
☎01 496 4616

Peter Walsh MIHCA
10 Beaumont Drive
Churchtown, Dublin 14
☎01 298 6015

Karen Ward MIHCA
35 Wicklow Court
South Great George's St
Dublin 2. ☎01 671 1455

Lena Ward MIHCA
122 Claremont Court
Glasnevin, Dublin 11
☎01 830 9770

Margaret Watts
MIHCA
15 Roselawn View
Castleknock, Dublin 15
☎01 821 2573

Patricia Wheeler MIHCA
3 Belisk Avenue
St Augustine's Park
Blackrock

Imelda Wilson MIHCA
Rathbeale Road, Swords
☎01 840 2852.

Co. Fermanagh
Gabrielle Tottenham
  MIHCA
Innish-Beg, Blaney
Enniskillen
☎08 01365 64525

Co. Galway
Bernie's Hair, Health &
  Beauty
Main Street, Oranmore
☎091 794 636

David Byrne MIHCA
Patrician Brothers
Kingston, Galway
☎091 68707

Jenny Clarke MIHCA
5 Dr Mannix Avenue
Salthill. ☎091 23133

Galway Ki Massage
Knocknacarra, Galway
Martin Daly Dips Ki
  Massage & Clinical
  Massage MIHCA
Jenny Clarke Dip Ki
  Massage MIHCA
☎091 528 982

Ann McDonagh IMTA
21 Mill Street, Galway
☎091 566 829

Ciaran Mannion MIHCA
10 Lakeview
Claregalway
☎091 798 521

Michael Nevin LCSP
  (Assoc)
15 Emerson Avenue
Salthill. ☎091 529 870/
087 617 171

Co. Kerry
Aspects of Beauty
4 Bridge Place, Tralee
☎066 20943

Draíocht Beauty Salon
Daly's Lane, Killorglin
☎066 62022

Paulette Ní Shé MIHCA
Whitehouse, Ross Road
Killarney. ☎064 34750

Noeleen's Beauty Salon
63 Main St, Castleisland
Noeleen Tangney CIDESCO
☎066 4 26 09

Co. Kildare
Alternative Treatment
  Centre
Ballytore, Athy
Mary O'Mara Dip
  HMT MIRI ITEC
☎0507 23221

Leo Cluxton MIHCA
41 Mount Carmel
Newbridge. ☎045 34560

Helen Dawed SRN
  SCM MIIR
2 Rye River Park
Dún Carraig, Leixlip
☎01 624 4604

Decleor Health &
  Beauty Salon Stand
The Curragh
☎045 434 298

Anthony Doody HM
  Dip MAHT
61 Esmondale, Naas
☎045 874 349

Adrian C. Doyle MIHCA
16 South Main Street
Naas. ☎045 71017 *or*
St David's Castle, Naas
☎045 874 350

Marian Fahey MIHCA
Cloneygath, Monasterevin
☎045 523 480

Margaret Halligan MIHCA
Broadfield, Naas
☎045 75925

Michael Nooney MIHCA
76 Monread Heights
Naas. ☎045 32757

Brigid Uí Chuanaigh
  MIHCA
8 Willowbrook Lawns
Celbridge. ☎01 628 8961

Co. Kilkenny
Seán Kelly MIHCA
Leggettsrath
Dublin Road, Kilkenny
☎056 22462/63874

Caroline Mason MIHCA
17 The Rise, Cashel Hills
Kilkenny. ☎056 52215

Maura Murphy IMTA
Buruchurch
Cuffes Grange
☎056 29040

Ellen Nolan MIHCA
Racecourse, Kells Road
Kilkenny. ☎056 29060

Co. Laois
Stephen J. Lowry
  MIHCA
26 Emmet Street
Mountmellick
☎0502 24755

Joan Ryan MIHCA
Newtown House
Castletown, Portlaoise
☎0502 32876

Co. Limerick
Castleoaks Country Club
Castleconnell
☎061 377 722

Liz Dowling IMTA
Limerick Natural
  Health Centre
65 Catherine Street
☎061 409 920

Marion Fenton IMTA
5 Alphonsus Terrace
Quin Street, Limerick
☎061 417 781

Nora Gleeson MIHCA
Ballinoe, Castlemahon
☎069 83119

M. McElduff Lic Ac
MAIC IHCA Dip TCM
Limerick. ☎061 227 601

Christina O'Driscoll
MIHCA
19 Elm Park
Ennis Road, Limerick

Helen O'Grady
MIHCA
Apt. A, 'Ardmore'
St Nessan's Road
Dooradoyle, Limerick
☎061 413 490

Co. Longford
Maureen Bracken MIHCA
Ballinalee. ☎043 23196

Co. Louth
Margaret Agnew
MIHCA
90 Meadowgrove
Dundalk. ☎042 31531

Frances Byrne MIHCA
44 Maple Drive
Drogheda. ☎041 31682

Jean Coyle
Irish Grange
Carlingford. ☎042 76596

Tom Dolan MIHCA
Chapel Road
Dromiskin. ☎042 38097

Kathleen Fay MIHCA
Ounvarra, Ardee Road
Dundalk. ☎042 35656

Mary C Hutton
Main St, Dunshaughlin
☎01 825 0355

Rose Laverty MIHCA
St Joseph's
Newtownbalregan
Dundalk. ☎042 32045

Anne Quigley MIHCA
Castleroche, Dundalk
☎042 77114/31575

Martin Slattery MIHCA
2 Mary Street
Drogheda. ☎041 39673

Co. Mayo
Bonnie Connolly
Newtown, Castlebar
☎094 22588

Ki Massage Clinic
Pearse Street, Ballina
Angela Halloran MIHCA
☎096 71149

Breege Mulhern MIHCA
Cuilagurrain, Castlehill
Ballina. ☎096 31430

Nuala O'Malley MIHCA
Shanvolahange
Dooleeg, Ballina

Co. Meath
Sylvia Braun MIHCA
Lobinstown, Navan
☎046 53146

Margaret Brosnan MIHCA
Cedar Lodge, Kilbride
Clonee. ☎01 821 1697

Mary & Plunkett Cromwell
MIHCA
31 Ferndale, Navan
☎046 71097

Geraldine Holton MIHCA
An Croí, Baltrasnaane
Ashbourne. ☎01 831 2156

Catherine Lynch MIHCA
Freffens, Trim
☎046 36296/453 7941

Mary Eileen Nolan MIHCA
Cruicerath, Donore
☎041 23573

Martin Regan
Millview, Station Road
Dunboyne. ☎01 825 5792

David Robinson
MIHCA
c/o Mary Hutton
Main St, Dunshaughlin
☎046 25628/088 590 473

Hannah Ruane MIHCA
208 Silverlawns. Navan
☎046 29923

Sean Shortt
Newcastle, Enfield
☎01 284 3660

Co. Monaghan
Ann Connolly MIHCA
Corleygorm, Broomfield
Castleblaney. ☎042 43645

Margaret Gillen
MIHCA
Carragill, Cloughvalley
Carrickmacross
☎042 61653

Bernard Murphy
MIHCA
14B O'Neill Street
Carrickmacross
☎042 62323

Rose Quigley MIHCA
Dooskey, Smithboro
☎042 44194

Co. Offaly
Mary Kellaghan MIHCA
Garrymore, Geashill
Tullamore
☎0506 43035

Claudia Krygel MIHCA
Pine Lodge, Scregan
Tullamore. ☎0506 51927

Co. Roscommon
Regina Spellman-Finneran
MIHCA
Deerpark, Boyle
☎079 62641

Co. Sligo
Bernie Burke MIHCA
7 Kestrel Drive, Kevinsfort
Strandhill Road, Sligo
☎071 61593

Pat McManus MIHCA
Mountemple
Moneygold, Grange
☎071 66195

Karen Stewart
Lower Quay Street
Sligo. ☎071 46270

Co. Tipperary
Teresa Breen MIHCA
Roesboro, Tipperary
☎062 51612

Catherine O'Dwyer
MIHCA
8 Slievenamon Road
Clongour, Thurles
☎0504 22448

Bernard O'Neill
MIHCA
48 Ard Fatima
Clonmel. ☎052 21116

Co. Waterford
John Bergin MIHCA
30 Highfield, Tramore
☎051 390347

Miriam Chestnutt
MIHCA
Winslow Moir Estate
Ballytruckle Road
Waterford. ☎051 72331

Church Street Clinic
19 Mary St, Dungarvan
☎058 44366

Catherine Fitzpatrick
MIHCA
Boatstrand, Annestown
☎051 396 393

Shay Fitzpatrick IMTA
Tigh Carraig, Kilcarragh
Ballygunner. ☎051 874 937

Agnes Kavanagh
MIHCA
2 Rosebank Terrace
Tramore. ☎051 381 226

Trudi Morrissey IMTA
Green Meadows
Ballymacmague
Dungarvan. ☎058 42128

Anne O'Brien MIHCA
35 Brookhurst Road
Collins Avenue
Waterford. ☎051 358 342

Geraldine Wells MIHCA
4 Cathal Brugha Street
Waterford
☎051 5155/72222

Co. Westmeath
Remedios Rodriguez
MIHCA
Carrickwood
Lough Ennell
Mullingar. ☎044 44898.

Co. Wexford
Miriam Bannon
MIHCA
25 Gorey Hill, Gorey

Centre for Nutritional
Therapies
16 George's Street
Wexford. ☎053 21363

Sandra Goodison
92 The Grove, Clonard
☎053 647 011

Laurence Maher
2 Mount Ross, New Ross
☎051 425 721

Kathryn Redmond IMTA
28 Lower Henrietta St
Wexford. ☎053 22527

Co. Wicklow
Carol Brunker MIHCA
11 Bellevue Heights
Greystones
☎01 287 5879

Maura Burke MIHCA
41 Ashton Wood
Herbert Road, Bray
☎01 286 0416

Kevin Clark ICR IMTA
Willow Grove, Delgany
☎01 287 6817

Brenda Connolly MIHCA
48 Rathdown Park
Greystones. ☎01 287 6054

Imelda Duffy MIHCA
45 Fairy Hill, Bray
☎01 276 0759

Michael Egan MIHCA
Mount Alvernia
41 Burnaby Park
Greystones. ☎01 287 6131

David Harris MIHCA
Riverdale, Templecarrig
Greystones. ☎01 287 6793

Kay Hudson MIHCA
'Longpine' Monastery
Enniskerry. ☎01 286 9448

Jason J. Kenna MIHCA
Ferguslea, Adelaide Rd
Bray. ☎01 286 8405

Jennifer Kiersey MIHCA
Lugduff, Tinahely
☎0402 38372

Claire Kingston IMTA
☎0404 47137

Catherine Loesken MIHCA
Maruna, Rathdown Rd
Greystones. ☎01 287 2126

JoJo Loftus IMTA
Royal Hotel, Bray
☎01 276 1206/282 9530

Margaret McDonald
MIHCA
188 Killarney Park
Bray. ☎01 2866223

Derek Madden MIHCA
42 Castlemanor Sea Rd
Newcastle. ☎01 281 0705

Susan Meade IMTA
Delgany. ☎01 287 3253

Paddy Mooney IMTA
8 Fr Colahan Terrace
Bray. ☎01 286 3971

Gillian Myler MIHCA
35 Connawood Green
Old Connawood, Bray
☎01 272 0642

Mary O'Brien MIHCA
'Jasmine', Herbert Road
Bray. ☎01 286 2165

Plexus Bio-energy &
Therapeutic Massage
Glencarrig, Eden Road
Greystones. ☎01 287 5416

Ruth Synott
The Harbour, Greystones
☎01 287 5944

Gretchen Thornton MIHCA
Carrigoona
Rocky Valley Drive
Kilmacanogue
☎01 286 2504

Deirdre Vallom MIHCA
67 Burnaby Heights
Greystones. ☎01 287 2514

Mari Warren MIHCA
49 Heathervue
Greystones. ☎01 287 7763

Meditation

Co. Dublin
Arts Unlimited
Mary Roden
☎01 281 1063

Astrea Psychic Services
33 Lr Pembroke Street
Dublin 2. ☎01 662 5669

Celtic Healing and
Natural Health Centre
117–119 Ranelagh
Dublin 6. ☎01 491 0689

Clanwilliam Institute
18 Clanwilliam Terrace
Grand Canal Quay
Dublin 2. ☎01 464 0628

Clondalkin Holistic
Healing Centre
Desmond House
Boot Road, Clondalkin
Dublin 22. ☎01 464 0628

Complementary
Healing Centre
91 Terenure Road North
Terenure, Dublin 6
☎01 492 9077

Divine Rainbow Centre
151 Celtic Park Avenue
Whitehall, Dublin 9
☎01 831 4976

Dublin Meditation Centre
23 South Frederick Street
Dublin 2. ☎01 671 3187

Holistic Healing Centre
38 Dame Street
Dublin 2. ☎01 671 0813

Irish Meditation Society
106 Templeville Drive
Templeogue, Dublin 6w
☎01 490 4313

Irish Spiritual Centre
30–31 Wicklow Street
Dublin 2. ☎01 671 5106

Moytura Healing Centre
2 Lr Glenageary Road
Dún Laoghaire
☎01 285 4005

Rigpa Meditation Centre
12 Wicklow Street
Dublin 2. ☎01 454 0480

Samye Trust (Buddhist)
Kilmainham Well House
56 Inchicore Road
Kilmainham, Dublin 8
☎01 453 7427

Mary Sartini Healing
Centre
☎01 451 1694

Shambala Meditation
Group (Non-religious)
☎01 453 9159/453 8488

T'ai Chi Chuan
Association
c/o St Andrew's
Resource Centre
114–116 Pearse Street
Dublin 2. ☎01 677 1930

T'ai Chi Energy Centre
Milltown Park
Sandford Road
Ranelagh, Dublin 6
☎01 496 1533/280 8400

Transcendental
Meditation Centre
14 Ontario Terrace
Ranelagh, Dublin 6
☎01 496 0762

The Studio, Rere 330
Harold's Cross Road
Dublin 6w. ☎01 492 3965

Co. Louth
Iomlánú
Roden Place, Dundalk
☎042 32804/27253

Co. Wicklow
Avon Park
Glendalough Road
Rathdrum. ☎0404 46610

Chrysalis
Donard. ☎045 404713

Metamorphosis

Co. Cork
Beara Circle
Castletownbere
Franzi Topf. ☎027 70744

Inner Healing Centre
46 Sheares Street
Cork. ☎021 278 243

Leonie Maria Smith
182 The Willows
Ballincollig, Cork
☎021 871 559

Co. Dublin
Harvest Moon Centre
24 Lower Baggot Street
Dublin 2. ☎01 662 7556

For referrals in your
area, contact:

Eithne O'Mahony
Metamorphosis Ireland
'Shiloh', Clondulane
Fermoy. ☎025 31525 *or*

Fermoy Natural Health
   and Chiropody Centre
Abbey House
2 Abbey Street, Fermoy
☎025 32966

Movement and Dance Therapy

Co. Dublin
Complementary
   Healing Centre
Hilltop, Station Road
Raheny, Dublin 5
Jacinta Burke
☎01 851 0077

Anna Craig
☎01 452 7789

Joan Davis
'The Studio'
Rere 330
Harold's Cross Road
Dublin 6. ☎01 287 6986

Johanna Harmala
73 Heytsbury Street
Dublin 8. ☎01 475 5265

Co. Wicklow
Ann O'Hanlon
Blessington. ☎045 401 641

Antoinette Spillane
☎01 295 3882

Northern Ireland
Angela Knight
c/o PO Box 4176
Dublin 1

Muscle Effect Therapy

Bobby MacLaughlin
33 Wellington Lane
Dublin 4. ☎01 668 0316

Music Therapy

Co. Antrim
Northern Ireland Music
   Therapy Trust
Graham Clinic
Purdysburn Hospital
Saintfield Road, Belfast
☎08 01232 705 854

Co. Cork
Judith Brereton/
   Una McInerney
c/o PO Box 4176
Dublin 1

Co. Dublin
Jim Cosgrove
c/o PO Box 4176
Dublin 1

The Irish Association of
   Drama, Art and
   Music Therapists
PO Box 4176, Dublin 1

Mary McCooey
Brookville, Westpark
Artane, Dublin 5
☎01 848 0603/848 1216

Co. Kilkenny
John Clark/Antoine Roulet
c/o PO Box 4176
Dublin 1

Northern Ireland
Ruth Walsh
c/o PO Box 4176
Dublin 1

Naturopathy

Co. Cork
Mystical Ireland for Women
Cloghroe House
Blarney. ☎021 382 382

Co. Dublin
Gerard Flynn
3 Merrion, Ailesbury Rd
Ballsbridge, Dublin 4
☎01 269 5525

Martin Forde ND DO
66 Eccles Street
Dublin 7. ☎01 833 9902

Co. Roscommon
Henry Evikeens
Boyle. ☎079 62114

Neuro Linguistic Programming (NLP)

Co. Dublin
Ardagh Clinic
32 Dawson Street
Dublin 2. ☎01 670 9799

Centre for Creative
   Change
14 Upr Clanbrassil Street
Dublin 8
Aidan Maloney
☎01 453 8356

Elizabeth Foxworth
   M Pract NLP, M Pract
   Time Line Management
   Adv Dip Hyp
69 Lower Baggot Street
Dublin 2. ☎01 662 5656/
087 234 0169

Natural Solutions
6 Clifton Terrace
Monkstown. ☎01 280 5506

Co. Wicklow
Holistic Therapy Clinic
Bray
Massan Ghorbani
☎01 286 4085

Nutrition

For referrals, contact one of the following:

Irish Health Culture Association
9–11 Grafton Street
Dublin 2. ☎01 671 2788

The Irish Nutrition and Dietician's Institute
Dundrum Business Centre
Frankfort, Dundrum
Dublin 14. ☎01 298 7466

Natural Living Centre
Walmer House
Station Road, Raheny
Dublin 5. ☎01 832 7859

Teach Bán
6 Parnell Road
Harold's Cross, Dublin 6
Patrick Duggan/Ann Currie
☎01 454 3943

Many healthfood shops have qualified nutritionists available for consultations.

Irish Association of Health Stores
Unit 2D, Kylemore Ind. Est.
Dublin 10. ☎01 623 6828

INDIVIDUALS

Co. Cork
Beara Circle
Castletownbere
Ulla Kinon. ☎027 70744

Natural Medicine Clinic
Main Street, Carrigaline
Dr Jennifer Daly MB MICGP Lic Ac MIRI
☎021 372 787

Co. Dublin
Deirdre Downs BSc HDip
☎01 286 8465

Dr Brendan Fitzpatrick
MB MRCPI DCH DO MF Hom
115 Morehampton Rd
Dublin 4. ☎01 269 7768

The Holistic Health Centre
197 Lr Kimmage Rd
Dublin 6w. ☎01 492 9279

A. Hughes
1 Leopardstown Drive
Dublin. ☎01 288 0352

Siobhan Kennedy ITEC Dip in nutrition
West Wood Club
Leopardstown Racecourse
Foxrock, Dublin 18
☎01 289 5665

Natural Health Clinic
The Mews, 154 Leinster Rd
Rathmines, Dublin 6
Catherine Brady
☎01 496 1316

Co. Galway
Clinic of Complementary and Natural Medicine
Forster Street, Galway
☎091 568 804

Co. Wexford
Centre for Nutritional Therapies
16 George's Street
Wexford. ☎053 21363

OTHER ADDRESSES

Dublin Food Co-op
St Andrew's Centre
Pearse Street, Dublin 2
and Carmichael House
North Brunswick Street
Dublin 7. ☎01 872 1191
Organically grown foods, wholefoods and environmentally friendly products. Talks on food nutrition and cooking demonstrations.

Wholefood Wholesales
Unit 2D
Kylemore Ind. Estate
Dublin 10. ☎01 626 2315
Information on organic foods and health products. Also Bioforce training course.

Osteopathy

For a listing of the members of the Irish Osteopathic Association (IOA), contact the IOA (number and address listed in Professional Associations directory pp. 208–10).

Co. Antrim
M.D. Agnew DO MUOA/B. Jackson DO MUOA/W.M. Ryan MGO (Lon), DO FUOA MIAH
215 Kingsway, Dunmurry
Belfast BT17 9SB
☎08 01232 301 202

Avril Gibson DO MRO MIOA
41 Finaghy Road South
Belfast BT10 0BW
☎08 01232 617 510

Geoffrey A. Hayhurst BDS DO LL.Ac
207 Belmont Road
Belfast
☎08 01232 656 664

Lifespring Centre
111 Cliftonville Road
Belfast BT14 6JQ
Mary Grant Associates
☎08 01232 753 658

Olympic Homecare
11 Great Northern Street
Belfast
☎08 01232 667 959

Evan Pamely DO MGO
123 Belmont Road
Belfast
☎08 01232 656 432

Co. Armagh
Oliver McAtamney DO
  FLCSP MGO MIOA
82 Church Street
Portadown BT62 3EU
☎08 01762 332 437

Co. Clare
Ian Milne DO MCO MICO
Ennis. ☎087 456 213

Co. Cork
Acupuncture, Allergy
  & Osteopathy Clinic
Rochestown/Douglas
☎021 292 737
Laurence Hattersley BSc DO
4 St Brigid's Street
Greenmount, Cork
☎021 316 496

Caille Laurent BSc
  (Hons) Ost DO MRO
Rochestown/Douglas
☎021 292 737

Natural Healing Centre
Thompson House
McCurtain Street, Cork
☎021 501 600

Noel O'Connor DO LCSP
  (Phys), MBEOA MIOA
Killross Clinic
Bishopstown Road
Cork. ☎021 342 042 *or*
2 Percival Street
Kanturk. ☎029 50899

Mary O'Leary DO MGO
Knocknagree ☎064 56010

Dr Kevin O'Sullivan
  MB MRCGP DO
  MRO Dip MSMed
The Surgery
South Douglas Road
☎021 365 013

Christopher Pardoe ND
  DO MIOA
29 Castle Close Drive
Blarney. ☎021 381 173

Co. Donegal
Dr Aidan Dunn MB BCh
  BAO MICGP MLCOM
Knather Road
Ballyshannon
☎072 51447

Bosco Reid MIOA DO
Ballymacarry Lower
Buncrana. ☎077 61513

Co. Down
W.L. Bell MBEOA
  MGO MIOA DO
Rockfield
89a Carnreagh
Hillsborough BT26 6LJ
☎08 01846 683390

Robert Boyd DO MCOA,
  MBEOA MIOA
15 Farnham Road
Bangor BT20 3SP
☎08 01247 270 626

Dr Carl V. Campbell
  MLCOM, MRO
19A Causeway Road
Newcastle BT33 ODL
☎08 013967 23145

A.E. Gibson DO MRO
45 Bryansford Road
Newcastle
☎08 013967 24627

Ralph M. McCutcheon
  ND DO MRO MIOA
150 High Street
Holywood BT18 9HS
☎08 01232 425 953

Tina McCutcheon
  MIOA DO
White House, Sand End
Ballywater BT22 2PE
☎08 012477 58069

Co. Dublin
Chris Campbell MIOA
  DO
18 Cromwellsfort Road
Dublin 12. ☎01 450 4432

Carysfort Clinic
11 Proby Square
Blackrock
Simon Curtis BSc
  MIOA DO MRO
☎01 288 6514

Dr James A. Dolan MB
  BAO BCh MA MIOA
  DO DCH
191 Howth Road
Killester, Dublin 3
☎01 833 5962 *or*
Suite 1b
Olympia House
62 Dame Street
Dublin 2. ☎01 677 3591

James M.P. Doyle
  MIOA DO MBEOA
17 Windsor Terrace
Portobello, Dublin 8
☎01 473 0828

Patrick Fahy MIOA DO
42 Sutton Park, Dublin 13
☎01 832 5572 *or*
1 Merrion Square
Dublin 2. ☎01 661 6143

Dr P.J. Finn MB MRO
  MIOA DO
Northside Surgery
Northside SC
Dublin 17. ☎01 848 3179

Gerry Flynn MIOA DO
  MRO
3 Merrion Court
Ailesbury Road
Dublin 4. ☎01 269 5525

Alexander Gibbs MIOA
  DO MRO
c/o 10 Winton Avenue
Rathgar, Dublin 6
☎01 269 5281

Sarah Hanrahan MRO
MIOA DO
'Breffni', 21 Church Road
Dalkey. ☎01 280 1925

John Harrington
6 Martello Tce, Sandycove
☎01 284 2294/284 3275

Michaela Kullack
MIOA DO
21 Church Road
Dalkey. ☎01 280 1925 *or*
18 Cromwellsfort Road
Walkinstown, Dublin 12
☎01 450 4438

Barra Lane MIOA DO
313 Templeogue Road
Dublin 6w
☎087 230 9808 *or*
Fairways Health Centre
2 Fairways, Rathfarnham
Dublin 14

Dr M.D. McCready
29 Pembroke Park
Donnybrook, Dublin 4
☎01 668 0342

Dr Goodwin McDonnell
MB MFHom
3 Upper Ely Place
Dublin 2. ☎01 661 6844

Anne Mangan RGN
DO MGO
18 Priory Hall
Stillorgan. ☎01 283 5566

Richard Mann BSc (Ost)
MRO MIOA DO/
Diana Smyth BSc (Ost)
MRO MIOA DO
1 Rus-in-Urbe Terrace
Lower Glenageary Rd
Dún Laoghaire
☎01 280 3890

Paula Marren MIOA DO
1 Merrion Square
Dublin 1. ☎01 661 6143

Bridget O'Brien
519 South Circular Rd
Dublin 8. ☎01 454 1170

The Osteopathic Centre
For Children
Dublin 12
☎01 450 2539

Pamela Synge MIOA DO
1 Merrion Square
Dublin 1. ☎01 661 6143

Teran Synge MIOA DO
MRO
1 Merrion Square
Dublin 1. ☎01 661 6143

Walkinstown
Osteopathy Clinic
18 Cromwellsfort Road
Dublin 12
Elizabeth O'Neill/
Rory Tope MIOA DO
☎01 450 4438

West Wood Club
Leopardstown
Racecourse
Foxrock, Dublin 18
Richard Mann BSc (Ost)
MRO MIOA DO/
Diana Smyth BSc
(Ost) MRO MIOA
DO
☎01 289 3208

Co. Fermanagh
Cherrymount Clinic
Drumcoo
D. Flanagan
☎08 01365 322622

Co. Galway
Acupuncture,
Osteopathy and
Allergy Testing Clinic
1 McDara Road
Shangalla
Galway. ☎091 522 631

Alan Brannelly DO
MGO MAFI
1 McDara Rd, Shantalla
Galway. ☎091 522 631

Dr Ray Doyle MB BCh
MRCGP MF Hom
33 Woodquay, Galway
☎091 562 165

Dr Aidan Dunn MB
BCh BAO MICGP
MLCOM
7 Upper Abbeygate St
Galway. ☎091 562 572

Karl Prendergast
MIOA DO
5 Devon Place
The Crescent
☎091 589417

Co. Kerry
Pamela Sheehan DO
MRO MIOA
The Gables, Milltown
☎066 67304

Co. Kilkenny
Carmel Farrell MIOA DO
MRO
Friary Court
Friary Street, Kilkenny
☎056 65221

Co. Laois
Margaret Hoey DO
MIPA
Clonmore
Daingean Road
Portlaoise. ☎0506 41095

Co. Louth
Paula Marren MIOA DO
48 Fair Street
Drogheda. ☎041 31620

Dr Eric Tobin MB DA
(London) MIAOM
Dunany House
Seatown Place
Dundalk. ☎042 32695

Co. Sligo
Dr Ray Doyle MB BCh
  MRCGP MF Hom
1 High Street, Sligo
☎071 46162

Co. Tipperary
Kieran English MIOA
  DO MRO
Mountain View
Mountain Road
Clonmel. ☎052 25309

Nenagh Osteopathic
  Practice
Arden House
Kenyon Street, Nenagh
Robert Scott Johnston
  DO MRO
☎067 32272

Co. Tyrone
James Myler MIOA DO
4 Church Street, Omagh
☎08 01662 45278

Co. Waterford
Power Patrick DO MGO
14 Grattan Square
Dungarvan
☎058 42903

Co. Westmeath
Spine, Sport & Limb
  Clinic
Longford Road
Mullingar
Dr Dennis Slattery MRO
☎044 42993

Co. Wicklow
Patrick D'Arcy DO
  MGO Phys
5A Castle Street, Bray
☎01 286 7025

Mary Kennedy O'Brien
  DO MGO
41 Glenthorn
Killarney Road, Bray
☎01 286 2054

Teran Synge MIOA DO
'St Jude's'
Dublin Road, Arklow
☎0402 32473

Co. Wexford
Denis Kinsella LCSP (Phys)
The Square, Ferns
☎054 66442

Psychodrama
Co. Antrim
Noelle Branagan
c/o Shaftesbury Square
  Hospital
116–120 Gt Victoria St
Belfast BT27BG.
*GP referral directly to
hospital and community
addiction team referrals.
For private consultations*
☎08 01232 649 557

Co. Cork
Stephen Flynn
c/o Southern Health Board
St Stephen's Hospital
Sarsfield Court, Glenville
*Referrals from SHB
senior social workers and
consultant psychiatrists.*

Catherine Murray
Newtown House
Doneraile. ☎022 24117

Co. Down
Claire Munroe
45 Kinnegar Drive
Hollywood BT18 9JQ
☎01 01232 422 587

Psychosynthesis
For a list of qualified
practitioners or for
individual referrals,
contact:
Eckhart House
19 Clyde Road
Dublin 4. ☎01 668 4687

Psychotherapy
See Counselling and
Psychotherapy.

Reality Therapy
To obtain the name of a
reality therapist in your
area (designated letters
RT Cert), contact:

Eileen Hearne
24 Glendown Court
Templeogue
Dublin 6w. ☎01 456 2216

INDIVIDUAL REALITY
THERAPISTS

Co. Dublin
Eileen Boyle
57 Upr Grand Canal St
Dublin 4. ☎01 660 4574

Marie Caulfield
51 Devinish Road
Kimmage, Dublin 12
☎01 492 1273

Lucy Costigan RT
  (Cert), Maynooth
  Dip. in Counselling,
  MIAH, Adv Dip in
  Clinical Hypnosis,
  Healer Mem (NFSH)
Irish Spiritual Centre
30–31 Wicklow Street
Dublin 2. ☎053 22923
*Sessions held at Irish
Spiritual Centre. Please
phone her Wexford
number for appointments.*

Mary Flynn
☎01 821 6807

Kathleen McGivern
☎01 492 9648

Co. Kildare
Angela Lane
56 College Park
Newbridge. ☎045 431755

Co. Wexford
Lucy Costigan RT
(Cert), Maynooth
Dip. in Counselling,
MIAH, Adv Dip in
Clinical Hypnosis,
Healer Mem (NFSH)
☎053 22923

Rebirthing

The following are
registered with the
Association of Irish
Rebirthers (AIR):

Co. Dublin
Michael Blake (Rebirther
in Training)
Templeogue
☎01 490 2261

Ann Curran (Rebirther
in Training)
Rathfarnham
☎01 493 9543

Catherine Dowling
(Reg. Rebirther)
Kilmainham
☎01 453 3166

Patsy Kavanagh (Reg.
Rebirther)
Clondalkin
☎01 455 7480

Lucy Mullee (Rebirther)
Dundrum
Dublin 14
☎01 295 6129

Co. Kildare

Margaret Dunne (Reg.
Rebirther)
Leixlip. ☎01 624 2799

Co. Tipperary
Mary Condren (Rebirther)
☎062 55102

Véronique Jalaber (Reg.
Rebirther)
☎067 28061

Sally McCormac
(Rebirther in Training)
☎062 55102

Eileen Peters (Rebirther
in Training)
☎067 33297

Co. Wicklow
Steve Gregory (Reg.
Rebirther)
Wicklow. ☎01 287 5330

The following are registered
with the Association of
Rebirther Trainers
International (ARTI):

Co. Dublin
Patsy Brennan (Trainer)
☎01 2841660

Brenda Doherty
Odyssey Healing Centre
15 Wicklow St, Dublin 2
☎01 677 1021/842 2460

Kathleen Hogan Purcell
30 Oakley Grove
Blackrock. ☎01 288 1725

Co. Wicklow
Majella Conway
Annamoe. ☎0404 45277

INDIVIDUALS
Assumpta Byrne
The Banks, Manor Kilbride
☎01 458 2407

Majella Conway
6 Clifton Terrace
Monkstown. ☎01 280 5506

Healing Arts Centre
International
46 Walnut Rise
Drumcondra, Dublin 9
Angela Gorman
☎01 837 0832/088 274 9701

Natural Solutions
6 Clifton Terrace
Monkstown. ☎01 280 5506

Reflexology

For lists of members of
the Irish Reflexologists
Institute (IRI) and the
Association of
Reflexologists (AOR),
contact the associations
(numbers and addresses
listed in Professional
Associations directory
pp. 208–10).

Co. Antrim
Andrea Palmer
Reflexology
14 Chichester Pk South
Belfast BT15
☎08 01232 776 358

Eileen Baille SRN RMN
SCM MAR MICR
AOR
10 Cairnshill Crescent
Belfast BT8 4RL
☎08 01232 703 012

Carole Caldwell
12 Dalways, Bawn Road
Carrickfergus BT38 9BY
☎08 01960 378 620

Complimentary Care
4 Glencroft Road
Newtownabbey
Gavin Devlin
☎08 01232 832 966

Fortwilliam Reflexology
537 Antrim Road
Belfast BT15
D. McDaniel BSc MIRI
☎08 01232 716 352

Brendan Glover BAM
Phil, MICR
17 Brucevale Park
Belfast BT14 6BQ
☎08 01232 743 717

Mary Grant Associates
Lifespring Centre
111 Cliftonville Rd, Belfast
☎08 01232 753 658

Hair & Scalp Clinic
32 Knockbreda Road
Belfast BT6 OJB
☎08 01232 692 511

Health & Relaxation Centre
30 Knowehead Road
Broughshane BT43 7LF
Lorna McCooke AOR
☎08 01266 862 060

Hilary Hoare-Doherty AOR
38 Ruskin Park
Lisburn BT27 5QN
☎08 01846 678 611

The House of Beauty
6A Mount Merrion Ave
Rosetta, Belfast
☎08 01232 492 315

Lifespring Centre
111 Cliftonville Rd, Belfast
☎08 01232 753 658

Sharon McMichael MIRI
19 Hawthornden Drive
Belmont, Belfast
☎08 01232 768 477

Marian MacPolin MIRI
13 Sydenham Gardens
Belfast BT4
☎08 01232 654 541

Mary Montgomery AOR
6 Finlaystown Road
Portglenone BT44 8EA
☎08 01266 821 438

Kathryn Rea AOR
4 Ruskin Park
Lisburn BT27 5QN
☎08 01846 677 806

Reflexology Clinic
34 Lucerne Parade
Stranmillis, Belfast BT9 5FT
Carole Wray AOR
☎08 01232 669 913

Jean Sage AOR
T/A Therapy Matters
The Trees
31 Fortwilliam Park
Belfast BT15 4AP
☎08 01232 777 830

Serena Sheppard AOR
4 Windslow Court
Carrickfergus BT38 9DP
☎08 01960 66100

Co. Armagh
Lynne Hanna AOR
114 Dromore Road
Donaghcloney
Craigavon BT66 7NH
☎08 01762 881 945

Co. Carlow
Mary Hogan
45 Monacurragh
Carlow. ☎0503 43388

Marianne Madden
 AOR
Nampara, Ballymurphy Rd
Tullow. ☎0503 51681

Co. Cavan
Christine McGuinness
Upper Main Street
Cavan. ☎049 61019

Co. Clare
Eileen Addley AOR
Swallow Hill
Rahenamore
Killaloe. ☎061 376 783

Noelette Keane RGN
Sláinte Car Park, Ennis
☎065 42019

Lisdoonvarna Spa Wells
 & Health Centre
Lisdoonvarna
☎065 74023

Miranda's Health &
 Beauty Clinic
Main Street, Killaloe
☎061 376 696

Scent of Beauty
31 O'Connell Street
Ennis. ☎065 21888

Co. Cork
Beara Circle
Castletownbere
Franzi Topf. ☎027 70744

Beauty Culture Ltd
123 Oliver Plunkett St
Cork

Maureen Murray ITEC
 CIBTAC CIDESCO
☎021 276 493

Blackrock Acupuncture
 & Reflexology Clinic
6 Clontarf Estate
Skehard Road
Blackrock. ☎021 358 777

The Bridge Clinc
8 Bridge Street, Cork
Lucy Fintan MAIR
☎021 551 263

Mary Collins ICNHS (Dip)
 Aroma MIIAA MAIR
104 Oliver Plunkett St
Cork. ☎021 274 130

Evergreen Clinic of
 Natural Medicine
79 Evergreen Rd, Cork
Nicola Darrell ITEC
☎021 966 209

Jacinta Fitzgibbon
 IMTA ITEC
Killowen, Enniskeane
☎021 338 170

Rosaire Harrington RGN
 MIINT MAIR Dip.
10 Parnell Place, Cork
☎021 278 593

Una Hayward AOR
22 Uam Var Grove
Bishopstown, Cork
☎021 346 103

Helen Holden Dip NTM
ITEC ISPA MAIR
Heathercroft
1 Castle Close Crescent
Blarney. ☎021 385 708

Inner Healing Centre
1st Floor
46 Sheare's Street, Cork
☎021 278 243

Irish Institute of
Natural Therapy
Croghta Park
Glasheen Road, Cork
☎021 964 313

Rachel Lacey-Porter AOR
The Commons
Inchigeelagh
☎026 49254

Ladysbridge
Reflexology Clinic
Ladysbridge
☎021 667 369 *and*
Ballymacoda
☎024 98198

Mary McCarthy IMTA
ITEC
Orchard Grove
Western Rd, Clonakilty

Carmel Madigan SEN
ONC MSRI
School Road
Whitechurch
☎021 385 942

Elizabeth Murphy
Fitzgerald House
74 Grande Parade, Cork
☎021 272 100

Matt Murphy MSRI
Ballinvarosig House
Carrigaline
☎021 372 693

Natural Healing Centre
Thompson House
McCurtain Street
☎021 501 600

Natural Health Centre
Hannah O'Brien MIRI
Inchnagree, Buttevant
☎022 24286

Natural Healthcare
Centre
17 Main Street, Kinsale
Agnes Beary AOR
☎021 774 907

Natural Medicine Clinic
Main Street, Carrigaline
Dr Jennifer Daly MB
MICGP LIC AC MIRI
☎021 322 787

Hannah O'Brien MIRI
Inchnagree, Buttevant
☎022 24286

Anne Ryan
Hillview House
Riverstick. ☎021 771 350

Léonie Maria Smith
182 The Willows
Ballincollig
☎021 871 559

Co. Derry
Patricia Broderick AOR
8 Mayogall Road
Magherafelt BT45 8PD
☎08 01504 42136

Dorothy Hardyway
AOR
27 Central Avenue
Portstewart
Derry BT55 9BS
☎08 01504 834 080

Olive McGarvey AOR
76 Strand Road
Portstewart BT55 7LY
☎08 01504 832 974

Co. Donegal
Joan O'Connell AOR
Airghialla, Lissadel Ave
Magheracar, Bundoran
☎072 41964

Co. Down
Sarah Boyd MISNT MIRI
28 Belfast Road
Holywood
☎08 01232 425 307

Christopher Cassidy AOR
15 Villa Grove
Warrenpoint BT34 3PQ
☎08 016937 52520

Avril Clarke MA
IIHHT Dip. Reflex
Dip. Massage
12 Rowantree Glen
Dromore BT25 1HB
☎08 01846 699 318

G. (Deena) M. Craig
D.Hy.FIHP Acc.Hyp.
IIHHT
33 Church Street, Bangor
☎08 01247 458 161

International Institute
of Reflexology
Lower Catherine Street
Newry. ☎08 01693 62567/
848904

Moira Reflexology Clinic
76 Main Street, Moira
☎08 01846 619 163

Judy Sinclair
60a Thornyhill Road
Killinchy
☎08 01238 542 252

Co. Dublin
Academy International
48 Upr Drumcondra Rd
Dublin 9. ☎01 836 8201

Mary Anderson
Hamilton House
Trafalgar Terrace
Monkstown .☎01 280 3635

Mary Beecham MSRI
MCSCH SRN SCM
Swan Shopping Centre
Rathmines
☎01 496 0330 *and*

25 Highland Avenue
The Park, Cabinteely
Dublin 18. ☎01 285 7294

Margaret Boland SRN
MIRI
Killiney. ☎01 285 2733

Geraldine Bolger RGN
MSRI
53 Coolnevaun
Stillorgan

Eileen Boyle
57 Upr Grand Canal St
Dublin 4. ☎01 660 4574

Miriam Brady ITEC
7 York Avenue
Rathmines, Dublin 6
☎01 496 7605

Clondalkin
    Acupuncture Clinic
Desmond House
Boot Road, Dublin 22
☎01 464 0050

Catherine Collins
136 New Cabra Road
Dublin 7. ☎01 868 1110

Bridie Connellan ITEC
    Dip MICR
70 Wellington Road
Ballsbridge, Dublin 4
☎01 600 0510

Amy Cronin
Blackrock Shopping Centre
Dublin 18. ☎01 288 5601

Rosaleen Dempsey MICR
126 Whitecliff
Dublin 16. ☎01 494 3533

Donnybrook Medical
    Centre
6 Main St, Donnybrook
Dublin 4
Patricia McWilliams
    ITEC/Audrey Ross ITEC
☎01 269 6588

Drumcondra Health
    Clinic
11 Sion Hill Road
Drumcondra, Dublin 9
☎01 837 8310

Margaret Duffy RGN
    MICR
16 Baggot Road
Dublin 7. ☎01 868 3141

Gillian Fox
29 South Anne Street
Dublin 2. ☎01 670 9324

Siobhan Guthrie AOR
34b Royal Terrace West
Dún Laoghaire
☎01 280 6092

The Hair & Beauty
    Clinic
Irish Life Mall
Talbot Street, Dublin 1
☎01 874 5106

Patricia Hanrahan
38 Tamarisk Heights
Tallaght, Dublin 24
☎01 452 0279

Olive Hayes
44 Whitecliff
Rathfarnham, Dublin 14
☎01 494 1257

Cathie Hogan IMTA
    ITEC
Sandymount
☎01 668 9242

Holistic Healing Centre
38 Dame Street
Dublin 2. ☎01 671 0813

The Holistic Health
    Centre
197 Lr Kimmage Road
Dublin 6w. ☎01 492 9279

Holistic School of
    Reflexology
2 Laurel Park Clondalkin
Dublin 22. ☎01 459 2460

International Institute
    of Reflexology (Irl)
Portmarnock
Mary Canavan MIIR MIRI
☎01 846 1514

The Irish College of
    Complementary
    Medicine
6 Main Street
Donnybrook, Dublin 4
☎01 269 6588

Peig Keane AOR
19 Selskar Rise
Townparks, Skerries
☎01 849 0020

Teresa Keating RGN
    CST MRSI
8 The Crescent
Limerick. ☎061 310 166

Valerie Keleghan MIRI
13 Vernon Heath
Clontarf, Dublin 3
☎01 833 0631

Caroline Kelly MIRI
35 Hampton Park
Booterstown
☎01 283 6338

Alison Larkin AOR
3 Oakwood Close
Finglas East, Dublin 11
☎01 834 0276

Anne McDevitt DRE
    BCAA
13 Wicklow Street
Dublin 2. ☎01 677 7962

Dolores McGuilligan
    MIIR
Donnybrook
☎01 269 5629

Maureen McLarnon
    MIRI
48 Castleknock Park
Castleknock
Dublin 15. ☎01 821 5121

Ethna McQuillan MIRI ITEC
140 Foxfield Gve, Raheny Dublin 5. ☎01 831 2008

Maeve Macken
11 Sion Hill Road Drumcondra Dublin 9. ☎01 837 8310

Margaret Mallon
126 Woodview Heights Lucan. ☎01 624 1632

MELT, Temple Bar Natural Healing Centre
2 Temple Lane South Dublin 2. ☎01 679 8786

Natural Living Centre
Walmer Hse, Station Rd Raheny, Dublin 5
Carol Donnelly AOR ☎01 832 7859/846 2574

Natural Solutions
6 Clifton Terrace Monkstown ☎01 280 5506

The Natural Therapy & Beauty Clinic
Coolmine Sports Complex Clonsilla, Dublin 15 ☎01 820 7172

Maureen Nightingale AOR
20 Auburn Drive Watson Estate, Killiney ☎01 285 7963

Dolores O'Neill
54 St John's Wood Clondalkin, Dublin 22 ☎01 457 1789

Yvonne O'Riordan AOR
St Jude's, Oldbridge Road Templeogue, Dublin 16 ☎01 494 7821

Laura O'Sullivan MIIR
Newtown Cross, The Ward ☎01 835 0566

Reflexology Centre
Lower Kimmage Road Dublin 6w. ☎01 490 9915

Mary Regan IMTA ITEC
47 Heatherview Lawn Aylesbury, Tallaght ☎01 451 4915

Sandycove Foot and Health Clinic
57a Glasthule Road Sandycove
John Peter Caviston ITEC Dip. IFR Dip Reflexology IMTA ☎01 284 5287

Joy Stone MIRI
128 Meadow Grove Dundrum, Dublin 16 ☎01 298 8168

Yvonne Townson AOR
33 Killiney Towers Killiney. ☎01 284 8606

Helen Varden MCSCh MICHO
18 Upper George's St Dún Laoghaire ☎01 284 3265

Walkinstown Osteopathy Clinic
18 Cromwellsfort Road Dublin 12
Elizabeth O'Neill ☎01 450 4438

West Wood Club
Leopardstown Racecourse Dublin 18 ☎01 289 5665

Co. Fermanagh
Body Language
72 Main Street Maguiresbridge Lisnaskea ☎08 013657 23313

Co. Galway
Marian Brady
Kilrainey, Moycullen ☎091 555 706

Mary Commins
5 Curralee, Sandyvale Lawn Galway. ☎091 762 476

Co. Kerry
Carmel Gornall
Mountcoal, Listowel ☎068 40173

Oakpark Medical Centre
Oakpark, Tralee
Áine McKivergan ☎066 26255

Timothy J. O'Riordan
The Village, Rathmore ☎064 58663

Marie Prendergast LIC, TCM AI ACU MAIR IASK
Caherdean House Ballyhar, Killarney ☎066 64114

Freddy Van De Wal MPRTCM
Cahirciveen. ☎088 608 511

Co. Kildare
Alternative Treatment Centre
Crookstown Ballytore, Athy
Mary O'Mara ☎0507 23231

Helen Dawed
2 Rye River Park Dun Carraig, Leixlip ☎01 624 4604

Catherine Dempsey
Kilbelin, Newbridge ☎045 436 992

The Footcare Clinic
Carlow Road, Kilcullen ☎087 443 474

Edwina Hanley MRSI
Hazeldene Green Road
Kildare. ☎045 521 294

Mary O'Mara Dip
    HMT MIRI ITEC
Ballytore, Athy
☎0507 23221

Co. Laois
Body Works CIBTAC SAC
Railway Street
Portlaoise. ☎0502 60610

Co. Limerick
Inches
Rossmoyne, Ennis Road
Limerick. ☎061 325 053

Limerick Natural
    Health Centre
65 Catherine St, Limerick
Liz Dowling IMTA ITEC
☎061 419 920

Mikelle Health Studio
153 Russell Court
Ballykeefe, Limerick
Geraldine Kenny AOR
☎061 227 981

Natural Harmony
26 William Street
Limerick. ☎061 419 455

J. O'Connell SRN Mem
    Ins PB Hons Dip Paris
18 Upper Mallow Street
Limerick. ☎061 413 528

Aileen O'Connor
2 Conty View Terrace
Ballincarra, Limerick
☎061 228 860

Susan O'Riordan
6 Meadowlawn
Raheen. ☎061 227 897

Co. Mayo
Heidi Brandt
Rathowen, Killala
☎096 32645

Martina Horan-Barrett AOR
20 Pontoon Drive
Castlebar. ☎094 23161

Maura Martyn
Corheens, Castlebar
☎094 24756

Tir na n-Óg Holistic
    Beauty Centre
The Square, Claremorris
☎094 62678

Co. Monaghan
Foot & Ankle Clinic
18 Glaslough Street
Monaghan
Eileen Dunwoody-
    Brennan BMedSci POD
☎047 71179

Co. Roscommon
Simon Lesley
Aughalustia
Ballaghaderreen
☎0907 61218

Co. Tipperary
Mary Clare Heffernan
1st Floor
34 O'Connell Street
Clonmel. ☎052 27155

Geraldine Lonergan
Silversprings Road
Clonmel. ☎052 26349

Co. Tyrone
Cookstown
    Physiotherapy &
    Sports Injury Clinic
28 Fairhill Rd, Cookstown
☎08 016487 61996

Eileen Kenny
12 Augher Rd, Clogher
☎08 016625 49509

Co. Waterford
Patricia McAvinue
1 Lower Yellow Road
Balybricken, Waterford
☎051 854 477

Trudi Morrissey IMTA
    ITEC
Green Meadows
Ballymacmague
Dungarvan
☎058 42128

Co. Westmeath
Aromaflex
Enterprise Centre
Mullingar
Britta Stewart MIRI
☎044 43444/66287

G. Killeen MIChO
    MRSI AMBRA
32 Mardyke Street
Athlone. ☎088 517 524

Co. Wexford
Centre for Natural
    Therapies
16 George's Street
Wexford. ☎053 21363

Laurence Maher
2 Mount Ross
New Ross. ☎051 425 721

Máire Stafford
Blackhall, Bannow
☎051 561 182

Co. Wicklow
Kevin Clark IMTA ITEC
Delgany. ☎01 287 6917

Valerie Lawrence AOR
Priestnewtown
Delgany, Greystones

Reiki

Most of the training
centres (see Training
and Workshops
directory, p. 211) also
provide referrals to
reiki practitioners.

Co. Cork
Alpha Holistic Centre
29 Parnell Place, Cork

The Bridge Clinic
2nd Floor, 8 Bridge St
Cork. ☎021 551 263

Kieran Corcoran
'San Roja'
Hawthorn Mews
Dublin Hill, Cork
☎021 301 935/894 949/
319 069

Rosaire Harrington RGN
MIINT MAIR Dip.
10 Parnell Place, Cork
☎021 278 593

Inner Healing Centre
46 Sheare's Street, Cork
☎021 278 243

Margaret Kruijswijk
Mourneabbey, Mallow
☎022 29102

Carmel Long
Cork. ☎021 371 377

Mary C. McCarthy
IMTA ITEC
Orchard Grove
Western Rd, Clonakilty

Hannah O'Brien
Inchnagree, Buttevant
Cork. ☎022 24286

Leonie Maria Smith
182 The Willows
Ballincollig, Cork
☎021 871 559

Co. Dublin
Miriam Brady
7 York Avenue
Rathmines, Dublin 6
☎01 496 7605

Helen Hand
Palmerstown, Dublin 20
☎01 626 9703

Hands of Light
Institute of Healing
160 Pembroke Road
Dublin 4 ☎01 668 1809

Healing Arts Centre
International
46 Walnut Rise
Drumcondra, Dublin 9
☎01 837 0832/
088 274 9701

The Holistic Health
Centre
197 Lr Kimmage Rd
Dublin 6w. ☎01 492 9279

House of Astrology
9 Parliament Street
Dublin 2. ☎01 679 3404

Caroline Kelly MIRI
35 Hampton Park
Booterstown
☎01 283 6338

Siobhán Kennedy
West Wood Club
Leopardstown
Racecourse
Foxrock, Dublin 18
☎01 289 5665

Ann Kenny
Sandymount
☎01 269 2346

Nuala Kiernan
22 Treesdale
Stillorgan Road
☎01 283 5648

Gwendolene MacGowan
Hamilton House
Turvey Avenue
Donabate. ☎01 840 7206/
087 448 545

MELT Temple Bar
Natural Healing
Centre
2 Temple Lane South
Dublin 2. ☎01 679 8786

Mary Roden
66 Lower Baggot Street
Dublin 2. ☎0404 61248

Sandycove Foot and
Health Clinic
57a Glasthule Road
Sandycove
John Caviston IMTA
ITEC
☎01 284 5287

Heidi Winston
Beechview, Kilteel Road
Rathcoole. ☎01 458 8394

Co. Limerick
Limerick Natural
Health Centre
65 Catherine Street
Limerick
Liz Dowling
☎061 419 920

M. McElduff Lic Ac
MAIAC IHCA Dip TCM
Limerick. ☎061 227 601

Co. Louth
Iomlánú
Roden Place, Dundalk
☎042 32804/27253

Co. Sligo
Rainbow's End Healing
Centre
Castlebaldwin
☎071 65728

Co. Wexford
Centre for Natural
Therapies
16 George's Street
Wexford. ☎053 21363

Laurence Maher
2 Mount Ross
New Ross. ☎051 425 721

Co. Wicklow
Avon Park
Glendalough Road
Rathdrum. ☎0404 46610

Paddy Mooney
8 Fr Colahan Terrace
Bray. ☎01 286 3971

Rolfing

Galway Rolfing Clinic
Pollnaclough
Moycullen, Co. Galway
Barry O'Brien BSc PhD
  Certified Rolfer
☎091 555 025

SHEN®

American Holistic
  Institute of Ireland
73 Claremont
Circular Road, Galway
☎091 525 941/01 848 1852

Shen Tao Acupressure

Information on
practitioners in your area
can be obtained from:

The Shen Tao
  Practitioners
  Association (SPA)
c/o Judith Hoad
Room for Healing
Inver, Co. Donegal
☎073 36406

Shiatsu

For the name of a
practitioner in your
area, contact:

Patricia O'Hanlon
12 The Cove, Malahide
Co. Dublin
☎01 845 3647

INDIVIDUALS

Co. Antrim
John McKeever
327 Antrim Rd, Belfast
☎08 018206 26941

Co. Cork
Margaret Kruijswijk
Mourneabbey, Mallow
☎022 29102

Co. Dublin
Anne McDevitt DRE BCAA
13 Wicklow Street
Dublin 2. ☎01 677 7962

MELT, Temple Bar
  Natural Healing Centre
2 Temple Lane South
Dublin 2. ☎01 679 8786

The Natural Health
  Clinic
The Mews
154 Leinster Road
Rathmines, Dublin 6
☎01 496 1316

T'ai Chi, Quigong and
  Shiatsu Treatment
  Centre
Dún Laoghaire
☎01 284 2662

Co. Limerick
Shiatsu and
  Acupressure Centre
8 The Crescent, Limerick
Teresa Keating RGN
  CST MRSI
☎061 400 431

Spinology

Co. Cork
Brigid McLoughlin FISI
Summerhill North
Cork. ☎021 509075

Martin Mulchrone FISI
c/o Institute of
  Spinologists in Ireland
4 Summerhill North, Cork

Co. Derry
Kevin Ginty FISI
☎08 01504 24540

Co. Donegal
Kevin Ginty FISI
Glencar, Letterkenny
☎074 24540

Co. Dublin
Dermot Kelly FISI
46 Fortfield Park
Terenure, Dublin 6
☎01 490 2565

Stephen M. Shaw FISI
6 Monkstown Grove
Monkstown
☎01 280 4821

Co. Galway
Ray O'Beara FISI
44 Lr Newcastle Road
Galway. ☎091 24093

Co. Kildare
Brian Moore FISI
Abbey St, Castledermot
☎0503 44396

Dermot Kelly FISI
10 Basin Street, Naas
☎045 79489

Co. Kilkenny
Brian Moore FISI
4 Castlecomer Road
Kilkenny. ☎0503 44396

Co. Laois
Patrick Kelly FISI
New Road, Portlaoise
☎0502 22994

Co. Wexford
Centre for Nutritional
  Therapies
16 George's Street
Wexford. ☎053 21363

Brian Moore FISI
IFA Centre, Enniscorthy
☎0503 44396

Co. Wicklow
Jean Doorley FISI
15 Cuala Road, Bray
☎01 286 8037

Dermot Kelly FISI
Hillview, Dunlavin
☎045 51267

Patrick Kelly FISI
Lemonstown Bridge
Hollywood. ☎045 64497

Spiritual Healing

For referrals to a
spiritual healer in your
area, contact one of the
following:

The National Federation
of Spiritual Healers
Old Manor Farm Studio
Church Street
Sunbury-on-Thames
Middlesex TW16 6RG
UK. ☎0044 1932 783164

Irish Spiritual Centre
30/31 Wicklow Street
Dublin 2
Sarah Branagan
☎01 670 7034
Lucy Costigan RT
(Cert), Maynooth
Dip. in Counselling,
MIAH, Adv Dip in
Clinical Hypnosis,
Healer Mem (NFSH)
☎053 22923
Clara Martin
☎01 280 0692
Brendan O'Callaghan
☎01 671 5106

OTHERS

Co. Dublin
Hands of Light
Institute of Healing
160 Pembroke Road
Dublin 4 ☎01 668 1809

The Holistic Health
Centre
197 Lr Kimmage Rd
Dublin 6w. ☎01 492 9279

Nuala Kiernan
22 Treesdale, Stillorgan Rd
☎01 283 5648

The Natural Health Clinic
The Mews
154 Leinster Road
Rathmines, Dublin 6
☎01 496 1316

The healing house
24 O'Connell Avenue
Berkeley Rd, Dublin 7
☎01 830 6413

Co. Limerick
Limerick Natural
Healing Centre
64 Catherine Street
Limerick. ☎061 400 431

Co. Wexford
Lucy Costigan RT
(Cert), Maynooth
Dip. in Counselling,
MIAH, Adv Dip in
Clinical Hypnosis,
Healer Mem (NFSH)
Wexford Town
☎053 22923

Traditional Chinese Medicine (includes Acupuncture)

For a list of members of
the Register of
acupuncture and
Traditional Chinese
Medicine practitioners
of Ireland (RTCMI),
contact ☎01 679 4216.

Co. Antrim
Aaron Acupuncture &
Physiotherapy Clinic
17 Hightown Road
Glengormley
Bob Granville Dip.Ac Dip.
Physio/Dr Lynn Dun-
woody PhD Dip Ac
☎08 01232 836 216/
0860 699 187

Belfast Chinese Medical
Clinic
80 Upper Lisburn Road
☎08 01232 600 600

Dr R.F.S. Cheah
463 Falls Road, Belfast
☎08 01232 243 593

Chinese Acupuncture
Clinic
14 Comber Road
Dundonald, Belfast
Dr James T.S. Lee
☎08 01232 489 644

Dr Stella Cullington,
MB ChB Mem BMAS
113 Station Road
Greenisland
Carrickfergus BT38 8UW
☎08 01232 863 852

Dr B. Gonsalves MB BCh
MBAS
72 Maryville Park
Malone Rd, Belfast BT9 6LQ
☎08 01232 662 729

Dr A. Maini MB ChB Lic
Ac MBAcC
12 Malone Meadows
Belfast . ☎08 01232 663 066

Natural Health Chinese
Medical Centre
401 Lisburn Road
☎08 01232 666 212

Dr K. Seetha-Unni
17 Jordanstown Road
Newtownabbey
☎08 01232 868 100

Co. Armagh
'Clonard' Acupuncture
Clinic
Batchelors Walk
Portadown
Mary Riley BA DPM
SEN SCM ONC Lic
Acupuncturist
☎08 01762 332 141

Dr Mary Nesbitt MB ChB
21 Tobermore
Magherafelt
☎08 01648 32713

Co. *Cavan*
Mathew Kennedy
RTCMI
Upper Main Street
Cavan. ☎049 61414

Co. *Clare*
Mary V. MacNamara
The Bungalow
Turn Pike Road, Ennis
☎065 39139/41280

Still Point Holistic
Health Clinic
Richard Healy Lic Ac
PRN MBAcC
Barrack Street, Ennis
☎065 20454

Co. *Cork*
Acupuncture, Allergy
& Osteopathy Clinic
Rochestown/Douglas
☎021 292 737

Bandon Acupuncture
Clinic
Laurel Walk, Bandon
Chantal Riordan Lic Ac
(China) Dip. AC
MAFI MRTCMI SRN
SRCN (France)
☎023 44186

Christine Beswick Lic
Ac MTAS (UK)
Courtmacsherry
Bandon. ☎023 46102

Blackrock Acupuncture
& Reflexology Clinic
6 Clontarf Estate
Skehard Road
Marian Flynn SRN
SCM Lic Ac MI Ac
☎021 358 777

Blarney Acupuncture &
Reflexology Centre
2 Sunset Place, Killeens
Cork. ☎021 381 280

Dr John Bourke MB BCh
BAQ LIC AC
Scarteen, Newmarket
☎029 60461 *and*
Liscarroll, Mallow
☎022 48340

Dr Audrey Bradley MB
BCh BAO LIC AC
Wrightville
Douglas Road, Cork
☎021 314 044

Cork Road Clinic
Dr S. and Dr M. Dunphy
Carrigaline
☎021 371 177

Betsy Didderiens Lic
Ac MAIA
Guangming
Townsend Street
Skibbereen. ☎028 22616

Dr A. Gravina MB BCh
MRC Physc. DPM
6 Block B, Harley Court
White Oaks, Wilton
Cork. ☎021 546 087

Niamh Hennessy RTCMI
Old Cork Road
Middleton. ☎021 13334

Dr Pierce A. Hennessy
TCM MWHO RTCMI
Lower Windmill Hill
Youghal. ☎024 93519
and
7A Old Cork Road
Midleton. ☎021 613 334

The Irish Institute of
Natural Therapy
Croaghta Park
Glasheen Road, Cork
☎021 964 313

Dr Patrick Lee MB
MICGP MRCGP
DAcup (Beijing)
1 The Square, Ballincollig
☎021 875 353

Gerard Lyons RTCMI
18 George's Quay, Cork
☎021 319 069

Millbrook Clinic
New Road, Bandon
Mary K. Ryan RTCMI
☎023 43577

Albert Muckey Lic Ac
TAS (UK)
East Ferry, Midleton
☎021 652 678

Gary P. Murphy Lic Ac
AMTAS MAI Ac
U1 Rossdale House
Medical Centre
Bishopstown, Cork
☎021 342 000

Dr Gerard Murphy MB
MRCGP MICGP
Gleann an Óir
Main Road, Ballincollig
☎021 873 640

Dr Patrick J. Murphy
11 Oliver Plunkett St
Bandon *and*
Main Street, Innishannon
☎023 42253

Natural Healing Centre
Thompson House
McCurtain Street
☎021 501 600

Natural Health Centre
Ashdale House, Blarney
Síle Hennigan RTCMI
☎021 382 151

Natural Medicine Clinic
Main Street, Carrigaline
Dr Jennifer Daly, MB
MICGP Lic Ac MIRI
☎021 372 787

Seán O'Brien RTCMI
17 Oakview, Douglas
☎021 893 504/363 312

Drs Diarmuid O'Connell
and Margaret Ryan
MB MRCGP D.AC
(Beijing)
Belvedere Surgery
Douglas Road, Cork
☎021 294 777

Dr Noel O'Regan
8 Arnica House
Langford Row, Cork
☎021 964 470

Chantal Riordan
RTCMI
'La Vanoise'
Laurel Walk, Bandon
☎023 44186

Bernadette Whelan
MBAcA
3 Ballyannon Court
Coolbawn, Midleton
☎021 631 119

Co. Derry
John O'Mahoney
Lic.Ac.MTAcS
18a Queen Street, Derry
☎08 01504 267 062

Co. Donegal
Letterkenny
Acupuncture/
Physiotherapy Clinic
Inverarie, Ramelton Rd
Ballyraine, Letterkenny
Dr Murrough
Birmingham MB BCh
Lic Ac MBAcA
☎074 24559

Co. Down
Ards Chiropractic Clinic
69 Frances Street
Newtownards
☎08 01232 826696

Vivien E. Bell MBAW
Ac Lic Ac
Rockfield
89A Carnreagh
Hillsborough
☎08 01846 683 390

Dr J. T-S Lee
14 Comber Road
Dundonald
☎08 01232 489644

Celine Leonard, PhD,
Lic Ac MBAC
25 Glenhill Park
Dublin Road
Newry BT35 8BU
☎08 01693 63663

The Lyclum Centre
12 Hamilton Rd, Bangor
☎08 01247 467467

Natural Health Chinese
Medical Centre
45 Cloghskelt Road
Ballyward, Katesbridge
☎08 018206 71213

Co. Dublin
Acupoint
2–5 Johnson's Place
South King St, Dublin 2
Irja Foley/Sharon Kirwan
Lic Ac (China) RTCMI
☎01 677 4114

Acupuncture & Allergy
Testing Clinic
59 Maywood Avenue
Raheny, Dublin 5
☎01 851 0285

Acupuncture & Chinese
Medical Clinic
2 Greythorn Pk, Glenageary
☎01 280 4821 *and*
2 Fairways, Rathfarnham
Dublin 14
Stephen Shaw/Leo
Traynor Lic Ac (Nanjing)
☎01 294 1534/088 628 394

Acupuncture & Herbal
Clinic
50 Sandycove Road
Dún Laoghaire
Nicholas Power Lic Ac
Dip Ac Nanjing
☎01 280 3505
087 429 745

Acupuncture and
Herbal Clinic
24 Main St, Blackrock
Áine Delaney
☎01 278 3547

Acupuncture and
Sports Injury Clinic
68 Old Bawn Road
Dublin 24. ☎01 451 3207

Acupuncture,
Homoeopathic and
Hypnotherapy Clinic
U6, Phisboro S.C.
Dublin 7
Dr Ranjith Lalloo MD
(MA) PhD (Sri Lanka)
☎01 830 9551

The Albany Clinic
Lower Fitzwilliam Street
Dublin 2
Jacqueline McDonnell
Lic Ac (Nanjing)
RTCMI
☎01 661 6029

Belgrave Acupuncture
Clinic
The Basement
17 Belgrave Square
Monkstown
☎01 284 5400

Carmel Bradley Lic Ac
CAc (Nanjing)
RTCMI
138 Philipsburgh Ave.
Fairview, Dublin 3
☎01 837 0543

Blackrock Acupuncture
Clinic
Seafield Avenue
Monkstown
Paul McCarthy RGN
RPN RNT Dip Ac Lic
Ac (China) MRTCMI
☎01 280 1950

Arlene Capot Lic TCM
27 Ranelagh Road
Dublin 6. ☎01 496 3484

Paul Carolan
13 Moatfield Park
St Brendan's Estate
Dublin 5. ☎01 867 0343

Dr Vincent J. Carroll
MB BCh BAO MPH
DCh RTCMI
Fairfield House
Newbridge Avenue
Dublin 4. ☎01 660 1487

Dr Palden Carson MAcA
(China 1976) MD D
Sports Med MBAcA (UK)
1 Walker's Cottages
Ranelagh, Dublin 6
☎01 496 2132

The Chinese Health
Clinic
1A Alma House
Prince of Wales Terrace
Sandymount Avenue
Dublin 4. ☎01 660 5057

The Chinese Medicine &
Acupuncture Centre
☎01 496 1533

Dr John C. Clement
70 Ranelagh Village
Dublin 6. ☎01 660 4810

The Clinic of Natural
Medicine
570 Howth Road
Raheny, Dublin 5
Michael Gygax
☎01 832 7399

Clinic of Wholistic
Medicine
Basement
50 Merrion Square
Dublin 2. ☎01 676 4640

Clondalkin
Acupuncture Clinic
Desmond Hse, Boot Rd
Clondalkin, Dublin 22
Bernadette Jewell Dip Ac
Lic Ac MRTCMI
RTCMI
☎01 464 0050/088 620 598

The Clonskeagh Clinic
36 Glenswood Drive
Clonskeagh, Dublin 14
Mary Gardiner SRN Lic
Acu (Nanjing)
RTCMI
☎01 260 0090

Michael Collins RTCMI
154 Leinster Road
Rathmines, Dublin 6
☎01 492 9492

Karen Costin
3 Craiglands, Dalkey
☎01 285 0874

Deirdre Courtney
RTCMI
2nd Floor, 66 Adelaide Rd
Dublin 2. ☎01 475 2006

The Crannagh Clinic
147 Rathfarnham Road
Dublin 14
Eileen O'Driscoll MCSP
MISCP Lic Ac MBAcA
☎01 490 5275

Noelle Cullinane Lic Ac
RTCMI
59 Hermitage Park
Rathfarnham
Dublin 16. ☎01 494 5628

Kate Curtis RTCMI
13 Hillcrest Heights
Lucan. ☎01 628 2220

Christopher Davala Lic
TCM MAIA
12 Clarinda Park North
Dún Laoghaire
☎01 280 1740

Áine Delaney SRN Lic Ac
RTCMI
77 Springhill Avenue
Blackrock. ☎01 289 5067

Aileen Donnelly
69 Marley Court
Rathfarnham
Dublin 14. ☎ 01 298 0763

Tina Dunne Lic Ac
MIHCA Reflex.
RTCMI
58 Old Finglas Road
Glasnevin, Dublin 11
☎01 837 4859 *and*
Over Chemist
Main St, Dunshaughlin
☎01 825 0007

Eileen Dunnelly RGN
Lic Ac RTCMI
69 Marley Court
Rathfarnham
Dublin 14. ☎01 298 0763

Dr Brendan Fitzpatrick
MB MRCPI DCH DO
MF Hom
115 Morehampton Rd
Dublin 4. ☎01 269 7768

Fitzwilliam Acupuncture
& Herbal Clinic
77 Lower Leeson Street
Dublin 2
Dr MS Khan MBBS C
Ac (China)
☎01 676 4912

Dr Josephine Freeney
5 Lakelands Drive
Kilmacud, Stillorgan
☎01 288 8174

Dr Noel M. Gallivan
MB BCh MF Hom
5 Lower Hatch Street
Dublin 2. ☎01 676 0311

Olive Gentleman Lic Ac
RTCMI
2 Laurel Park
Clondalkin, Dublin 22
☎01 459 2460

Tony Hartin BSc Lic Ac
CAc (Nanjing)
RTCMI
27 Hermitage Drive
Rathfarnham, Dublin 16
☎01 494 3328/088 551 271

Margaret Hennessy Dip
Ac Lic Ac (China)
RTCMI
15 Old Rectory, Lucan
☎01 628 3795

The Holistic Health Centre
197 Lr Kimmage Rd
Dublin 6w. ☎01 492 9279

Anthony Hughes BSc
Lic TCM
1 Leopardstown Drive
Stillorgan. ☎01 288 0352

Institute of Alternative
Medicine
6 Martello Terrace
Sandycove
☎01 284 3275

The Irish College of
Traditional Chinese
Medicine
100 Marlborough Road
Dublin 4. ☎01 496 7830

Mary Keilthy RTCMI
35 Turnberry, Baldoyle
Dublin 13. ☎01 839 3480

Ena Kellett RTCMI
22 Burnell Park
Castleknock, Dublin 15
☎01 820 8539

Phil Kelly RTCMI
68 Old Bawn Road
Tallaght, Dublin 24
☎01 452 2205

Dr Khan RTCMI
80 Aungier Street
Dublin 2. ☎01 475 6975

Dr S. Khan MBBSC Ac
CHerb (Nanjing)
9 Upper Fitzwilliam St
Dublin 2. ☎01 662 3525

Dr Ranjith Laloo
Unit 6 Phibsboro SC
Dublin 7. ☎01 860 0561

Alison Larkin RTCMI
3 Oakwood Close
Finglas East, Dublin 11
☎01 834 0276

Dr Catherine Larkin MB
FRCR C Ac (China)
61 Wilfield Road
Sandymount, Dublin 4
☎01 260 0826

Joy Lennon
Ashfield, 66 Kincoro Rd
Dublin 3. ☎01 833 4356

Celine Leonard PhD
Lic Ac MBAcC
24 Hamilton Street
Dublin 8. ☎01 454 2140

Seamus Lynch Lic Ac.
MTAcS
17 Alma Rd, Monkstown
☎01 284 6073

Michael McCarthy M
Lic Ac C (Nanjing) D
Tuina RTCMI
65 Kenilworth Square
Dublin 6. ☎01 497 8958

Ros McFeeley BSc Lic
Ac (Nanjing) RTCMI
18 Oaklands Drive
Sandymount, Dublin 4
☎01 668 4574

Edel MacGinty Lic TCM
Clin Ac (Beijing)
2 Brighton Rd, Foxrock
Dublin 18. ☎01 289 4393

Beverley McGovern RTCMI
59 Maywood Avenue
Raheny, Dublin 5
☎01 851 0285

Susan Meagher MCSP
Lic Ac
3 Lr Pembroke Street
Dublin 2. ☎01 662 1211

Medical Acupuncture
5 Lower Hatch Street
Dublin 2. ☎01 676 0311

MELT, Temple Bar
Natural Healing Centre
2 Temple Lane South
Dublin 2. ☎01 679 8786

Mulvany Medical Centre
10 Cherry Lawn
Carpenterstown
Castleknock
☎01 820 2155

Siobhán Murphy
RTCMI
Channel Road, Rush
☎01 843 8545

The Natural Health Clinic
154 Leinster Road
Rathmines
Michael Collins
☎01 492 9492

Northside Acupuncture
Herbal Clinic
87 North Circular Road
☎01 662 3525

Dr Ann O'Rourke MB DA
30 Iona Crescent
Dublin 9. ☎01 830 6438

Pain Care Clinic
Manor House
Brennanstown, Dublin18
Áine Delaney
☎01 278 3547

Peking Acupuncture
Clinic
126 Mount Merrion Ave
Blackrock. ☎01 288 9838

Deirdre Phelan Lic Ac
RTCMI
12 Willow Gardens
Glasnevin, Dublin 9
☎01 836 8187

Mrs Su Pin OMB ACA
SAC CRI (Shang)
62 Dame St, Dublin 2
☎01 677 3591 *and*
12 Wood Dale Grove
Firhouse, Dublin 24
☎01 493 8141

The Priory Clinic
Stillorgan
Deirdre Courtney
☎01 283 5566/283 5756

Professional Register of
Acupuncture and
TCM Practitioners of
Ireland
2–5 Johnson's Place
South King Street
Dublin 2. ☎01 838 8196

Professional Register of
Traditional Chinese
Medicine
100 Marlborough Road
Dublin 4. ☎01 496 7830

Pu-Shan Chinese
Medicine Centre
Suite 14, 24/26 Dame St
Dublin 2. ☎01 679 9753

Sandycove Clinic
50 Sandycove Road
Nicholas Power RTCMI
☎01 280 3505/087 429 745

Shape Up
13 Hillcrest Heights
Lucan
Kate Curtis RGN LicAc
☎01 628 2220

Angela Shaw D Ac Lic
Ac RGN RM RNT
FFRCSI
23 Church Road
Dalkey. ☎01 280 6419

Skerries Healing Centre
85 Strand St, Skerries
Gary Westby RTCMI
☎01 849 1741/088 517 345

Noeleen Slattery DAc
Phyp
Main Street, Rathcoole
☎01 458 9672

Paul D. Smyth Dip Ac
Lic Ac (China)
RTCMI
Chinese Medicine &
Acupuncture Centre
3 Castleknock Road
Dublin 15
☎01 820 9181 *and*
196 Upper Rathmines Rd
Dublin 6. ☎01 496 1533

Sports Injuries Clinic
Apollo Building
Dundrum, Dublin 14
Adam Bux. ☎01 298 8127

Sports Injury Clinic
564 Howth Road
Raheny, Dublin 5
☎01 851 0285

Philip Staveley Lic Ac
(China)
Shamrock Cottage
Balkill Road, Howth
☎01 832 6670

Annette Tallon
6 Martello Terrace
Sandycove
☎01 284 2294/284 3275

T'ai Chi, Quigong & Shiatsu
Treatment Centre
Dún Laoghaire
☎01 284 2662

TCM Centre
Main Street, Rathcoole
Deirdre Courtney
☎01 458 9672/458 9705

Leo Traynor
2 Fairways, Rathfarnham
Dublin 14. ☎01 494 1534

Turner Clinic of
Alternative Medicine
Dr Ronald J. Turner Ac
Dublin Road, Stillorgan
☎01 288 4327

Stephen Vaughan D
Acu, Lic Ac (China,
MRATMI
Odyssey Healing Centre
15 Wicklow St, Dublin 2
☎01 677 1021/087 235 6377

Gary Walsh Lic Ac Dip
Ac (Nanjing)
85 Strand Street
Skerries. ☎088 517 345

James Walsh Lic Acu
RTCMI
111 Walkinstown Road
Dublin 12. ☎01 450 8232

Dr Ye Wu
8 St James' Terrace
Malahide. ☎01 845 0407

Co. Galway
Acupuncture,
Osteopathy and
Allergy Testing Clinic
1 McDara Rd, Shantalla
Alan Brannelly RTCMI
Galway. ☎091 522 631

Martin Aherne
Cosmona, Loughrea
☎091 842 762

Marian Brady BA MSc
MIRI Lic Ac RTCMI
Kilrainey, Moycullen
☎091 555 706

Clinic of Complementary
& Natural Medicine
Kiltartan House
Forster Street, Galway
Dr Hussain Bhatti
☎091 568 804

Clinic of Wholistic
Medicine
34 Upper Abbeygate St
Galway
Nora O'Connell-Keane
RTCMI
☎091 567 416/087 439 758

Geraldine Flannery
2 Bellair Drive, Tuam
☎093 25180

Kerry Hanbury RTCMI
Rusheen Bay
Barna Road, Galway
☎091 591 937

Linda Heffernan Lic Ac
6 St Brendan's Road
Woodquay, Galway
☎091 561 676

Darina Joyce Lic Ac
MAFIR RTCMI
Árd Rí House
Lower Abbeygate St
Galway. ☎091 563 329

Thomas Joseph Shanahan
5 Devon Place
The Crescent, Galway
☎091 581 575

Co. Kerry
Peter Curran
Creevaghbeg, Quin
☎065 25801

Tony McGinley MAIA
9 Westcourt, Tralee
☎066 24694

P.J. O'Neill
2 Denny Street, Tralee
☎066 20121

Catherine Overhauser
M Ac Cert ZB
The Balance Point
Kenmare . ☎064 41215

Marie Prendergast Lic
TCM AI Acu MAIR
IASK
Caherdean House
Ballyhar, Killarney
☎066 64114

Fiona Maxwell Smith
33 Main St, Castleisland
☎066 42317 *and*
38 New Street
Killarney. ☎064 35995

Traditional Chinese
Medicine Clinic
Upper Bridge Street
Killorglin
Alan Sheehy MPRTCM
☎066 62344

Freddy Van De Wal
Cahirciveen. ☎088 608 511

Co. Kildare
Acupuncture and
Chinese Herbal Clinic
Garadice, Kilcock
Mary Furlong MB Ac A
MCSP. ☎0405 57428

Anne Campbell Lic Ac
12 Rye River Gardens
Duncarrig, Leixlip
☎01 624 6255

Complementary
Medical Centre
Rathasker Square
Kilcullen Road, Naas
Monica Teahan Lic Ac
MRCM SRN Clin. Cert
☎045 876 687

Peg Cronly RTCMI
'Annagh', Central Park
Clane. ☎045 868 015

Dr Paul Gallagher MB
DAcu MRTCMI
39 The Grange
Newbridge. ☎045 431 766

Bridget Heavey Dip Ac
Lic Ac
Lower Eyre Street
Newbridge. ☎045 431 022

Bernadette Jewell
RTCMI
Whole Earth
Lower Main Street
Celbridge. ☎01 627 4411

Naas Physiotherapy
Clinic
Elizabeth Kent MISCP
Lic Ac MBAcA
☎045 866 075

Co. Kilkenny
Friary Court Medical &
Dental Centre
Friary Street, Kilkenny
Anne-Marie Mollereau
ICCAM RTCMI
☎056 65613

Kilkenny Acupuncture
& Reflexology Clinic
26 Upper John Street
Kilkenny
Anne O'Donoghue
SRN SCM Dip Psych
Dip Micrb Lic TCM
☎056 62196

Co. Limerick
A.C.T. Centre
64 Catherine Street
Limerick
Dr John Le Boeuf DC
☎061 419 920

Marion Fenton SRN Lic
TCM AIA
5 Alphonsus Terrace
Quin Street, Limerick
☎061 417 781

Mary Keating BSc Lic
  Ac MAIA
Bishop St, Newcastlewest
☎088 530 432 *and*
Broadford. ☎063 84040

M. McElduff Lic Ac
  MAIAC IHCA Dip TCM
Limerick. ☎061 227 601

Derry O'Malley RTCMI
34 Catherine Street
Limerick. ☎061 317 670/
1800 61 1177

Co. Longford
Gerald Ward
Corboy, Mostrim
☎043 46993

Betty White RTCMI
'Carbery', Clonrollagh
☎043 459 431

Co. Louth
Acupuncture Clinic
  RTCMI
Irish Street, Ardee
Gemma Dillon/
  Carol Small
☎041 56263

Acupuncture Clinic
84 West Street
Drogheda. ☎041 43162

Co. Mayo
Margaret P. Deffely
Glenisland, Castlebar
☎094 22940

Co. Meath
Acupuncture & Chinese
  Medicine Clinic
Abbey House Medical
  Centre
Navan
Charles Morton/
  Frances Lee Lic Ac
  MBACA MISCP
  RTCMI
☎046 22126/21186

Athboy Beauty Centre
O'Growney St, Athboy
Sandra Glennon RTCMI
☎046 32855

Dolores McEntee Lic
  Ac RGN RSCN
Crickst'n Curragha
Ashbourne. ☎01 835 2409

Natural Medicine Centre
14 Ludlow Street
Navan
Gemma Dillon/
  Carol Small RTCMI
☎046 27156

Co. Offaly
Peg Cronly RTCMI
Kilbride Street
Tullamore. ☎0506 41851

Co. Roscommon
Ronan Donnelly
  RTCMI
Cloongarvin
Strokestown. ☎078 37151

Eileen Kennedy RTCMI
9 Kildallouge Heights
Strokestown
☎078 33237

Michael Lennon
  RTCMI
Galway Road
Roscommon
☎0903 26023

Co. Tipperary
Anne-Marie Lovett Dip
  Ac Lic Ac (China)
  RTCMI
Altona, Dromin Road
Nenagh. ☎067 31585

Celine O'Connor Casey
  RGN Lic TCM
  MRCM
Rockbarton, Bruff
☎061 382 151
Nenagh. ☎088 612 941

Emer Purcell Lic Ac
  MAIA (Beijing)
The Lodge
Marlfield House
Clonmel
☎052 22297/088 528 859

Co. Waterford
Dungarvan
  Acupuncture Clinic
47 Main Street
Dungarvan
Kevin Power Lic TCM
  MRTCM
☎058 44299

Katherine Foran
  RTCMI
Jury's Leisure Centre
Jury's Hotel
☎051 51038 *and*
63 Morrison's Avenue
☎051 71595

Omni Health Clinic
47 The Quay, Waterford
☎051 874 520

Nona Taylor Dip Ac
  MBAcC
Mountain View
Mountain Rd, Clonmel
Waterford. ☎052 25309

Co. Westmeath
Acupuncture Clinic
32 Mardyke Street
Athlone
Maureen Feely BSc
  (Hons) Lic TCM
☎0902 73848

The Acupuncture Clinic
Church Street, Athlone
Siobhan Meehan
☎0902 37454

The Clinic of Wholistic
  Medicine
Church Street, Athlone
☎0902 78750

Natural Therapies
   Clinic
Dublingate Street
Athlone
Mathew Kennedy
   RTCMI
☎0902 72965

Co. Wexford
Centre for Natural
   Therapies
16 George's Street
Wexford. ☎053 21363

Dr Derek Forde MICGP
Toorak Lodge, Oulart
Wexford. ☎053 36333

Physiotherapy &
   Acupuncture Clinic
McCauley Chemists
Wexford
Clare McCormack Dip
   Ac MISCP MSOM
☎053 22669

Co. Wicklow
Katharine Curtis
   RTCMI
16 High Street, Wicklow
☎0404 66321

Greystones
   Acupuncture Clinic
Triton House
The Harbour, Greystones
Paul McCarthy RGN
   RPN RNT Dip Ac Lic
   Ac (China) MRTCMI
☎01 287 5944

John Kelly Lic Ac C Ac
   (Nanjing) RTCMI
17 Rectory Slopes
Herbert Road, Bray
☎01 286 8183 *and*
Milltown North
Rathnew. ☎0404 67020

Dr Khan RTCMI
Seaview, Bray
☎01 282 8194

David Morrisroe
   RTCMI
Briar Cottage
Knockfadda, Roundwood
☎01 281 8215

Ann Prendergast
   RTCMI
32 Seacourt, Newcastle
☎01 286 6611

Shape Up
Adare House
Killincarrig, Greystones
Kate Curtis RGN LicAc
☎01 287 3166

Ship Shape RTCMI
The Mall Centre
Wicklow. Paul McCarthy
☎0404 69267

Vega Test

For the names of
trained vega-test
practitioners, contact:

Clinic Support Services
Dublin. ☎01 460 0203

Nature's Way offers a
short vega test for food
sensitivity at the
following locations:

Co. Cork
Paul Street Centre
☎021 270 729

Merchant's Quay
   Centre
☎021 275 989

Wilton Centre
☎021 544 284

Co. Dublin
Blackrock Centre
☎01 288 6696

Donaghmede
☎01 867 1174

Ilac Centre
☎01 872 8391

Northside Centre
☎01 847 8028

The Square
Tallaght
☎01 459 6268

St Stephen's Green Centre
☎01 478 0165

Co. Kilkenny
Market Cross Centre
☎056 65896

Co. Limerick
Arthur's Quay Centre
☎061 310 466

OTHERS

Co. Cork
Beara Circle
Castletownbere
Sinéad Murphy
☎027 70744

Co. Dublin
Acupoint
2–5 Johnson's Place
South King Street
Dublin 2
Irja Foley Lic Ac (China)
☎01 677 4114

Voice Therapy

For information, contact:

Co. Dublin
Joan Davis
'The Studio'
Rere 330 Harold's Cross
Dublin 6. ☎01 287 6986

Kalichi. ☎01 497 3097

Co. Wicklow
Chrysalis, Donard
☎045 404 713

Yoga

Dublin Yoga Centre
19 Upper Mount Street
Dublin 2. ☎01 284 3445

The Holistic Health
Centre
197 Lr Kimmage Road
Dublin 6w
☎01 492 9279

Irish Association of
Holistic Medicine
9–11 Grafton Street
Dublin 2. ☎01 671 2788

Irish Yoga Association
108 Lr Kimmage Road
Harold's Cross
Dublin 6w. ☎01 492 9213

Temple Bar Natural
Healing Centre
2 Temple Lane
Dublin 2. ☎01 679 8786

YOGA CLASSES

Co. Cork
Beara Circle
Castletownbere
Patricia Farrell
☎027 70744

Brahma Kumaris
Bishopstown
☎021 341 297

Marianne Gabriel
Myrtlegrove House
Old Cork Road
Bandon. ☎023 41841

Macroom Yoga and
Reflexology Centre
Rockborough
Macroom. ☎026 41641

Regina O'Mahoney
8 Kilmoney Heights
Carrigaline
☎021 372 519

Satyananda Yoga
Centre
Liberty House
2 Liberty Street, Cork
☎021 545 207

Tony Quinn Health Centre
20 Academy Street
Cork. ☎021 276364

Co. Dublin
Dublin Meditation Centre
23 South Frederick St
Dublin 2. ☎01 671 3187

Dundrum Family
Recreation Centre Ltd
Meadowbrook
Dundrum, Dublin 16
☎01 298 4654

Holistic Healing Centre
38 Dame Street
Dublin 2. ☎01 671 0813

Mella Murphy
20 Churchview Road
Killiney. ☎01 285 0465

Natural Health
Training Centre
1 Parklane East
Pearse Street, Dublin 2
☎01 671 8454

Natural Solutions
6 Clifton Terrace
Monkstown. ☎01 280 5506

The Raja Yoga Centre
36 Lansdowne Road
Dublin 4. ☎01 660 3967

Sandymount TM Centre
Dublin 4. ☎01 288 7171

The T'Ai-Chi Ch'uan
Association
St Andrew's Resource
Centre
114 Pearse Street
Dublin 2. ☎01 677 1930

Teresa's Inspiring
Living Health Shop
8 Main Street, Raheny
Dublin 5. ☎01 832 9464

Tony Quinn Health Centre
66 Eccles Street
Dublin 7. ☎01 830 4998

Co. Galway
Galway Yoga Centre
Church Yard Street
Galway. ☎091 844 449

Co. Kerry
P.J. O'Neill
Denny Street, Tralee
☎066 20121

Co. Limerick
Limerick Natural
Healing Centre
64 Catherine Street
Limerick. ☎061 400 431

The Yoga Centre
Old Crescent College
O'Connell Street
Limerick. ☎061 330 534

Co. Mayo
Brahma Kumaris World
Spiritual University
'Om Niwas'
Mountain View
Castlebar. ☎094 25503

Co. Westmeath
Keating Yoga Centre
7 Retreat Heights
Athlone. ☎0902 78015

Zero Balancing

Co. Dublin
The Family and
Counselling Centre
46 Lr Elmwood Avenue
Ranelagh, Dublin 6
Freda Roche
☎01 497 1188/497 1722

Seamus Lynch (Certified
Zero Balancer)
☎01 284 6073

Co. Kerry
Catherine Overhauser
MAc Cert ZB
The Balance Point
Kenmare. ☎064 41215

Helplines and Useful Addresses

AIDS Helpline Dublin. ☎01 872 4277

AIM Group (*Family Law Information and Mediation Centre*)
6 D'Olier Street, Dublin 2. ☎01 670 8363

Alcoholics Anonymous
109 South Circular Road, Dublin 8. ☎01 453 8998. (After-hours: 01 679 5967/679 6555)
Community Centre, Monkstown Ave.
☎01 280 8723

Al-Anon Family Groups, and **Alateen** (*Support group for families and teenage children of alcoholics*)
5 Capel Street, Dublin 1. ☎01 873 2699

Augustine Fellowship (*Sexual/Romantic Addiction*)
PO Box 3935, Dublin 1

Aware Helpline (*Depression*)
☎01 679 1711

Barnardos (*Childcare and Adoption*)
Christchurch Square, Dublin 8
☎01 453 0355

Body Positive (*Aids Organisation*)
53 Parnell Square, Dublin 1. ☎01 872 0554

Body Whys (*Self-support group for those with eating problems, anorexia etc.*)
☎01 493 7576

BUPA Ireland
12 Fitzwilliam Square, Dublin 2. ☎01 662 7662; Fax: 01 662 7672
Mill Island, Fermoy, Co. Cork. ☎025 42121

Cairde (*One-to-one befriending for those with HIV-positive or AIDS*)
25 St Mary's Abbey (off Capel Street), Dublin 7. ☎01 873 0006

CARI Foundation (*For abused children*)
110 Drumcondra Road, Dublin 9. ☎01 830 8529

Cherish (*Association of one-parent families*)
2 Lower Pembroke Street, Dublin 2. ☎01 662 9212

Childline
c/o ISPCC, 20 Molesworth Street, Dublin 2. Freefone 1800 666 666

Cot Death: Irish Sudden Infant Death Association
Carmichael House, 4 North Brunswick Street, Dublin 7
☎1800 391 391 (Freefone) or 01 873 2711 (General enquiries)

Cura (*Pregnancy Advice*)
30 South Anne Street, Dublin 2. ☎01 671 0598

Drug Treatment Centre Board
Trinity Court, 30–31 Pearse Street, Dublin 2. ☎01 677 1122

Dublin AIDS Alliance
53 Parnell Square West, Dublin 1. ☎01 873 3799/873 3065/373 3480

Dublin Lesbian Line
Carmichael House, Brunswick Street, Dublin 7. ☎01 872 9911

Dublin Well Woman Centre (*Women's Health Centre and Family Planning Clinic*)
73 Lower Leeson Street, Dublin 2. ☎01 661 0083/661 0086
35 Liffey Street, Dublin 1. ☎01 872 8051/872 8095
9 Main Street, Bray, Co. Wicklow. ☎01 282 9331
Family Mediation Service
Irish Life Centre Block 1, Floor 5, Lower Abbey Street, Dublin 1. ☎01 872 8277
Federation of Services for Unmarried Parents and Their Children
36 Upper Rathmines Road, Dublin 6. ☎01 496 4155
Focus Point
14a/15 Eustace Street, Dublin 2. ☎01 617 2555/677 6421/670 5226
Dublin 7. ☎01 838 6054
Focus Point Day Activity Centre
5 John Street West, Dublin 8, ☎01 677 0691
Friends of the Suicide Bereaved
c/o Lynn Hallman. ☎021 294 318
Gamblers Anonymous
Carmichael House, North Brunswick Street, Dublin 7. ☎01 872 1133
Gay and Lesbian Federation, National
6 South William Street, Dublin 2. ☎01 671 0939
Gay Switchboard Dublin (*Counselling information*)
Old Doctor's Residence, Richmond Hospital, Dublin 7. ☎01 872 1055
Gingerbread (*Association for one-parent families*)
29 Dame Street, Dublin 2. ☎01 671 0291
Grow Community Mental Health Movement
167A Capel Street, Dublin 1. ☎01 873 4029
Haven House (*Women's night shelter*)
Dublin 7. ☎01 873 2279
Hospital Savings Association (HSA)
Hambledon House, Andover, Hants SP10 1LQ, UK. ☎0044 264 358 977
Dublin Contact ☎01 840 3500
Homeless Persons
(*Eastern Health Board out-of-hours emergency accommodation for adults*)
☎1800 724 724 (Freefone)
Hospital Saturday Fund
Health Plan, 1 Lower O'Connell Street, Dublin 1. ☎01 874 2136/874 2432
Irish Cancer Society
5 Northumberland Road, Dublin 4. ☎01 668 1855/Freefone 1800 200 700
The Irish Hospice Foundation
9 Fitzwilliam Place, Dublin 2. ☎01 676 5599
Irish Still Birth and Neonatal Death Society
4 North Brunswick Street, Dublin 7. ☎01 295 7785/872 6996/821 1238
Life Ireland (*Pregnancy support service*)
29 Dame Street, Dublin 2. ☎01 679 8989/Callsave 1850 281 281
Narcotics Anonymous
Dublin 1. ☎01 830 0944 (24-hour)
National Association of Widows in Ireland
12 Upper Ormond Quay, Dublin 7. ☎01 677 0977

Overeaters Anonymous
PO Box 2529, Dublin 5. ☎01 451 5138
Parents Alone Resource Centre
Community Project, 325 Bunratty Road, Coolock, Dublin 17. ☎01 848 1116
Parental Equality (*The Shared Parenting and Joint Custody Support Group*)
1 Muirhevna, Dublin Road, Dundalk. ☎042 33163
Parentline (*Organisation for parents under stress*)
Carmichael House, North Brunswick Street, Dublin 7. ☎01 873 3500
Post-Natal Distress Association of Ireland
Carmichael House, North Brunswick Street, Dublin 7. ☎01 872 7172
Rape Crisis Centre
70 Lower Leeson Street, Dublin 2. ☎01661 4911/661 4564
Freefone 1800 778 888
Samaritans
112 Marlborough Street, Dublin 1. ☎01 872 7700/1850 609 090 (Callsave)
Simon Community
119 Capel Street, Dublin 1. ☎01 872 0188
Night Shelter, 25 Usher's Island, Dublin 8
Residential houses. ☎01 679 2391
Victim Support
29 Dame Street, Dublin 2
☎01 679 8673 (General Enquiries)
☎054 76222 (24-hour)
The Voluntary Health Insurance Board (VHI)
20 Lower Abbey Street, Dublin 1. ☎01 872 4499/874 9171
35 Lower George's Street, Dún Laoghaire, Co. Dublin. ☎01 280 0306
Admissions Office, Beaumont Hospital, Dublin 9
Women's Aid Helpline
☎1800 341 900
Women's Refuge (Aoibhneas)
☎01 867 0701/867 0805
Women's Refuge (Eastern Health Board)
Rathmines, Dublin 6. ☎01 496 1002

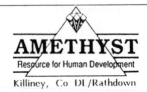

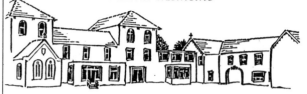

beara circle ltd.
Natural Medicine

Castletownbere,
Co. Cork.
Tel. (027) 70744
Fax (027) 70745

- Electro-acupuncture diagnosis
- Allergy testing and therapy
- Homoeopathy, supplements, variety of massages

Bach-Flowers, emotional clearing, colon hydrotherapy

- Proven candida and mycosis treatment
- Workshops and workshop facilities
- Accommodation, wholefood, sauna, yoga and meditation

Please see Residential Healing Centres for full listing.

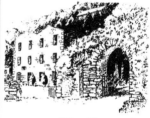

Cloona Health Centre

Westport Co Mayo

Ireland's longest established Health Farm.

We offer a unique and carefully structured programme
from Sunday to Friday.

We aim to promote health and well-being
through a process of relaxation, stress reduction,
body awareness and a de-tox diet.

Enjoy a week of rest and recovery in a beautiful
and peaceful environment.
A GIFT TO YOURSELF !

The organised daily schedule includes yoga, guided walk, sauna,
massage, cleansing diet. Optional therapies also available.

For brochure, e-mail to: cloona@jazzybee.ie or phone: (098) 25251.

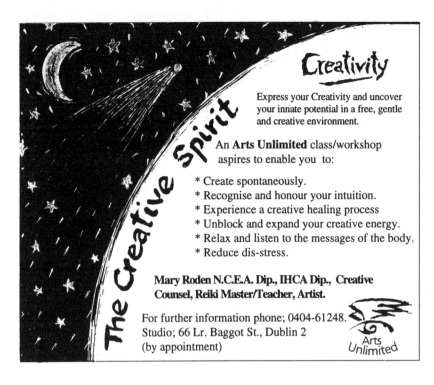

Creativity

Express your Creativity and uncover your innate potential in a free, gentle and creative environment.

An **Arts Unlimited** class/workshop aspires to enable you to:

* Create spontaneously.
* Recognise and honour your intuition.
* Experience a creative healing process
* Unblock and expand your creative energy.
* Relax and listen to the messages of the body.
* Reduce dis-stress.

Mary Roden N.C.E.A. Dip., IHCA Dip., Creative Counsel, Reiki Master/Teacher, Artist.

For further information phone; 0404-61248. Studio; 66 Lr. Baggot St., Dublin 2 (by appointment)

Arts Unlimited

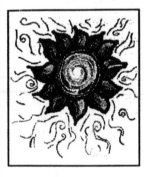

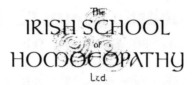

The IRISH SCHOOL of HOMOEOPATHY Ltd.

Venue for Courses and Seminars:
Milltown Park College, Sandford Road, Dublin 6.

The Irish School of Homoeopathy is committed to homoeopathic education in Ireland and to this end we provide regular weekend workshops as an introduction to the philosophy and practical use of homoeopathy. Our four-year part-time professional training course in Homoeopathic Studies & Practice includes 12 weekend seminars with 12 supervised regional tutorials following each seminar. Clinical training is an essential part of the course. The Milltown clinic offers hands-on experience in the treatment and management of patients; thus preparing the student to commence Homoeopathic Practice upon fulfilling the final-year assessment criteria. The Licentiate of the school is awarded in recognition of a student's ability to commence safe and competent practice of homoeopathy within an appropriate ethical context. This Licentiate is recognised by the Irish Society of Homoeopaths.

The Four-Year Part-time Course Syllabus is summarised as follows:

HOMOEOPATHIC PHILOSOPHY & METHODOLOGY
The principles and theories associated with homoeopathic prescribing; Clinical training; Casetaking & prescribing skills; Therapeutics of degenerative pathological states; Homoeopathic obstetric management; Long-term patient management; Dietary support for patients; Clinical diagnostic skills; Proving methodology; Patient/Practitioner relationship.

HOMOEOPATHIC MATERIA MEDICA
The practical application of the main remedies used in acute and chronic homoeopathic prescribing; Remedy "families"; Commonly used small remedies in therapeutic practice.

HUMAN SCIENCES
Lectures on human anatomy and physiology; Lectures on pathological processes in order to inform clinical decision-making and referral activities.

PERSONAL DEVELOPMENT & COUNSELLING SKILLS MODULE
Forwarding address for above course and workshops

Irish School of Homoeopathy
Administration, 47 Ratoath Estate, Dublin 7.
Tel/Fax: (01) 868 2581.

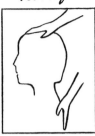
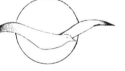

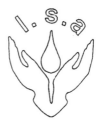

Daniel Tanguay

Biodynamic Psychotherapist & Radionics practitioner

Biodynamic Psychotherapy

Depressed, anxious, stressed. In need of a breakthrough in your personal life? Biodynamic psychotherapy could help you unlock your life energy and make it work **for** you instead of **against** you.

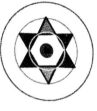

Radionics(psycho-physics)

Radionics analyses and help to reharmonize the physical body (organs) and the energetic bodies (aura) by tuning in to the subtle electronic vibrations found in all living beings. Radionics can help in many areas from detoxifying the body to restructuring our auric field

For information & appointment
phone 091 794028
Galway

Trainings are also offered in Radionics certified by the Psycho-Physics Academy London

---

Chinese Medicine & Acupuncture Centre / The T'ai Chi Energy Centre
Acupuncture - Herbs - T'ai Chi - Qi Gong - Dietary Therapy.
Paul D. Smyth Dip. Ac., Lic. Ac., MRTCMI - All medical problems treated.
Clinics at Upr. Rathmines Road, D6. & Castleknock Road, D15.
Tai Chi / Qi Gong - Weekly classes, Weekend Workshops - All Levels
Classes at Milltown Park, Sandford Road, D6.
Tel. 496 1533

DR. HAUSCHKA

Tir Na nÓg
Holistic Beauty Centre
The Square, Claremorris, Co. Mayo. Tel: 094 62678.
Reflexology & Aromatherapy. Dr Hauschka Cosmetics.
Proprietor: Donna Flatley I.T.E.C. C.I.D.E.S.C.O. M.I.R.I.

STEPHEN VAUGHAN
D.Acu., Lic.Ac.(China), MRATMI.
Acupuncture & Tuina Massage

Odyssey Healing Centre, 15 Wicklow Street, **Dublin 2**
Donnybrook Medical Centre, 6 Main Street, **Donnybrook**
Phone 01 677 1021. Mobile 087 235 6377

Backpain
Sports Injury
Stress
Sinusitis
Asthma
Skin
Digestive
Gynaecology
Arthritis
General Health

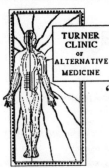
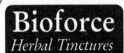
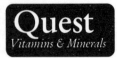
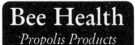
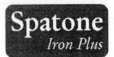
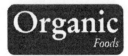

IRISH INSTITUTE OF COUNSELLING & HYPNOTHERAPY
Director: Dr. Sean Collins, B.A. (Psych), D.C.H.

COUNSELLING & THERAPY TRAINING

- Two-Year Diploma & Foundation Skills Certification Courses in Counselling, NLP and Ericksonian Hypnotherapy

- City & Guilds & BTEC Certification

- NLP Practitioner Certification

- Clinical Application of Behavioural Medicine & Complementary Healthcare Programme Management
(Foundation Skills Certification - Levels 1 & 2)

at Milltown Park, Dublin 6

Information from IICH, 118 Stillorgan Rd, Dublin 4, Tel: (01) 260 0118
Fax/Data: (01) 260 0115, CIS: 100553,2036, e-mail: therapy@iol.ie

List of Advertisers

Another exciting title from Wolfhound Press

Campaigns and How to Win Them!

Clare Watson, Mícheál Ó Cadhla, Cristíona Ní Dhurcáin
Foreword by Adi Roche

Arising from the authors' own wide experience of campaigning, this handbook
is for those setting up or already running a campaign – local or national, large
or small. *Campaigns and How to Win Them!* is easy to read, contains plenty of
practical tips and covers a wide variety of topics from fund-raising, working
with the media, accessing information, political lobbying to organising public
protests, legal and planning issues and promoting the group and its message.

'...an essential read for the experienced and novice campaigner alike. It
offers plenty of practical advice about how to run a smooth and effective
campaign. I wish I could have read a book like this when I first became
involved in campaigning.'
– Patricia McKenna, MEP

'...the perfect activist handbook. It gives to anyone wishing to run a
lobbying campaign all the best and most practical advice in
easy to follow stages.'
– Senator David Norris

ISBN 0 86327 554 0
£7.99